Quality control of veterinary vaccines in developing countries

Edited by
Noel Mowat

Published by arrangement with the
Food and Agriculture Organization of the United Nations
by
Daya Publishing House®
A Division of
Astral International Pvt. Ltd.
New Delhi - 110 002

"This book was originally published by the Food and Agriculture Organization of the United Nations (FAO) as Quality control of veterinary vaccines in developing countries, FAO Animal Production and Health Paper, 116".

"The designations employed and the presentation of material in this publication do not imply the expression of any opinion, whatsoever on the part of the Food and Agriculture Organization of the United Nations concerning the legal status of any country, territory, city or area or of its authorities, or concerning the delimitations of its frontiers or boundaries."

'The designations 'developed' and 'developing' economies are intended for statistical convenience and do not necessarily express a judgment about the stage reached by a particular country, territory or area in the development process.'

First Indian Edition, 1998
Reprinted, 2016
ISBN: 978-81-7035-211-2

Published by : **Daya Publishing House®**
A Division of
Astral International Pvt. Ltd.
– ISO 9001:2008 Certified Company –
4760-61/23, Ansari Road, Darya Ganj
New Delhi-110 002
Ph. 011-43549197, 23278134
E-mail: info@astralint.com
Website: www.astralint.com

Printed at : **Chawla Offset Printers,**
Delhi-110 052

CONTENTS

INTRODUCTION

With an expanding global population the demand for foodstuffs in the future will become ever greater, resulting in increased pressures on the agriculture and livestock industries for higher levels of production. In the case of livestock, control of the major epizootic diseases will be a prime requirement if increased production is to come from exploiting the potential for animal husbandry in the developing world.

Veterinary vaccines are a major factor in programmes to bring the economically important diseases under control. To achieve that goal vaccines have to be effective, consistent in performance and economically affordable. With these needs in mind an Expert Consultation was held at FAO Headquarters, Rome during the 2nd to the 6th December 1991 on the subject of "Quality Control of Veterinary Vaccines in Developing Countries".

The purpose of the Consultation was to bring together experts in various aspects of vaccine production and quality control, to consider present problems and likely future developments in the application of vaccines to the control of animal disease - and to make recommendations for further improvements in this important field.

The programme for the Consultation was based upon the following broad range of topics:

- Veterinary vaccine production and quality control with special emphasis on developing and less advanced countries
- Major vaccine producers and their role in technology transfer to developing countries
- Modern trends in veterinary vaccinology and prospects of their application in developing countries
- Quality control of vaccines in major vaccination campaigns
- Role of postvaccinal sero-monitoring in quality assessment of applied veterinary vaccines

The work of the Consultation was divided into 6 major Sessions in each of which, papers were presented and there were opportunities for general discussion of the topics raised. These are recorded in the following pages of this report. Towards the end of the Consultation, Working Groups were formed and asked to formulate recommendations for improvements related to specific topics on the agenda. These recommendations are also recorded here.

The Consultation was formally opened by Dr H de Haen, Assistant Director-General, Department of Agriculture, FAO - who welcomed all those attending the Consultation. Dr de Haen in his opening address emphasised the importance of work on the quality control of veterinary vaccines and made the following comments:

"Veterinary vaccines are a safeguard against numerous viral and bacterial diseases as well as some parasitic infections. They are used in an attempt to protect 4 billion livestock globally and nearly 12 billion poultry. Vaccines are the basic element in disease control campaigns presently underway or in the course of preparation at national and international levels. These include the rinderpest campaigns (PARC, WAREC and SAREC) in 53 countries on 3 continents. Also the control of foot and mouth disease in Asia, Africa, the Middle East and Latin America; similarly rabies control in Europe, Asia, Africa and the Americas is dependant on the use of effective vaccines, as is the control of Newcastle disease of poultry in the same areas.

The potency and safety of vaccines has to be assured through quality control procedures of manufacturers and independent laboratories at national and regional levels in accordance with international requirements. Without efficient quality control procedures there is a risk that costly vaccination campaigns may be carried out in vain without achieving the intended results.

In Africa alone there are 23 national laboratories producing nearly 30 types of veterinary vaccines - manufactured at different technological levels. Since 1986 through the agency of the Pan African Veterinary Vaccine Centre (PANVAC), FAO has been strengthening its member countries' capacities to improve standards of production through strict quality control methods. The quality of rinderpest vaccines has been of major concern to the Organization, particularly in relation to the Global Rinderpest Eradication Programme. FAO's concern and involvement in rinderpest vaccine quality control was made clear by the holding of an Expert Consultation on Rinderpest Diagnosis, Vaccine Production and Quality Control in Rome in 1984 and also the Expert Consultation on Global Strategy for Control and Eradication of Rinderpest again in Rome in 1987. Similarly, the production and quality control of Swine Fever vaccine was the subject of an Expert Consultation in Rome in 1984.

Again, quality control of foot and mouth disease vaccines has been discussed during numerous sessions and meetings held under the aegis of the FAO's European Commission for the Control of Foot and Mouth Disease.

During the last decade FAO through national and regional projects has contributed to improving the quality standards of vaccines by the provision of expertise to individual laboratories, assistance with the setting up of networks, co-operation with international organisations on the standardisation of particular products and by the holding of regional training courses on vaccines and their associated technologies.

In addition to the conventional vaccines in present day use, quality control procedures in the future will also have to cover the newly emerging bio-engineered products. FAO is already involved in this work and participated in the OIE Expert Consultation on the Requirements for Vaccinia Vector Recombinant Vaccines in Paris in 1989. It is now arranging with some of those research centres undertaking this type of work, for the preliminary testing of prototype candidate recombinant vaccines.

The recent Meeting of Near East countries held at FAO in November 1991 in relation to the rinderpest emergency situation in Turkey and its neighbouring countries, drew attention to the critical importance of proper quality control of rinderpest vaccines. The countries involved have agreed to seek FAO technical assistance and co-ordination on the subject.

It is hoped that during the present Consultation there will be fruitful discussions on the application of modern methods of vaccine production, technology and quality control in the context of the developing and less advanced countries and the problems associated with the transfer of such technology to those countries.

It is anticipated that the Consultation will identify constraints and requirements regarding standardisation of vaccine quality control methods and institutional, organisational and training needs. It is also hoped the discussions will help to define FAO's policies on this topic. There may also be an opportunity for discussion of the format of the FAO Manual on Quality Control of Veterinary Vaccines to be published in 1993.

I am very happy to see among the participants of this Consultation, internationally recognised specialists on veterinary vaccines as well as representatives from the international organisations and private industry. I hope that during the course of the Consultation it will be possible to arrive at useful conclusions on some of the more important professional aspects of the subject and to define strategies urgently needed for the further development of reliable veterinary vaccines.

It is to be hoped that our joint efforts will help in the future to protect farmers in the developing countries from the effects of poor quality veterinary vaccines and contribute to the welfare of their livestock - as well as the global control of animal disease.

LIST OF PARTICIPANTS

BOTSWANA	Dr M Mannathoko Botswana Vaccine Institute (Pty) Ltd Broadhurst Industrial Estate Private Bag 0031 Gaborone 312711
CAMEROON	Dr N Zoyem Head, Viral Vaccine Production Laboratoire National Veterinaire (LANAVET) B.P. 503 Garoua
CHINA	Professor T Guiyun Deputy Director National Control Institute of Veterinary Bioproducts and Pharmaceuticals 30, Baishiqiao Road Beijing
ETHIOPIA	Dr G Y Mebratu Deputy Director National Veterinary Institute Debre-Zeit
FRANCE	Dr R M Lombard Chef de Produit Rhone Merieux Lyon
	Dr P Lefèvre Head of Laboratory Institut d'Elevage et de Medecine Veterinaire des Pays Tropicaux (IEMVT) 10, rue Pierre Curie 94704 Maisons Alfort Paris
GERMANY	Professor O Thraenhart Director Instituts für med. Virologie and Immunologie Universitat Essen (IMVI) Hufelandstrasse 55 D-4300 Essen 1

INDIA	Dr P N Bhat Director Indian Veterinary Research Institute (IVRI) Izatnagar Bareilly, Uttar Pradesh
INDONESIA	Dr S B Siregar Director Veterinary Drugs Assay Laboratory (VDAL) Gunung Sindar Bogor 16340
ITALY	Dr Maria Tollis Istituto Superiore di Sanita Viale Regina Elena 299 00161 Rome
KENYA	Dr S Chema Director Agricultural Research Foundation (AGREF) P O Box 39189 Nairobi
MALAYSIA	Professor A L Ibrahim Dean University Pertanian Malaysia 43,400 UPM Serdang Selangor Darul Ehsan
POLAND	Professor Z Pejsak Head of Laboratory Instytut Weterynarii (Pulawy) Al Partyzantow 57 24-100 Pulawy
SYRIA	Dr G Khoury Chief of Bacterial Vaccine Production Central Veterinary Laboratories Damascus
UNITED KINGDOM	Dr F G Davies Consultant, Veterinary Vaccines G2, The Court St Mary's Place Shrewsbury Shropshire SY1 1DY

Dr T R Doel
Head, Vaccine Research Department
Pirbright Laboratory
AFRC Institute for Animal Health
Ash Road
Pirbright
Woking
Surrey GU24 ONF

Dr L K Nagy
Consultant, Veterinary Vaccines
8, Malmains Close
Beckenham
Kent BR3 2SE

Dr J M Rutter
Director and Chief Executive
Veterinary Medicines Directorate
Woodham Lane
New Haw, Weybridge
Surrey KT15 3NB

UNITED STATES OF AMERICA

Dr C A Mebus
Chief of Laboratory
United States Department of Agriculture
Animal and Plant Health Inspection Service
National Veterinary Services Laboratory
Foreign Animal Disease Laboratory
P O Box 848 Greenport
New York 11944

Professor L Carmichael
Director
James A Baker Institute for Animal Health
New York State College of Veterinary Medicine
Cornell University
Ithaca, N.Y. 14853

Professor T Yilma
Director
Laboratory of Molecular Biology for Tropical Disease Agents
FAO Collaborative Laboratory on Biotechnology
University of California
Davis

PAN AMERICAN HEALTH

Dr Raul Casas Olascoaga
Consultant

ORGANISATION
c/o Centro Panamericano de Fiebre Aftosa
PAHO
Caixa Postal 589
2001 Rio de Janeiro
Brasil

RAPPORTEUR
Dr G N Mowat
Veterinary Adviser
46, Boxgrove Avenue
Guildford
Surrey GU1 1XQ
U.K.

INVITED SPEAKERS

OUA-IBAR
Dr Y Cheneau
c/o OAU-IBAR
P O Box 30786
Nairobi
Kenya

OFFICE INTERNATIONAL DES EPIZOOTIES
Dr Y Ozawa
Principal Scientific Adviser
Office International des Epizooties
Tokyo
Japan

UNIDO
Dr A Atgar
Industrial Development Officer
Pharmaceutical Industries Unit
Chemical Industries Branch
United Nations Industrial Development Organisation
Vienna International Centre
P O Box 300
A-1400 Vienna
Austria

WHO
Dr P Sizaret
Scientist, Biologicals Dept.
World Health Organisation
20, Avenue Appia
CH-1211 Geneva 27
Switzerland

THERMOPAC, SWEDEN	Dr A Blom Managing Director THERMOPAC Industricentrum S-972 00 Gallivare
	Professor B Karlsson Scientific Adviser University of Linkoping Sweden
KEVEVAPI, KENYA	Dr R Korir Managing Director P O Box 53260 Nairobi Kenya

FAO HEADQUARTERS SECRETARIAT

Agriculture Department	Dr H de Haen Assistant Director-General
Animal Production & Health Division	Dr E P Cunningham Director
Animal Health Service	Dr P Stouriatis Secretary European Commission for the Control of Foot-and-Mouth Disease
	Dr J De Ryke Animal Health Officer (Bacteriology)
	Dr V R Welte Animal Health Officer (Disease Intelligence)
	Dr K J Wojciechowski Animal Health Officer (Virology) (Secretariat)
	Mrs J Street-Ciarroca Secretariat

FAO EXTERNAL STAFF

Dr M Jeggo
Animal Production and Health
Joint FAO-IAEA Division of Nuclear Techniques
in Food and Agriculture
Wagramerstrasse 5
A-1400 Vienna
Austria

Dr M Sasaki
Regional Animal Production and Health Officer
Regional Office for Asia and the Pacific
Maliwan Mansion
Phra Atit Road
Bangkok 10200
Thailand

Pan African Veterinary Vaccine Centre (PANVAC)

Dr M Rweyemamu
Project Manager, UNDP/RAF/88050
PANVAC
Debre-Zeit
Ethiopia

Dr V Palya
Microbiologist, PANVAC

Dr D Sylla
Project Manager, RAF/88050
PANVAC
Dakar
Senegal

Dr F L Musisi
Project Manager, GCP/RAF/297/NET
Lilongwe
Malawi

Dr V Rozkosny
Virologist, UTFN/LIB/025
Veterinary Services Support, Phase IV
Tripoli
Libya

CONCLUSIONS

A. GENERAL

1. Discussions at this meeting have repeatedly highlighted duplication of recommendations and procedures from international organisations. WHO, OIE and FAO have previously prepared guidelines and recommendations for various aspects of animal vaccine preparation and quality control. There appears to be a lack of co-ordination or co-operation in undertaking these activities.

2. There are wide variations in the effectiveness of standardisation and or regulatory procedures for veterinary immuno-biologicals between and within Regions.

B. TRANSFER OF TECHNOLOGY

Newcastle Disease Oral (or Feed Based) Vaccines

Newcastle Disease (ND) is a major constraint to village poultry production in developing countries and vaccination is the sole safeguard against it. Recently, a new technology has been developed by Australian and Malaysian scientists to vaccinate village chickens based on the use of the Australian lentogenic V4 strain which has been rendered heat-tolerant. A number of countries in South East Asia are investigating the use of this technology. It could also be utilised in Africa for the same purpose.

Industrial Vaccine Production

The meeting recognised the role private industry can play in the transfer of technology, in addition to the public institutions such as universities and national and international centres.

After completion of the transfer of technology, there needs to be adequate contractual arrangements between the transferring and the recipient institutions in order to ensure smooth operation of the transferred technology.

Continued technological support on a contractual basis from the transferring institutes is deemed essential for sustainability of technology transferred.

International organisations such as UNIDO may be able to help in the implementation of these technologies.

C. REGIONAL

Africa

In Africa, several protozoan and rickettsial vaccines are produced which pose special problems in quality control. They are prepared from donor animals or from homogenised ticks which have fed upon them. There are very real dangers that potential pathogens may contaminate these vaccines and a wide range of safety tests are necessary.

Asia - Middle East - Pacific

The meeting recognised that there is a real need to upgrade the quality control and standardisation procedures currently used in the countries of these Regions.

Europe - the Non EEC Countries

Each of these countries has its own system of quality control and licensing of veterinary biologicals. These systems vary widely.

The Americas

The meeting recognised that the strengths of the system for the production of veterinary vaccines in the Americas are related to the availability of good laboratories and networks established for diagnosis, disease monitoring and training in addition to a strong private sector that acts in harmony with Governments and Regulatory Agencies.

In addition to national and international centres for the promotion and control of these activities the Grupo InterAmericano Cooperacion Salud Animal (GICSA) serves to harmonise the activities of several groups to prevent duplication and achieve standardisation in disease control activities including vaccine production, quality control and solution of regional issues. Organisations with whom GICSA interacts include: PAHO, FAO, OIE, IICA, OIRSA, USAID, USDA, JICA (observer), BID.

The successful Latin American experience could be a model that would be expected to benefit other developing countries engaged in regional disease control efforts. Successful examples of international co-operative efforts in the Americas include: FMD Control Programme, ASF eradication, Bovine Brucellosis control in several countries and rabies control in urban areas.

Notwithstanding the achievements of Latin and North American countries to cope with important diseases that threaten the Continental herds, much remains to be done.

RECOMMENDATIONS

A. GENERAL

This meeting recommends that a closer co-operation be established with other international organisations to develop a more coherent approach on guidelines for vaccine quality control and to this end urges FAO to take the initiative.

The meeting recommends that FAO, WHO and OIE work jointly with developing countries to agree priorities and carry forward regional participation in standardisation including development of appropriate laboratory facilities and post-licensing surveillance. This should include participation at national level and within regions and require those countries with no procedures to begin standardisation and regulation unless a decision has been taken to accept standards agreed by other countries or regions. Procedures to be recommended for developing countries should take account of differing requirements and conditions.

It is recommended that regional repositories of master seed stocks of vaccine strains and cell lines and challenge strains should be established to aid the attainment of uniform quality of vaccines.

There is a need for establishment of regional vaccine banks for emergency use. FAO should encourage member countries in the regions to establish such banks on a cost sharing basis.

The meeting recognised the value of the activities of PANVAC and recommended that FAO and OAU/IBAR should solicit appropriate regional and international support for the conversion of PANVAC to the status of a long term programme Institute with appropriate facilities and support.

To save limited resources there should be common structures for controlling vaccines for human or veterinary use independently from and additionally to those of manufacturers.

Situations in which such possibilities should be explored, are those in which:

1. Tests required by the national authority to licence or release vaccines are identical or similar - (eg tests for sterility, safety and potency relating to vaccines) and,

2. Experts for conducting inspections of Good Manufacturing Practise (GMP) are available for either human or veterinary vaccines.

B. TRANSFER OF TECHNOLOGY

1. Rinderpest Recombinant Vaccines

Rinderpest recombinant vaccines should be as efficacious as referenced by OIE with respect to the Tissue (or Cell) Culture vaccine.

All rinderpest recombinant vaccines should comply with the WHO and OIE recommendations on products obtained by biotechnology or genetic engineering. Emphasis should be put on the OIE recommendations that stipulates that all rinderpest recombinant vaccines should be evaluated before release to producing laboratories.

2. Newcastle Disease Oral (or Food Based) Vaccine

The Meeting recommended:

a) that a pilot trial be conducted in Africa under the supervision of PANVAC.

b) that FAO request the support of the Australian Centre for International Agricultural Research (ACIAR) and/or the Malaysian Government to acquire the master seed virus and the vaccine necessary for the pilot study.

c) that FAO seek technology transfer from the Australasian Newcastle disease vaccine network (Australia and Malaysia) with a view to assisting the PANVAC network countries.

d) that FAO request the assistance of the Australian and Malaysian Governments in further training activities required in the control of ND in village chickens.

3. Industrial Vaccine Production

The need and extent of technology transfer should be clearly defined by the developing country. It should be adapted to meet national and regional needs.

To be sustainable in the long term, production should be cost effective and along commercial lines. The technology should preferably be easy to adapt and apply.

C. REGIONAL

Africa

The meeting recommended that countries be encouraged to develop a common approach and criteria for the licensing of veterinary vaccines. It recommended that IBAR be strengthened so as to be able to stimulate adequate and responsible licensing procedures by member countries through an appropriate licensing authority. Some guidance on the suitability of safety tests for protozoan and rickettsial vaccines is clearly needed and to that end the meeting urged FAO to look into this matter and draw up the appropriate recommendations for guidelines.

In Africa, trade barriers should be reviewed in order to allow free movement of veterinary medicines and immuno-biologicals between countries where appropriate.

Asia - Middle East - Pacific

The Meeting recommended that FAO sponsored collaborating centres be identified to promote training in quality control and standardisation of veterinary vaccines - one to be located in the Middle East and two more in Asia.

Europe - the Non-EEC Countries

Apparently there is no need to create new specific veterinary regulations for these countries - however, they should be encouraged to introduce the methods and systems of control of biological products already approved and in operation in the EEC member countries. The same regulations for this purpose should be applicable to all European countries.

The EEC countries should be asked through the agency of the FAO to assist in introducing the minimal EEC requirements for biological products into the Non-EEC countries.

Future improvements or upgrading of licence requirements and other appropriate regulations should be a joint responsibility for both EEC and Non-EEC countries.

The Americas

The Meeting recommended that:

There should be development of cost effective mechanisms to expand regional control of disease. Regional laboratories are needed to produce critical reagents for existing priority diseases as well as those diseases that have been brought under control.

It should be recognised that for the control of important diseases in the Americas, there are constraints in terms of inadequate funding, technical capabilities, reagents and expertise such as proved necessary in the successful FMD campaigns in South America and Mexico.

Efforts should be made to continue the integration and harmonisation of national and international agencies concerned with animal disease control in the Americas.

Overview on Veterinary Vaccines for Developing Countries

REGIONAL HARMONIZATION OF VACCINE QUALITY STANDARDS AND STIMULATION OF VACCINE TECHNOLOGIES IN DEVELOPING COUNTRIES

by

M M Rweyemamu, D Sylla and V Palya

INTRODUCTION

Effective control of major epizootics through vaccination demands an integrated availability of 4 pre-requisites defined in 1982 by Henderson[1] as:

i A well planned, well organized and well financed field campaign based on the results of studies of the systems used in animal production, the scale and extent of the movement of animals and the epidemiology of the disease, all in the local situation.

ii A well trained, well equipped staff, adequate in disciplines and numbers supported by efficient laboratory service.

iii The vaccines used must be of the highest quality.

iv Good international collaboration with programmes running in parallel within epidemiological areas.

Developing countries are characterised by the deficiencies in one or more of the above pre-requisites. It should be noted at the outset that such deficiencies are not always financial.

An important role of the international community, therefore, is to help both in the identification and in the plugging of such gaps. A major objective of an Expert Consultation, such as the present one, is to define the most efficient and cost-effective ways for the countries/regions in need to overcome these obstacles.

VACCINE QUALITY

It is now generally accepted that vaccines are medicinal products and, as such, should be manufactured according to *Good Manufacturing Practices*. Also, it is accepted that quality is not defined simply by the result of testing of the final product. The following definition, given by the UK Veterinary Medicines Directorate, seems to command universal acceptance:

"Medicines must be manufactured with appropriate *Quality Control Procedures* in Premises that are inspected and licensed; the Ingredients must be of appropriate purity, in the correct

[1] Henderson W.M. 1982. Proc. 16th Conference of the OIE Commission for Foot and Mouth Disease Vol 1 p 399.

proportions and correctly processed, the Containers must be robust with secure closures; the Labelling must be accurate and informative." Rutter[2], 1990

In many developing countries, however, there is, generally, no clear awareness of such a definition. The fact that, in such countries, vaccines are produced by research laboratories of the veterinary departments, makes it difficult to take effective action for implementing the implied requirement of this definition.

TRENDS IN THE INDUSTRIALIZED WORLD

The definition of quality given above, nowadays provides the yardstick for quality assurance in the industrialized countries. Good Manufacturing Practices and Quality Assurance are fully integrated in all aspects of vaccine manufacture: from the design of the manufacturing plant, the specifications of all raw materials, the manufacturing process and in-process controls, right through the testing, presentation and marketing of the final product. The over all objective is to ensure the *continual* and *consistent* preparation of *quality* vaccines through the implementation of an appropriate series of pre-established and systematic measures intended to ensure that the required *QUALITY* will be obtained.

An important outcome of adherence to these principles has been the evolution of an efficient vaccine manufacturing industry and a gradual withdrawal from the market of the less efficient small units with no capacity to adhere cost-effectively to the above requirements.

Another outcome is that with the ever expanding free trade areas in America and Europe there has been an increasing emphasis on institutional and regulatory harmonization of vaccine quality standards. In the USA, inter-state movement of vaccines is subject to quality criteria, licensing and testing by federal laboratories and inspectors of the USDA-APHIS. Progressively the Canadian and American federal vaccine quality criteria are being harmonized to virtual identity.

In Europe, traditional emphasis has been on co-ordination through such agencies as the European Pharmacopoeia. However with increasing economic and political integration of European countries, emphasis has been on evolving common legislation governing vaccine quality and common quality control criteria.

There also seem to be trends for either designation or even construction of EEC biological standardization laboratories for execution of functions related to common quality control and biological standardization. There has been a growing tendency for diminishing the role of purely national quality control standards in favour of European standards.

Although the American and European Pharmacopoeias differ in matter of detail, they are both based on the same premise. The tendency is that gradually the difference will become blurred.

---

[2] Rutter J.M. 1990. Paper presented at the Mtg. of Directors of National Vaccine Laboratories in Africa, Nairobi September 1990 - PANVAC Vaccine Bulletin Vol. 1 No. 1 p 38.

TRENDS IN SOUTH AMERICA

The most important animal disease in South America is foot and mouth disease. Vaccine against this disease constitutes the largest biological product in the world. In South America it is estimated that some 400 million doses of FMD vaccine are produced every year. Thus, the largest vaccine production plants in the world are to be found in South America. There are many features in the development strategies for both vaccine production and quality control technologies from which other regions of the developing world, and particularly Africa, can fully benefit.

Realising the significance of FMD on their trade, the South American countries through the Organization of American States (OAS) set up in 1951 the Pan American Foot and Mouth Disease Centre (Centro Panamericano de Fiebre Aftosa - CPFA) in Rio de Janeiro, Brazil, to co-ordinate their technical programmes for controlling FMD. Within a few years, the OAS requested the Pan American Health Organization (PAHO), which now forms the Western Hemispheric Organization of the WHO, to finance and carry out the programme of the CPFA. Until now, the CPFA is still financed and directed by PAHO. This Centre has had a tremendous impact on harmonization and standardization of FMD vaccine production technologies. Also vaccine quality test methods, approaches and criteria and vaccination strategies, in a manner which South America could not have expected by pure reliance on awareness of externally based inventions. The CPFA now stands as an important pillar in FMD control, whose significance extends well beyond South America.

Whilst specific technical papers will be presented from South America, it is important to reflect on some of the key achievements of the CPFA in relation to the quality of FMD vaccine in South America and its use, thereby posing an implicit question to the Expert Consultation as to what extent the South American experience is relevant to other developing regions of the world.

a) CPFA's Role in Vaccine Production Technologies

Almost from its earliest days, the Centre has had a small pilot vaccine plant for *in situ* study of appropriate FMD vaccine production technology, for training of South Americans, and for adaptive research in vaccine production. Through this initiative the following have been achieved:

i South American countries of Argentina, Uruguay and Brazil were encouraged to adopt the new technology of the Frenkel system almost at the same time as it was being developed into an industrial process in Europe.

ii When the BHK cell culture technology was developed at the Pirbright Institute, the CPFA quickly changed its pilot unit from Frenkel to BHK. It is now difficult to find any FMD vaccine production plant in South America whose staff have not had some form of training in FMD BHK cell culture technology by the CPFA. Also this unit has influenced the design of several vaccine production plants in South America.

iii Through their adaptive research programme, the CPFA has evolved a BHK suspension cell sub-line with virus susceptibility and sedimentation characteristics which are reputed to be superior to the original Capstick and Telling P3 BHK cell. Many producers in South America have benefited from this. One corollary is that the South American stainless steel industry has become very efficient in the construction of fermenters and fermentation plants.

iv First order kinetics inactivation of FMD virus by acetyl-ethylene-imine (AEI) was discovered by Brown and others a Pirbright. This was quickly and universally applied by the Wellcome Foundation in all their FMD vaccine plants. The CPFA's adaptive research programme subsequently discovered a safer system of generating the aziridine inactivant through a binary process. Now the use of BEI has virtually replaced AEI as the safer first order kinetics inactivant of FMD virus.

v Concerned with the shortcomings of aqueous adjuvants, particularly aluminium hydroxide, the CPFA developed an oil-emulsion formulation for FMD vaccines and an appropriate emulsification process. Thus collaboration with the stainless steel industry in Brazil has led to the design of an in-line Silverson type emulsifier, which for preparation of oil-emulsion vaccine is superior to either an in-situ Silverson or an in-line sonicator. Incidentally, the stimulus

exerted by the CPFA for oil vaccine has catalysed other research groups in improving aqueous adjuvants such as those based on saponin (e.g. quil-A) and even synthetic adjuvants such as avridine.

b) <u>CPFA's Role in FMD Vaccine Quality Control</u>

It would be no exaggeration to state that the CPFA has revolutionized FMD vaccine Quality Control in South America at the government, regulatory and industry level. The following can be cited as developments which can be attributed to the direct influence of the CPFA in the South American zone.

i Every country in which FMD vaccine is produced has a national Quality Control laboratory for independent QC testing of every batch of vaccine sold irrespective of whether it is produced in a commercial or a government owned laboratory. The government officer responsible for the national Quality Control laboratory must have undergone training by the CPFA.

ii Every country has specific regulations for quality of FMD vaccine including minimum standards for manufacturing premises, inspection of manufacturing premises, licensing and quality control minimum tests.

iii Every manufacturer is required to submit a detailed technical dossier before being licensed. Every time a significant change in the process is introduced (e.g. a new adjuvant or inactivation process - even a change from AEI to BEI) requires a new licence application backed by a detailed technical dossier.

iv Every manufacturing plant is required to designate an officer responsible for quality control (i.e. *Tecnico Responsavel*), plus a deputy. Both must be veterinarians and must have undergone a successful training programme in Quality Control Procedures at the CPFA. Thus all officers with responsibility for Quality Control Procedures either in government or in industry are required to have undergone similar training by the CPFA.

v Accordingly, every vaccine manufacturing plant is required to have an in-house independent quality control unit. In most countries it is a requirement that either the *Tecnico Responsavel* or his deputy must be physically present on the premise during the manufacture of FMD vaccine. Also when submitting the final bottled vaccine to the national quality control laboratory (usually the vaccine is collected by a government quality control inspector), the manufacturer is required to submit results of all in-process control tests plus descriptive details of the manufacturing process for each batch.

vi The CPFA has either accelerated the introduction to South America of new in-process or final product testing procedures or even developed tests or criteria to suit the South American conditions. For example, the CPFA played a crucial role in the introduction of cattle challenge testing in Argentina, Brazil, Colombia and Paraguay in the 1980's. This has had a dramatic effect on the level of potency of the vaccine produced in South America and apparently on the success of the FMD control campaigns.

The mouse protection test using sera of vaccinated cattle was developed by the CPFA and has been shown to correlate well with protection, interestingly, even with the recently developed synthetic peptide candidate vaccines. The data generated in South America with both the mouse protection test and other forms of neutralization test is now so large that for most situations, control authorities can confidently replace the direct in vivo challenge with neutralization tests.

viii Although each country uses its own criteria, it has developed such QC criteria with the active participation of the CPFA.

ix The CPFA, being the hemispheric reference centre for FMD, holds reference vaccine seed viruses and antisera. In this regard, it is remarkable how the CPFA has effectively changed attitudes in South America from the use of a plethora of so-called homologous, local vaccine strains to a few well characterised strains of proven vaccine performance and antigenic appropriateness. Being strategically placed in the FMD endemic zone, the CPFA has had some remarkable innovative ideas in the assessment of the role of antigenic variation to vaccine quality.

c) The Role of the CPFA in Design of Vaccination Regimens

Right from its beginning, the CPFA has played a leading role in the design of vaccination regimens which are appropriate for South America. Thus all South American countries have traditionally adopted a 4-monthly vaccination frequency to take account of the specific epidemiology of the disease in South America. Recently, these programmes are being modified on a country by country basis to take into account epidemiological data on the different ecosystems as well as the use of better adjuvanted vaccines.

d) A Framework for Regional Co-operation

The impact of the CPFA in the areas defined above has been aided particularly by two agencies, besides the role of the regional OIE and FAO commissions. The first is the South American Commission for FMD (Comision Sud-Americana para la Lucha Contra la Fiebre Aftosa - COSALFA) which brings together all the National Directors of Veterinary Services and FMD Control Co-ordinators, with the Director of the CPFA functioning as the ex-officio Secretary. The second organ is the Ministerial Council of OAS Member Countries responsible for animal health, which meets bi-annually.

TRENDS FOR THE ASIAN CONTINENT

This is the largest and most diverse continent. It is probably unrealistic that the single uniform approach of South America is readily applicable to Asia. The Expert Consultation can consider Asia in 3 inter-linked segments:

a) The Middle (or Near) East stretching from Turkey to Afghanistan.

b) South Asia for countries of or around the Indian subcontinent.

c) The South Asian or Pacific zone.

Each of these zones has enough internal financial resource to be able to develop an institutional and/or regulatory framework conducive to evolving modern attitudes for vaccine quality and biological standardization. There are already elements within each of these zones upon which regional approaches can be built. An example is the Biological Standardization and Quality Control Division of the Indian Veterinary Research Institute.

TRENDS FOR AFRICA

Africa is the poorest continent. In Africa, animal epizootic diseases constitute the single most important constraint to livestock development. It should be noted also that Africa has a negative balance in the supply of animal protein, although there is a large population of livestock, particularly cattle, in Eastern and Southern Africa. The development question for Africa has to be how to optimize the utilisation of the meagre internal resources as well as the impact of financial and technical aid from the donor community. There are several developments in Africa which are so similar to those in South America during the 1950/60's, that Africa could probably benefit a lot in learning from the experience of the CPFA model.

Firstly, there exists a political continental framework, the Organization of African Unity (OAU), which soon is expected to embrace every state on the continent. Secondly, there are serious steps being taken for long-term evolution of an African economic community. Thirdly, within the veterinary field, there exists a nucleus, the *Inter-African Bureau for Animal Resources* (IBAR) of the OAU, that can be developed into an effective co-ordinating agency in matters of harmonization of regulatory and inspection services for vaccine quality.

As in South America where FMD has provided the single most important catalyst, in Africa this is provided by rinderpest. Thus in the 1960/70's, with the co-operation of OAU member states and the financial plus technical assistance of the donor and international community, IBAR was able to co-ordinate a Joint Programme (JP15) for the control of rinderpest in Africa. This succeeded in dramatically reducing the impact of this disease. In recent years, IBAR has been co-ordinating a similar programme, known as the Pan African Rinderpest Campaign (PARC). This programme contains new features in that it aims at:

i control and eradication of major epizootic diseases - rinderpest being the first one.

ii policy reforms of veterinary services to build them to a sustainable basis.

iii harmonization of the quality of vaccine used in the campaign.

The third element is what has given impetus to the programme of the Pan African Veterinary Vaccine Centre (PANVAC). The mandate of PANVAC - which will be expounded during the Expert Consultation - relates to priority vaccines. These have been defined by the Directors of National Laboratories and the Directors of Veterinary Services as *rinderpest, contagious bovine pleuropneumonia, Newcastle disease, foot and mouth disease* (for Eastern and Southern Africa), and a *bacterial vaccine* to be agreed on a regional basis.

The Ministers responsible for livestock development among OAU Member States have resolved to urge the Secretary General of the OAU to seek the technical and financial assistance of the FAO, OIE, UNDP, EEC and other donor agencies in order to convert the programme of PANVAC from a short term project base to a long-term institutional base. The resolution has been endorsed by the OAU Council of Ministers as strengthening the technical capability of IBAR. Therefore, it now forms part of OAU policy.

In matters of vaccine quality and vaccine technology for Africa, it seems that PANVAC can fulfil this role in a manner akin to the way the CPFA has operated in relation to FMD vaccines in South America.

Global strategies for veterinary vaccine development and quality assurance

A major issue for this meeting is likely to be: what are the priority vaccines for which international, concerted effort is required. Some examples of these could be:

Foot and Mouth Disease
Rinderpest
Contagious Bovine Pleuropneumonia
Newcastle Disease
Rabies
Aujeszky's Disease (Pseudorabies)
Brucella
Anthrax
Clostridials

The issue would be, should there be a global FAO/OIE initiative for such identified vaccines similar to the WHO Immunization Programme? Also, should FAO seek to stimulate some co-ordinated research along the lines of the WHO/UNDP Research Programme on priority vaccines? If such an initiative were to arise out of this meeting, what would be the most cost-effective way to ensure rapid but responsible transfer to the developing countries? The funding and co-ordination of such research could take on elements of:

- Discovery research - largely in the industrialised world
- Development and/or Product Improvement/Adaptive Research - largely by such regional centres as the CPFA and PANVAC, as well as industry (in industrialized or developing countries) and leading national laboratories of developing countries.
- Clinical trials and Production - by commerce and national laboratories of developing countries.

Another global issue for developing countries has to be the role of government departments in the production of vaccines and assurance of their quality.

The role of government in the developing countries, in vaccine quality assurance cannot be in any doubt. But it has to be questionable as to whether government veterinary departments of developing countries should be encouraged to continue in the production of vaccines. Is this not likely to compromise quality and, in the long term, can sustainability of production of high quality vaccines be effectively safeguarded in this way? Should developing countries be encouraged to transfer vaccine production to the commercial sector, be it entirely private or partially parastatal or completely parastatal?

Quality cannot be compromised between industrialized and non-industrialized countries. The FAO and OIE work towards global harmonization of quality standards. In this regard, it is expected that the present meeting will advise on some specific measures that will encourage developing countries to take appropriate steps towards acceptance and implementation of modern concepts of *QUALITY* and *QUALITY ASSURANCE.*

For these concepts to evolve effectively in developing countries, it would appear that the attitudes of international agencies will also need to be geared towards corporate commitment to quality. This Expert Consultation may wish to examine such aspects as:

i. The strengthening of such regional agencies as IBAR in Africa or regional commissions, such as COSALFA in South America, in their capacity to stimulate appropriate legislation in member countries and harmonization of the same, including the setting up of appropriate inspection services.

ii. The strengthening of appropriate regional laboratories - for example, CPFA and PANVAC - that will develop and harmonize regional quality standards, provide technical support to regional agencies or commissions in monitoring the implementation of quality assurance requirements.

iii. Encouraging or strengthening economically viable vaccine production units that can implement concepts of quality assurance.

iv. Encourage regional free trade of vaccines in developing countries of the same region.

It is our understanding that the results of this Consultation will impact on development strategies for the 21st century. Therefore, this paper has sought to pose some issues rather than propose specific solutions.

PROFILES OF VETERINARY VACCINE PRODUCTION AND QUALITY CONTROL IN DEVELOPING AND LESS ADVANCED COUNTRIES: VACCINES FOR LIVESTOCK

by

P C Lefévre

INTRODUCTION

Since the situation may vary greatly from one country to the other, it is difficult to draw an exact picture of the production of veterinary vaccines in the developing countries. Moreover, the author's experience has been limited to the Sub-Saharan countries and he therefore knows little of the situation in the other continents.

Nevertheless it is possible to give a list of the main constraints that the laboratories are facing at present.

A. AT THE PRODUCTION LEVEL

General considerations

For political reasons that are easy to understand, most of the developing countries have decided to build their own vaccine producing units. Unfortunately, this was done, often without any previous economical and/or marketing studies. The number of producing laboratories has increased in a very irrational manner - from 7 in 1960 to 25 in 1990 in Africa, south of the Sahara (including South Africa and Madagascar).

As a result it is not surprising that production is widely distributed, only few laboratories having a complete range of vaccines.

In 21 African laboratories:

	3	laboratories produce	1 vaccine,
	6	" "	2 to 5 vaccines,
	7	" "	6 to 10 vaccines,
	4	" "	11 to 15 vaccines,
and	1	" "	more than 16 vaccines.

This leads to difficult economic situations for most of these Units.

Buildings and equipment

While some of the laboratories are new and built according to modern considerations, others are rather old (more than 30 years) and improvements have never been undertaken to adjust them to the latest requirements. Among the technical problems they are facing, the most acute are concerned with water and power supplies.

In the old production units, even the basic principles, relating to the proper use of buildings are not respected:

i) diagnostics, research and vaccine production are frequently carried out in the same building and,

ii) separation between the infected area and the sterile one does not always exist.

A similar comment can be made relating to large laboratory equipment. Many laboratories have to rely on international aid to obtain new equipment. Even when it is possible to buy new equipment, the situation is not always improved since new and modern apparatus will not necessarily solve the problems of the whole production chain.

More importantly the chronic problem, for these units is the lack of maintenance and spare parts. This is linked to two characteristics of the producing laboratories: the lack of financial assets and manpower management.

Administration and finances

Many of the producing laboratories are specialized services of a Ministry (Agriculture, Rural Development, Livestock ...) and are therefore not autonomous. This is specially true where money is involved. Three reasons can explain the poor financial situation of these laboratories:

1. No payment by customers for the vaccines that are sold (the Ministry being often the main, if not the only customer for its national vaccination campaigns).

2. The totally unrealistic prices of the vaccines. The technicians working in the laboratories are paid by the government and their salaries are not included in the price. No real study of the production costs has been made recently. After a rough estimation, it can be said that the prices should be 3 to 5 times higher than the present ones. The latter have not been re-evaluated, in Africa, for the last 20 years. Rinderpest vaccine, for example sold at 15 CFA francs per dose, in the 70s, is still sold at the same price.

Moreover, in some countries in which the currency is under central control, laboratories have, like all other companies, to obtain permits every time they want to import reagents, spare parts, etc, and this can be a major obstacle to normal production.

3. The absence of financial autonomy of some laboratories.

Human resources

Three categories of personnel are involved in vaccine production: the scientists in charge of supervision, the laboratory technicians and the maintenance personnel.

In many cases, if not always, the scientists are highly trained persons and PhDs are not rare in the laboratories of developing countries. Unfortunately, they often have little time to spend on bench or control work since they are asked to deal with administrative or financial problems. Frustrated by the lack of means and the burden of problems they have to solve, many of them dream of going abroad to work again on scientific topics.

Usually, the laboratory technicians are not trained in specialized schools but are taught by the scientists themselves or by their colleagues. This "at the bench training" may be dangerous since it ignores the main principles and the importance of respecting good laboratory practice.

Concerning the maintenance personnel, it is usual to see well-trained technicians in electricity or refrigeration technology leave once they have been trained, to join private companies where they are offered higher salaries.

Technical problems

The technical problems are mainly the consequences of all the other constraints already reviewed: poor quality of water, inadequate buildings, deep-freezes or lyophilisors and other machines in poor condition, production techniques that are not properly followed, etc.

However in addition to these problems, it has to be admitted, that guidelines and good manufacturing practices for veterinary vaccine production are not always available. Norms for all the vaccines have not yet been published and where they exist are unknown or unavailable to the technicians, who do not know how to obtain them.

The lack of scientific and technical information is therefore an important constraint.

B. AT THE CONTROL LEVEL

In addition to the constraints previously listed for vaccine production, two more problems are specific to control work:

1. Usually, the production and the control activities are implemented in the same building, if not by the same person. If controls by the producer are necessary during production and on the final product, additional control should be undertaken by an impartial organisation.

   Regarding this problem, the creation of the 2 FAO/PANVAC laboratories, in Debre-Zeit (Ethiopia) and in Dakar (Sénégal), in October 1990, must be considered as a great success.

   To the best of knowledge, this is the first time that vaccine control work has been organized at a regional level. Dealing only with rinderpest vaccine for the present, the PANVAC laboratories should extend their control activities to other vaccines.

2. In many cases, laboratories have no opportunity to obtain the animals necessary for inocuity or efficacy tests. Farms for large animals are expensive and small animal facilities require skill to maintain laboratory animals under difficult climatic conditions.

CONCLUSIONS

Listing all the constraints of vaccine production in developing countries is of no interest and may even appear as sterile criticism, if no recommendations are given.

Five steps could be taken to improve the situation:

1. Laboratories should be given financial autonomy and should be able to reconsider the prices of vaccines. An analysis of the real production costs would permit a more realistic sale price to be made, in order not only to maintain the situation but also to improve the equipment and techniques and finally the quality of vaccines.

2. Training courses should be organized especially for the bench technicians and if the demand is great enough, technical schools could be created on a regional basis.

3. More attention should be paid to the salaries of personnel in order to avoid the loss of technicians once they have been trained.

4. The production and control of vaccines should be carried out by two different organisations. If vaccine production can be done by a private or parastatal company, quality control should remain in the hands of the State.

5. The International Organisations should publish and distribute, for each vaccine, details of good manufacturing practice as well as the norms for vaccine production and quality control.

PROFILES OF VETERINARY VACCINE PRODUCTION AND QUALITY CONTROL IN DEVELOPING AND LESS ADVANCED COUNTRIES: VACCINES FOR POULTRY

by

A L Ibrahim and L H Seng

INTRODUCTION

The poultry industry in most of the developing countries in Asia can be classified into two types of production:

a) commercial poultry farming and

b) traditional village based farming.

During the last 2 decades the development of the poultry industry in the developing countries is expanding very rapidly. Countries such as Malaysia, Thailand and Singapore are self sufficient in poultry, meat and eggs and the industry is moving into a state of progress and development with the establishment of modern poultry processing plants and of breeding farms. In countries such as Indonesia and Philippines the industry is predominantly village based. Diseases remain the greatest threat to the poultry industry. Almost all the known poultry diseases can be found in many of the developing countries in Asia. Among the major diseases encountered are: Newcastle disease (ND), Infectious bronchitis (IB), Fowl pox (FP), Mareks disease (MD), Avian encephalomyelitis (AE), Lymphoid leukosis (LL), egg drop syndrome (EDS), Infectious laryngotracheitis (ILT), Infectious bursal disease (IBD), Pullorum disease, coccidiosis, chronic respiratory disease (CRD), fowl cholera, Infectious coryza aspergiliosis and Leukocytozoonosis.

VACCINE PRODUCTION

Vaccines play a very important role in the prevention and control of many poultry diseases. In commercial farms vaccination is carried out routinely for most of the diseases mentioned above ie ND, MD, FP, IB and AE. Some farmers vaccinate for other diseases as well. Backyard poultry is vaccinated with ND and FP vaccines. Parenteral and non parenteral methods of administration are employed for vaccination. Most vaccine development deals with the improvement of existing products to increase potency or to improve safety, purity and production facilities. Table 1 shows vaccines that are produced by some of the countries of South East Asia.

Table 1: <u>Poultry Vaccine Production in South East Asia</u>

1.	<u>Malaysia</u>	1)	<u>Newcastle Disease Vaccine</u>
			a) lentogenic F
			b) mesogenic Mukteswar
		2)	Fowl pox Vaccine - Beaudette strain
1.	<u>Singapore</u>	1)	<u>Newcastle Disease Vaccine</u>
			a) lentogenic F
			b) mesogenic Mukteswar
		2)	Fowl pox Vaccine - B. strain
3.	<u>Thailand</u>	1)	<u>Newcastle Disease Vaccine</u>
			a) lentogenic F
			b) mesogenic Mukteswar
		2)	Infectious bronchitis vaccine - local strain
		3)	Fowl pox vaccine - Weybridge strain
		4)	Fowl cholera vaccine - <u>Pasteurella</u> <u>multocida</u> serotype A, formalinised
		5)	Duck plaque vaccine - Jensen's strain
4.	<u>Indonesia</u>	1)	<u>Newcastle Disease Vaccine</u>
			a) lentogenic F
			b) lentogenic B1
			c) lentogenic La Sota
			d) mesogenic Komarov
		2)	Fowl cholera vaccine (bacterin)
		3)	Infectious coryza-vaccine (bacterin)

5. <u>Philippines</u>

1) <u>Newcastle Disease Vaccine</u> - PD-1B (Philippines/Duck) strain

2) Fowl pox vaccine

3) Pigeon pox vaccine

4) Fowl cholera

Sometimes the improvement is one of an alternative mode of delivery such as the food based ND vaccine which was developed in Malaysia. Such a vaccine has been demonstrated to be very effective in the control of ND in the rural areas.

Many of the developing countries still rely on imported vaccine for the control of poultry disease. The decision to import vaccine depends on three factors:

1) the lack of trained manpower and facilities to produce such vaccine

2) financial constraints and

3) evidence that the disease is causing important losses and the proposed vaccine would significantly reduce those losses.

QUALITY CONTROL

In many of the developing countries vaccines are produced by government laboratories. These countries have developed their own standards based on one or all of the following documents:

1. European Pharmacopoeia

2. British Pharmacopoeia

3. USDA Code of Federal Regulation Title 9 Chapter 1 on Animal and Animal Products Part 101-107.

Quality control is usually carried out by the same laboratory that produces the vaccine. Tests are made from time to time to ensure that vaccines meet the standards of purity, safety and potency set by the laboratory. For example, in Malaysia in addition to tests of safety, immunological tests on animals for the presence of adventitious organisms other than the vaccine itself are required. Table 2 shows the range of tests carried out in chickens.

Table 2: Tests Carried Out for Poultry Vaccines

Bacteria, Fungi and Mycoplasma	Tests
Salmonella spp	AGPT and Isolation
Mycoplasma galisepticum	Antigen Agglutination
Mycoplasma synoviae	Antigen Agglutination/HI
Escherichia coli	Isolation
Staphylococcus spp.	Isolation
Aspergillus fugimatus	Isolation

Viruses	Tests
Avian adenovirus	AGPT
Avian encephalomyelitis virus	Embryo susceptibility/SNT
Avian Reovirus	AGPT
Fowl pox virus	SNT/COFAL
Infectious bronchitis virus	AGPT
Avian leucosis virus	SNT/COFAL
Marek's disease virus	AGPT
Newcastle disease virus	HI/Isolation/ELISA
Infectious bursal disease virus	SNT/AGPT
Adenovirus (EDS 76 virus)	AGPT/HI

The development of standardised procedures for quality control in developing countries is a very complex issue. Different countries have different interests, needs and organization structures. Often the authority for the registration of vaccines is not vested with the Department of Veterinary Services. For example, in Thailand the registration of veterinary vaccines is handled by the Food and Drug Administrator of the Ministry of Public Health, while the Department of Livestock Development carries out the quality control tests.

DISCUSSION

Vaccine development and production in the developing countries will continue to be the responsibility of governments in the future. Governments have an obligation to improve current products and evaluate available commercial vaccines. It is important that the evaluation of products and production methods be done by two separate laboratories. Developing countries should set up national quality control standards based on known documented standards, taking into account the country's needs, interests, resources and capacity. There is a need to adopt common acceptable quality control standards on a regional basis. This will encourage the development of technology in the quality control of veterinary vaccines for the purpose of registration and certification. A good example of regional co-operation on the formulation of quality standards is the ASEAN Vaccine Standard established by the ASEAN Co-ordinating Group on Livestock. At present, standard requirements for 17 poultry and 11 mammalian vaccines have been established and accepted by the ASEAN region.

VETERINARY VACCINE PRODUCTION AND QUALITY CONTROL IN DEVELOPING AND LESS ADVANCED COUNTRIES

by

F G Davies

INTRODUCTION

The response of veterinarians in the developing and less advanced countries to the major animal diseases has reflected considerable credit upon the members of the profession involved. The tissue culture rinderpest vaccine developed by Plowright is recognised as one of the most effective and successful vaccines ever used in the history of human or livestock medicine. Several other vaccines which were developed many years ago have proved to be remarkably effective in controlling animal disease. Notable amongst these have been the anthrax spore vaccine and the sheep pox vaccine of Borrel.

However, vaccination is not the only answer to the problems posed by infectious diseases. An acute observation of the natural history of African swine fever in the early days of the century, prompted Eustace Montgomery to propose a simple inexpensive control strategy. This consisted of a statute controlling the management of domestic pigs, in which they were required to be held in pens and housing of a certain specification. This was designed to prevent any contact with wild pig populations. It remains some 80 years later, as the best method of control in enzootic areas.

VACCINES FOR LIVESTOCK

1. First Generation Vaccines

Veterinarians in the developing world were faced by dramatic epizootics causing huge losses of stock over comparatively brief periods, and persistent sporadic problems where diseases were enzootic. These were identified and characterised and efforts to control them resulted in the first generation of veterinary vaccines, many of which are still widely used today, and have often been very successful. These vaccines were prepared by physical modification of the organisms, inactivation, modifications of virulence by cultivation in artificial media or alternate hosts systems. Many suffered quite serious disadvantages, which were, however, acceptable in the face of the enormous disease problems which were being faced. By todays standards, the safety and quality control testing left much to be desired.

Problem Areas

The pathogenicity of the vaccine strains was frequently found to differ considerably when they were used in Bos taurus rather than Bos indicus cattle, and often there were different reactions in different breeds of the same species. The caprinised rinderpest vaccine furnishes a good example of this.

The production systems frequently used donor animals of the same species for which the vaccine was intended. This creates an ideal system for the transmission of any other contaminating organism which may be present in the donor. History shows many instances where this has occurred. Lumpy skin disease virus was inadvertently transmitted when blood from donor animals was used to immunise against protozoan diseases. The transmissible agent of scrapie was once present in a batch of vaccine prepared from louping ill infected sheep brain. Much clinical disease followed these incidents.

A word of caution might be given here, of the inherent dangers involved in the preparation of the antigen for the simultaneous infection and treatment methods now in wider use for heartwater (Cowdria ruminantium) and East Coast fever/Corridor disease (Theileria spp). Ground up tick emulsions (GUTS) from specimens collected from laboratory held donor cattle or field collections, on occasion, are inoculated into cattle. Such GUTS are likely to contain viruses of the Bunya, Flavi or Orbivirus families, many of which are animal and human pathogens. One of these, Congo-Crimean Haemorrhagic fever (C-CHF) is a lethal human pathogen. Accidents have occurred handling this tick in the laboratory, where aerosols are created by homogenisation, and by accidental needle inoculation. The dangers to the people involved in the preparation and use of such vaccines are clear. Effective safety testing of all GUTS is necessary.

Despite the many defects of first generation vaccines, they still have an important role to play. In many developing countries, they are often the only means available to maintain productive animals in area enzootic or epizootic for these diseases. However, the safety and control procedures which are available today, can greatly reduce the dangers which were encountered when they were first introduced. It is in this area, with such vaccines that most improvements in quality control may be achieved.

2. Second Generation Vaccines

The great improvements in laboratory technology, particularly in virology with the development of tissue culture systems, was accompanied by the appearance of a new generation of veterinary vaccines. These allowed the cultivation of vaccine organisms to be made in better controlled production systems. The trend was, for example, to cultivate viruses in tissue culture systems and replace the previous donor or laboratory small animals. The development of Specific Pathogen Free units provided pathogen free embryonated eggs for vaccine production purposes. Many possible sources of contamination of vaccines were eliminated and safety and quality control procedures were made much easier.

The reduction of the pathogenicity of many viruses was achieved by serial passage in tissue culture systems, and was the source of many modified live virus strains for vaccine production. Rinderpest vaccine is probably the most successful example. There is now a wide range of tissue culture vaccines which are in regular use against animal disease in many parts of the world. Further, high titre yields of viruses from culture are concentrated and inactivated to produce totally safe antigens, which are acceptable to the most critical animal owners or intensive animal production systems.

The success of this generation of vaccines has been considerable. Diseases such as rinderpest have been eradicated from many countries and JP 15 came very close to eliminating it from the whole of Africa. Vaccines prepared against rabies have successfully reduced the incidence of the disease to minuscule proportions in previously heavily infected enzootic areas. In the companion animal field, of great importance to small animal veterinary practitioners, canine distemper and infectious canine hepatitis have been greatly reduced. There are many other examples.

Problem Areas

The tissue culture cell substrates which are used in the preparation of these second generation vaccines, have often been the primary or secondary culture of animal cells. These are frequently of the same species as the host in which the vaccine is to be used. In addition, the sera used to grow and maintain the cultures has been obtained from the same animals. Clearly there is a considerable danger that the cell cultures may contain contaminating viruses, as also may the serum. These viruses may not produce a cytopathic effect or may not replicate to a point where the contamination becomes evident in the cultures, until they have been passaged beyond that level at which vaccine is produced. The vaccine will however contain the virus. Some contaminants may not produce any cytopathic effects and only be detected by immunofluorescence or peroxidase testing after further passages of the production cell cultures.

The screening procedures used initially may have been inadequate to detect such contaminants, nor may they have been detected by the in vivo animal safety testing. Despite such defects, comparatively few problems have been encountered following the extensive use of vaccines prepared in this manner. They have occurred however. The Theileria annulata vaccine, suffers the same disadvantages as those of the other tissue culture vaccines described above.

A major problem in the developing countries is the supply of serum for tissue culture purposes. Many utilised sera from donor animals held in isolation pens at their laboratories. This gave opportunities for screening of the sera but was not always safe. Others collected sera from local slaughter houses which was also not satisfactory, but at least furnished sufficient sera for production purposes. The importation of sera with no antibody to the diseases prevalent in the country (as from New Zealand) for example has been an answer to this persistent problem. The purchase of foetal calf serum for production purposes in developing countries is not a practical proposition. The commercial costs of such preparations are prohibitive.

The more widespread use of continuous cell cultures or cell lines, on which a great deal of work has been carried out to ensure freedom from contaminating agents and which are non-permissive for many animal pathgens is highly desirable. There are moves to extend the use of Vero cells for rinderpest vaccine production and efforts are being made to define a suitable cell substrate for the cultivation of the sheep and goat pox vaccine strains and for lumpy skin disease. This will be a great improvement and remove the dangers arising from the use of primary and secondary sheep or calf cells for production purposes.

More advanced technology has been applied to these vaccines with carrier and suspension culture systems for viruses, bacteria and Mycoplasma. Foot and mouth disease and rabies vaccines are often produced in suspension or with carrier culture systems, and

Clostridial vaccines for the various sheep Clostridial toxaemias are produced with large industrial plant systems.

These vaccines have also been accompanied by the widespread use of freeze drying technology. The use of various protein/carbohydrate stabilizers in buffered solutions has allowed products to be made which retain their potency for long periods of time. Temperature tolerance has remained a problem and cold chains are required. Reconstitution has been a problem, where specifically prepared diluents have not been supplied with the vaccine. Despite the logistical problems and cost, it is strongly recommended that this be done wherever possible. Disastrous results often follow the use of unsatisfactory diluting fluids and account for much of the alleged poor immunogenicity of vaccines.

Adjuvants have also made a dramatic improvement in the efficacy of this generation of vaccines. Many of the culture produced toxoid whole organism and viral vaccines have greatly improved immunogenicity with the latest adjuvants. The water in oil emulsions which are used with the Clostridial and poultry vaccines have greatly improved the results obtained.

The improvement in the production systems of these vaccines, has allowed the quality control procedures required to be less exacting than is required for the first generation of vaccines prepared in animal systems. The first generation vaccines were usually subject to potency and safety testing at the same Institute, although different sections may have been carrying out the various tests. Increasingly separate quality control laboratories are being established, which operate independently from production laboratories and on a countrywide scale. They carry out testing of all vaccines whether imported or home produced. This is clearly a desirable development. A further recent change has been to establish a regional facility for quality control, and this has been done in Africa for the PARC OAU/ECC Rinderpest Programme, which has two quality control laboratories, one in Ethiopia and one in Senegal. They are a key to the success of the operations.

3. <u>Third Generation Vaccines</u>

These are the various protein antigens or other immunogens developed by the latest molecular biological techniques. This is an area of frenetic activity in the developed world which produces extremely encouraging results in certain instances. However, it is many years since genetically engineered foot and mouth disease vaccines were prepared, and we have yet to see any such preparations employed in the developing countries.

Many other important animal diseases are the subject of intensive work in this area. Encouraging results are being obtained with rabies and vaccines which use pox virus carrier systems. The further dissemination of vaccinia in the environment should be opposed and it is suggested that Capripox strains would be more suitable for ruminant use.

VACCINES FOR POULTRY

The early poultry vaccines were usually formalin inactivated bacterial cultures or embryonated egg material, such as those for fowl cholera, typhoid and Newcastle disease.

Later the mild strains of Newcastle disease virus grown in embryonated eggs, both lentogenic and mesogenic, were widely used and found to be extremely valuable vaccines. They had an important impact upon the occurrence of Newcastle disease in the developing countries where the mesogenic strains were used in village and mixed farming systems. The development of a more sophisticated industry with breeding flocks maintained under intensive conditions, led to an additional requirement for the safer inactivated vaccines, as the disadvantages of the more pathogenic mesogenic vaccines became apparent.

The mild Beaudette strain of fowl pox was also widely used throughout the developing world where pox was often a significant problem when transmitted by insect vectors.

There has always been an awareness of the dangers of contaminating live virus poultry vaccines with agents present in the seed cultures or eggs used for production. Early precautions were to use only eggs obtained from tested Minimal Disease Free flocks maintained under optimal hygienic conditions in isolation. Little trouble was experienced in many countries adopting such precautions. The advent of the Specific Pathogen Free poultry systems was a major development. Such high technology and extremely expensive plant could not be immediately adopted by most countries in the developing world, however much they would like to have them.

This is the major area where improvements can be made in the developing world today. Whether such improvements should be initiated by Government or paid for by the private sector is a question to be answered by individual countries. The latter option may be the most desirable.

VACCINES FOR WILDLIFE AND COMPANION ANIMALS

Vaccines are not widely used in wildlife populations unless very special circumstances occur. A situation where enzootic stability prevails is more desirable. Vaccine has been used as a necessary adjunct to animal health eradication policies, where the final reservoir for a disease is found in the wild animals. Such a situation has occurred with bison and the Brucella organism. Oral rabies vaccine has an important role to play in limiting the extension of rabies in countries where fox populations are responsible for propagation of the virus in parts of Europe. Great improvements have been made in these oral vaccines. In much of the developing world, the dog populations play the major role in rabies virus transmission and wildlife are generally only involved as accidental disease hosts.

The first generation of rabies vaccines were of considerable value in controlling the disease in dog populations when they were first introduced. Allied with strict policing operations, the rabies incidence in dog populations was often reduced to insignificant levels in many developing countries. Both the inactivated brain tissue and low egg passage Flury strains were used to achieve this. Problems were encountered with the incomplete inactivation of the brain material, which was often not detected by routine safety testing. The Flury vaccine was highly immunogenic in dogs, with an immunity which persisted for 3 years.

The second generation of rabies vaccines included the first tissue culture products such as the ERA vaccine in Canada, which used a modified live virus strain and also the inactivated vaccines produced in cell cultures. These were more acceptable to companion animal owners but as they gave a shorter period of immunity, were less suitable than the Flury strain in the developing countries, where the prime purpose was to reduce the public health problem. This was also a cheap vaccine to produce and while it was not as acceptable to pet owners, had many advantages for developing countries. Most of the tissue culture vaccines are still comparatively expensive.

A new generation of rabies vaccines prepared by molecular biological techniques is expected to appear shortly, so far experimental results are encouraging. What the level of application will be in the less developed countries, where the rabies problem is usually the greatest, remains to be seen.

4. Regional Issues

Livestock Populations

The distribution of livestock and husbandry practices are very much a regional characteristic and relate to the climatic and ecological factors which prevail. These will influence which vaccines are most important.

In South America, for example, there is an extensive large cattle population and because of its export markets, great attention is paid to foot and mouth disease control. Production of this vaccine is a major industry. In some parts of Asia, pigs and poultry are kept in large numbers and the demand for vaccines is high. In the Middle East there are extremely large poultry populations, and Newcastle disease vaccines are in great demand. In Africa, extensive cattle populations are kept on the bushed and wooded savannahs and vaccines for cattle diseases have been of prime concern.

Prevalence of Epizootic Diseases

Certain diseases are of far greater importance in some continents than others. Bovine pleuro pneumonia and rinderpest are still important problems in Africa and much vaccine production effort is directed to their control. Rinderpest is still important in the Middle East and Asia. Poultry vaccines are required in large quantities in some regions and are of less significance in others. Sheep and goat pox virus diseases assume greatest importance in the Middle East and parts of Asia and Africa. Vaccine production to control them has some considerable degree of priority.

There are periodic extensions in the range of many vector borne diseases from where they have been enzootic and epizootic for many years. Rift Valley fever, Lumpy skin disease, ephemeral fever, bluetongue, Akabane and African horse sickness have all extended their range beyond that with which they have traditionally been associated. There is some evidence to show that these extensions have occurred at earlier periods in history. When such diseases do extend, they create an emergency demand for the supply of vaccines for their control. Laboratories in the enzootic areas may be hard put, to produce sufficient to meet such demands, since they may be unable to meet even their own requirements.

There exists a need for the establishment of strategic reserves of vaccine or concentrated antigen to meet such emergencies. The means to achieve this must also be planned. In many instances these vaccines are of the first generation, while effective, they are often not suitable for use beyond enzootic areas. Improved vaccines are required and the resources for their development are also very necessary.

National or Regional Centres

It is the aim of most individual countries to establish and improve their own National Vaccine and Quality Control Laboratories. Regional Laboratories may be more cost effective however. A regional Quality Control system has been established in support of the PARC where FAO have supported two laboratories, one in Debre Zeit in Ethiopia and the other in Dakar in Senegal. This has resulted in a general improvement in the rinderpest vaccines being used in the campaigns, and most national centres have received valuable help with production problems.

Standardisation

There is a strong case for attempting to standardise production methods for different vaccines on a regional basis. Many laboratories use the same vaccine seeds but a variety of different production methods. The pooling of knowledge and experience could provide a common protocol which would probably improve standards generally. Most national laboratories in a region whether for vaccine production or diagnosis, probably share the same problems. A regional approach to the standardisation of methods would be a desirable trend.

DISCUSSION

Dr Doel thought that the transfer of vaccine production from Government agencies to the private sector might result in such price rises that farmers could not afford to buy vaccines. As a consequence, the size of the market would diminish to the point where commercial organisations would no longer be prepared to invest in development of products or facilities. He was of the opinion that the most important question for Governments to consider was the balance to be achieved between what is needed and what can be afforded.

Dr Lefevre agreed that this was an important point but in his experience in African countries, if the protection of livestock was sufficiently important, farmers would find ways of purchasing vaccine - eg by the sale of one or two cattle. By this type of approach the farming community could obtain the benefit of commercial production. He thought that PARC was a good example of a cost effective system.

Dr Cheneau pointed out that the markets in Africa for veterinary vaccines represented only some 3% of the global market and this explains why commercial interest in the development of new products for this part of the world is so poor. It may be that for some time to come the only solution to the control of important epizootics will be to subsidise the production and application of the appropriate vaccines. As a result the subsidisation of other vaccines of less importance and some drugs will not be possible.

Dr Mannathoko asked why Governments ever allowed small vaccine production units to start up, when in some cases it is possible to import high quality vaccines at acceptable prices. Small units which are not efficient and financially self-supporting should be allowed to collapse and the funds previously devoted to them should be directed towards more urgent needs such as the support of vaccination work in the field. He suggested that the funds provided by Aid Donors for the setting up of small units such as he had described were being misdirected.

Dr Mowat described the funding of animal health schemes provided by the National Dairy Development Board in India within the context of a national plan known as Operation Flood. For the control of foot and mouth disease in designated areas, vaccine produced by Indian Immunologicals is initially provided free and as the benefits of freedom from disease become more apparent the subsidy on the cost of vaccine is gradually reduced until the farmer is responsible for its entire cost. He suggested this might be a method of financing vaccination schemes in other countries.

Dr Chema was also convinced that farmers in Africa would pay for vaccines if the benefits to be derived from freedom of disease could be clearly demonstrated.

Dr Lefevre expressed the opinion that in terms of improvement of the livestock industries, the use of vaccines should be regarded as only one component of an overall plan and other measures such as the use of more productive breeds, albeit, in relatively smaller numbers must be introduced.

As the discussion came to an end, Dr Nagy in agreement with an earlier speaker emphasised that the proliferation of separate small production units was not the answer to the provision of vaccine on any significant scale and that perhaps a better and more rational approach would be the procurement of supplies on a Regional basis. Not only would this give advantages in the commercial negotiations on price etc, but would promote active collaboration between member countries within the region on international disease control schemes. Bulk procurement for a region might be seen as a stage in the long term development of a regional disease control strategy.

Veterinary Vaccine Production and Quality Control Facilities in Different Regions of the World

Country Reports:

AFRICA

1. ERADICATION POLICY OF FOOT-AND-MOUTH DISEASE IN BOTSWANA

by

M Mannathoko

INTRODUCTION

In Botswana, a country exporting beef to Europe, the livestock situation poses one of the most important concerns of the Veterinary Services Authorities, particulary in preventing Foot-and-Mouth Disease.

Measures taken for the prevention of Foot-and-Mouth Disease date back to the beginning of the 1950s and has required, among others, vaccination since 1964.

The vaccines available on the market proved ineffective in controlling the outbreaks of Foot-and-Mouth Disease which then appeared, so in 1977 the Government of the Republic of Botswana decided to build and exploit its own Institute for the production of Foot-and-Mouth Disease vaccines in collaboration with the company RHONE MERIEUX.

In 1978, in order to cope with the urgent situation and to put at the disposal of Botswana effective vaccines adapted to local virus strains, the co-operation agreement proceeded in two phases.

> Phase I - aimed at studying the different strains of Foot-and-Mouth virus and producing a limited quantity of vaccines.
>
> To carry out this plan as soon as possible, a fully equipped laboratory was sent by air and was made functional within one week.
>
> Phase II - aimed at building an industrial laboratory with a capacity of 21 million monovalent doses per year.

Owing to the excellent collaboration between the Botswana authorities and the French technical team, as well as the prompt availability of funds from the EEC, in less than 5 months after the signing of the agreement on the 12th of May 1978, the first vaccine was put into use and 6 months later, semi-industrial production was launched with a capacity of 200,000 doses per week.

Industrial production started in October 1981, with a capacity of 600,000 doses per week.

These installations allowed the study of FMD virus strains in the region, the development of effective vaccines against these strains after studying the serological and immunological relationships, and the control of the virus strains that could appear at borders or in neighbouring countries with close collaboration with the veterinary authorities of these countries.

Since the end of 1980, no case of Foot-and-Mouth Disease has been reported in Botswana.

At present, the Botswana Vaccine Institute has become the main supplier of Foot-and-Mouth Disease vaccine for Southern Africa. In 1985, it was designated the Regional Reference Laboratory for Foot-and-Mouth Disease.

The Eradication Policy

Between 1977 and 1980, several outbreaks of Foot-and-Mouth Disease were reported in the country.

The isolated virus strains were:

SAT1 type	BOT 1/79
	BOT 8/79
SAT2 type	BOT 8/78
	BOT 7/79
	BOT 11/79
	BOT 2/80
	BOT 4/80
	BOT 9/80

No SAT3 strain was isolated during this period (the last SAT3 strain was isolated in 1965).

One of the first research studies was to isolate these strains from the field, to adapt them to culture on cells and on bovine tongue epithelium (FRENKEL technique).

The antigenicity and immunological relationship of the viruses were studied after preparation of hyperimmune sera typical of each virus in guinea-pigs and the use of controlled vaccine in cattle.

These studies allowed the selection of virus strains best adapted to the epidemiology of Foot-and-Mouth Disease in Botswana for the preparation of vaccines.

Vaccines are prepared from industrial viral cultures inactivated with ethylenimine. The formulation of vaccine is completed by the addition of aluminium hydroxide and saponin as adjuvants.

Epidemiologic Supervision of FMD in Southern Africa

Botswana has 2.3 million head of livestock. The vaccine was only used in the Northern part of the country, starting in 198l, ie in the region where cattle might be in contact with wildlife. The amount of vaccine required for this has not been sufficient to ensure a long life for the Botswana Vaccine Institute, despite diversification to rinderpest vaccine production.

The major part of production is exported to other parts of Southern Africa (Zimbabwe, Namibia, Zambia, Mozambique, Malawi, South Africa). These countries also face problems related to contact with wildlife.

One of the primary responsibilities of the laboratory is the study of viruses from outbreaks in these countries, which have a common border with Botswana. These studies aim to include the currently used vaccine strains into investigations of the field epidemiology, and to supply to requesting countries, vaccines adapted to their needs.

Studies of virus strains comprise:

- typing by the 100% complement fixation method (KOLMER) and by ELISA;

- serological studies for the establishment of relationships between the virus subtypes included in vaccines;

- immunological studies by seroneutralisation on cattle sera obtained with the vaccine strains and potency control in cattle by vaccination and cross challenge.

Since the creation of the laboratory in 1978, the strains studied following these techniques are:

43 SAT1 strains

79 SAT2 strains

15 SAT3 strains

6 A strains

4 O strains

In the near future, the laboratory will be able to characterise virus strains at the molecular level by the development of sequencing of viral ribonucleic acid. These analyses will allow continuous work on the epidemiology of Foot-and-Mouth Disease in Southern African countries.

CONCLUSION

Following the creation in 1978 of the Botswana Vaccine Institute, the outbreaks of Foot-and-Mouth Disease which seriously affected Botswana's territory were brought under control within two years.

This was made possible due to an epidemiologic study of existing strains in the field, which allowed the production of vaccines adapted to those strains. The development of close collaboration with other Southern African countries has not only allowed the country to remain free from Foot-and-Mouth Disease, but has also brought international recognition of the role of this Institute which in 1985 became the OIE Regional Laboratory for Foot-and-Mouth Disease.

For the continuation of development and control of scientific techniques for vaccines at international level and to ensure good economical management, regular investments are still made in materials as well as in the training of technicians in co-operation with RHONE MERIEUX.

2. PRODUCTION AND QUALITY CONTROL OF VACCINE AT THE NATIONAL VETERINARY LABORATORY, GAROUA (CAMEROON)

by

N Zoyem

The National Veterinary Laboratory (LANAVET) of Garoua - a public institution, produces a range of 17 different types of vaccines (7 viral vaccines, 8 bacterial vaccines and 2 mixed vaccines). All these vaccines are controlled locally following international norms; certain vaccines are also dispatched to PANVAC (PanAfrican Regional Centre for Quality Control) in Dakar (Senegal) where they are submitted to a second quality control.

LANAVET which has a large production capacity endeavours to keep abreast with modern technology; consequently emphasis is placed on training and refresher courses for staff as well as contact with international organisations.

Financial difficulties attributed to lack of subvention, inability to sell vaccines on a large scale following market restriction and maintenance of equipment, constitute at the moment, problems for which solutions need to be found.

The development of new products, the search for new markets and financial and technical assistance from international organisations could boost the activities of LANAVET in the near future.

3. VACCINE PRODUCTION AND QUALITY CONTROL IN ETHIOPIA

by

G Y Mebratu

INTRODUCTION

Ethiopia has an agroclimate best suited for livestock production and that is why the country has the largest livestock population in Africa and ranks tenth in the world. Nevertheless, as in many developing countries animal health is claimed to be one of the constraints to increased productivity and a stumbling block to livestock exports.

The National Veterinary Institute - Debre Zeit (NVI) which came into existence in 1963 produces 9 types vaccines against some major infectious diseases.

Organization and Function of the Institute

The National Veterinary Institute (NVI) is the only vaccine producing Institute in the country. It is totally state owned. The Institute which is part of the Ministry of Agriculture and Environmental Protection is under the direction of the Animal and Fishery Resources Main Department.

The production capacity of the Institute has now reached a level of 50 million doses per year, which is sufficient for local consumption as well as for export.

The Institute vaccine production laboratories have no physical connection with the Research and Diagnostic laboratories. More over, it has its own supply of water with a softening system. Two standby electric generators are available for emergency purposes in case the town supply fails. There is a high security laboratory within the quarantine area of the Institute where handling of virulent and dangerous material as well as the test of vaccines can be carried out.

The Institute has a research laboratory where the development of vaccines is undertaken.

A specific pathogen free poultry breeding unit is available. It has been possible to produce SPF embryonated eggs. This has helped to minimize the importation of eggs, thus lowering the vaccine production costs. There is a laboratory animals breeding section where the national requirements for vaccine production, diagnostic and research purposes is met.

The Institute has its own laboratory maintenance workshop where much of the equipment is repaired.

In addition to vaccine production buildings other important facilities include warehouses for raw materials and finished goods, (+4°c, -20°c with adequate back up refrigeration equipment), freeze drying and packaging area, and laundry.

After satisfying local demands for veterinary vaccines it has been possible to export to some African countries (Uganda, Sudan, Somalia, Tanzania, Burkina Faso, Angola, Cameroon, Chad, Djibouti) and Oman.

Besides producing veterinary biologicals, the National Veterinary Institute is involved in providing training to professional staff of various countries (Africa, Asia) on vaccine production and quality control. Senior scientists of the Institute also provide consultancy services to international organizations.

The National Veterinary Institute was actively involved during the creation of a regional center, for the control of veterinary vaccines in Africa. At present it has been possible to host the Pan African Vaccine Center (PANVAC), which we highly estimate for its services to the region.

Technologies and Quality Control Methods

The National Veterinary Institute produces 9 types of vaccines. These are against Rinderpest, African Horse Sickness, Sheep pox, Newcastle Disease, Contagious Bovine Pleuropneumonia, Anthrax, Blackleg, Bovine Pasteurellosis and Ovine Pasteurellosis.

All viral, Anthrax and Contagious Bovine Pleuro Pneumonia vaccines are produced in a freeze dried form. The rest are in fluid form and are inactivated. Production and quality control technologies are mostly transferred from I.E.M.V.T. (France) and some have been developed within the Institute.

Cell culturing technology (primary cell cultures and cell lines) is fully utilized to produce viral vaccines with the exception of avian vaccines where SPF embryonated eggs are used. Bacterial vaccines (live and killed) are produced in media prepared within the Institute.

Manufacturing of vaccines is carried out on the seed lot system. Reference Master Seed Banks are received from known and recommended origins. Master Seed Banks in the National Veterinary Institute are prepared from the Reference Master Seed Bank (Manufacturer's Master Bank). Working Seed Banks are derived from the Manufacturer's Master Bank. In process quality control is done for all vaccines as recommended by O.I.E., WHO, FAO by applying the standard operating procedures.

Application of National Quality Control Norms and Standards

Standard operating procedures (S.O.P.) are prepared by the National Veterinary Institute. Production procedures are in line with International standards and norms for biological products.

Quality Control of vaccines is handled by the production laboratory and counter checked by the Technical Director of the Institute. It is intended that within the vaccine manufacturing facilities, there will be a separate quality control section.

Application of International Quality Control Norms and Standards

The production laboratory of the Institute strictly adheres to the International norms and standards. Vaccines for exportation and for local vaccination campaigns (Rinderpest and CBPP) are tested and certified by PANVAC.

Quality Control of Vaccines and Biologicals Imported into Ethiopia

Most of the vaccines of national importance are produced and supplied by the National Veterinary Institute. Nevertheless, there are a few vaccines (Foot and Mouth disease, Rabies) which are imported into the country. No quality control is done on these vaccines. All imported biologicals should possess a Quality Control certificate from the country of origin.

Access to New Technologies 'Know How' on Vaccine Production and Quality Control

Access to new technologies 'know how' on vaccine production and quality control is a major problem for Ethiopia and many developing countries. The transfer of 'know how' for the production of Foot and Mouth disease and rabies vaccines in Ethiopia is estimated to cost about 60% of the total cost of the plant production. This is a good example of how difficult it is to have access to modern technologies.

Level of Computerization

The National Veterinary Institute is starting to introduce computerization which at present is not available in the Institute. It is appreciated that training needs to be given to some professional staff on the management and application of data bases.

Major Financial, Technical and Socioeconomic Constraints

a) Shortage of local and foreign currency.

The local budget allocated to the National Veterinary Institute is not sufficient to run routine production activities. Since vaccines are not produced under commercial (ie. parastatal or private) conditions, no income from the sale of vaccines is available. Foreign currency for the purchase of biologicals, chemicals, laboratory equipment and spare parts is one of the major problems faced by the Institute.

b) Shortage of specialized personnel.

Specialized personnel on the production of biologicals and on maintenance and operation of laboratory equipment is one of the problems encountered in the Institute. This is mainly due to lack of adequate remuneration and incentives in order to be able to retain their services on a long term basis.

c) Lack of spare parts.

It is difficult to buy spare parts for equipment which is of vital importance to vaccine production (freeze dryer, autoclaves, distillers etc.)

It has been found that such equipment often remains unrepaired for months.

Development Strategies

Development of production institutions is only possible when there are adequate financial sources backed by highly qualified personnel. This can only be achieved if new strategies are formulated.

Therefore steps are being taken to allow vaccines to be produced under commercial (ie. parastatal or private) conditions, and the Institute should be able in the future to sell vaccines and keep the funds thus generated, and subsequently attain financial autonomy.

The National Veterinary Institute will be having two more vaccine production laboratories ie. Foot and Mouth disease and Rabies, in the future. The establishment of these two plants will enable the Institute to acquire more modern production technologies.

It is planned that progress should be made towards acquiring biotechnology which is accepted as appropriate for the production of more effective vaccines in the future.

The Institute is also planning an infrastructural development so as to have industrial production capacity. By doing this it will be possible to meet all regional demands for veterinary vaccines.

4. THE KENYA VETERINARY VACCINE PRODUCTION UNIT (KEVEVAPI)

by

R Korir

Kenya Veterinary Vaccine Production Unit (KEVEVAPI) is the national production facility. It has recently acquired parastatal status and is now required to function on a self-sustaining financial basis. So far this approach has been successful, at least for the past three years.

With a range of some 14 vaccines in production it now has a staff of 67 persons made up of 8 graduates, 18 technologists and 41 technicians. Significantly, of the 8 graduate staff some 5 are employed in the Research and Development and the Quality Control Departments.

Design capacity of the production unit is considerable. At present some 20 million doses of foot and mouth disease vaccine are taken up, however, there is potential to produce up to 50 million doses per year. Similarly, there is the possibility of expanding the present annual production of 2 million doses each of rinderpest and Newcastle Disease vaccines to 7 million and 5 million doses respectively.

Present production capacity is more than sufficient to meet national requirements and the opportunity has therefore been taken to export vaccines to some 14 other countries mainly located within Africa. However, the Unit does not have production and export of vaccines as a prime objective.

Quality control of all veterinary vaccines manufactured by KEVEVAPI is fully carried out before they are released for use in disease control programmes. The full range of check tests are undertaken and include:

1. Assessment of raw materials.

2. In process controls - sterility, infectivity assays, type identification, growth potential, antigen assays and serological evaluations.

3. Innocuity and Safety tests.

4. Potency tests.

The standards and norms adopted for quality control work at KEVEVAPI follow those accepted internationally. As a result of research and development, 'in house' standards have been developed and this work continues with the objective of further improving the vaccines under production. A close collaboration with PANVAC has built up on the quality control of vaccines.

5. VACCINE PRODUCTION IN WEST AFRICA - SENEGAL AND MALI

by

D Sylla and M Rweyemamu

INTRODUCTION

Disease constraints has impeded for a long time the development of the livestock industry in Africa. Until the 1950's the greatest mortality was caused by rinderpest, CBPP, hemorragic septicemia, anthrax and blackleg. Stock owners were periodically threatened by outbreaks which wiped out most of the herds. This was because prophylactic measures were and still are difficult to apply in the wide open areas of the Sahel, where the wind blows constantly during the transhumance.

The large gatherings of livestock at the water points and on grazing lands play an important role in the transmission of diseases. Three to four decades ago, the veterinary services of West Africa were overstretched and had little to offer except compulsory vaccination imposed with the assistance of police forces. This lasted until stock owners realized the benefits of vaccination.

Rinderpest Vaccine

In the 1940's vaccination teams were used to take fire brigade action when outbreaks were declared in a district. Inactivated vaccine was prepared in the field, using virulent virus injected into susceptible calves in the herd. The temperature was monitored daily and the calves were slaughtered when it reached 41°C to 42°C. The blood, lymph nodes and spleen were collected, ground and inactivated with formalin, and then mixed with aluminium hydroxide gel. Vaccination teams proceeded from village to village in non infected areas. This vaccine well known in the francophone countries as VGA (vaccin au gel d'alumine) has been highly valued for a long time.

In the 1950's, the live caprinised vaccine and the lapinised vaccine were prepared by dessication of spleen and lymph node pulp under a glass bell. The product was reduced to powder, weighed and dispensed in ampoules to be sealed. This vaccine with its residual virulence was used only on Sahelian zebu cattle and produced long lasting immunity. This vaccine produces very severe reactions in NDama cattle and European breeds.

The live tissue culture vaccine (TCV) was introduced to West Africa during the JP 15 campaign in the early 1960's. In West and Central Africa, the vaccine was produced in Dakar, Bamako, Niamey, Vom and Farcha and in East Africa in Kabete and Muguga.

At the beginning of the JP 15 campaign this vaccine was not accepted by zebu herders because it did not produce any visible reactions in vaccinated animals. It took time to substitute it for the goat vaccine.

ANIMAL HEALTH STRATEGY IN FRANCOPHONE AFRICA

Before independence, veterinary services were organised on the basis of a federal system in West and Central Africa.

1. West Africa: 10 countries: Senegal, Guinee, Soudan (Mali), Mauritanie, Niger, Haute Volta (Burkina F.), Cote d'Ivoire, Dahomey (Benin), Togo. With Federal Veterinary Services centred in Dakar and the Federal Laboratory in Dakar, with a subunit in Bamako. The Federal Veterinary School was located in Bamako.

2. Equatorial Africa: 6 countries: Congo, Tchad, Gabon, Oubangui Chari (CAR), Cameroun. The Federal Veterinary Services were based in Brazzaville and the Federal Veterinary Laboratory in Farcha.

The emergence of new independent states in 1960 has created a need for restructuring of the system and the creation of national laboratories and new veterinary schools. Several states continue to be supplied with vaccines from Dakar; others meet their own requirements. The vaccine producers are now located at Dakar, Kindia, Bingerville, Bamako, Niamey, Farcha, Vom and Garoua. However, in the present economic context, not all of these laboratories are sustainable. They are no longer viable, but their existence is a matter of national pride. It is a fact that a number of laboratories have been obliged to stop vaccine production because of multiple constraints. A few of them cannot meet the standards required for good quality vaccines. The meeting of the Directors of national laboratories (27-28 September in Nairobi) was endorsed by the IIIrd Conference of Ministers responsible for livestock development in the OAU Member States. The Central African Economic Community (CEEAC) is also moving in this direction and has considered the regionalization of vaccine production in its project RAF/88/049 - granted by UNDP. It is opportune that this expert consultation may give a guideline on the subject.

VACCINE PRODUCTION UNITS IN WEST AFRICA:

LNERV DAKAR-HANN

Physical structure

One building for viral vaccine production and one building for bacterial vaccine production. In both buildings, vaccine production and research and diagnosis are performed. This does not comply with GMP rules. The vaccine quality control service is incorporated in the research service.

Equipment

The equipment is in working condition and maintained routinely.

Staff

World bank and IMF pressure on government economic policy has imposed a reduction of staff, thus reducing the level of activities.

Budget

There is more and more budget restriction. The funds from vaccine sales is not returned to the LNERV. The administrative linkage to ISRA is rather a constraint and an unnecessary burden to LNERV which has difficulties of its own in ordering chemicals and equipment for vaccine production.

Vaccines produced

Approximately fifteen types of vaccines are produced, the most important being rinderpest and CBPP vaccines. Only vaccines for export are submitted to PANVAC for quality control. LNERV holds a PARC rinderpest vaccine bank which has been tested by PANVAC, but is not under PANVAC's custody.

Maintenance service

This is managed by a dedicated national engineer who has not enough staff or funds. There is a need for more trained staff, equipment and resources.

The Sangalkam farm of experimental animals 30 km distant is not properly maintained.

The facilities for in vivo testing of vaccines also needs some improvement.

CENTRAL VETERINARY LABORATORY, MALI:

This laboratory built by the US-AID was designed by the Virus Department of the Veterinary School at Cornell University.

Buildings

There are separate buildings for vaccine production, research, diagnosis, workshop and stores etc. A farm for clean animals is located 2 km from the laboratory premises. A water treatment plant located at the farm is connected to the city water supply.

Equipment

In general good modern equipment is available. However, the freeze dryers are old and need to be replaced. Among all African laboratories the CVL MALI is particularly well equipped in computers.

Staff

There is a good training program under the US-AID technical assistance. Most Heads of Divisions have been trained in US Universities.

Budget

The research budget is supported from the livestock sector development project. Vaccine production is financed from the national budget and is insufficient. The CVL used to have financial autonomy but this has been cancelled recently; hence it is no longer possible to use the funds from the sale of vaccines. Long procedures for budget allocation makes it difficult to purchase equipment, chemicals and supplies from overseas.

Vaccines

Five types of vaccines are produced: RP, CBPP, HS, anthrax and blackleg. A new building has been set up for the production of avian vaccines in 1992. Vaccine production and quality control services are completely independent and located in separate premises. In addition to 'in house' quality control, rinderpest vaccine batches are tested by PANVAC on regular basis.

Maintenance service

The maintenance service is well equipped and well organized. Staff members have received training in the USA with companies manufacturing freeze dryers, steam engines, generators, etc.

Farm

Forty ha. of land on the riverside is used for cattle, horses, small ruminants and laboratory animals.

LANAVET GAROUA:

This is the most recent laboratory - having started vaccine production in 1985. As far as GMP and quality assurance are concerned, LANAVET is the best laboratory in this part of the Continent. The staff is well trained and competent. However, because of the country's financial constraints and because of the uncertainty of the vaccine market, the long term sustainability of this institution is seriously in doubt. The regionalization of vaccine production will be of help in maximising the use of the facilities of LANAVET.

Other laboratories of minor importance are located at Farcha and Niamey. The laboratories of Bingerville (Cote d'Ivoire) and Kindia (Guinee) have stopped producing vaccines.

QUALITY OF VACCINES PRODUCED IN WEST AFRICA

International quality control standards were introduced in 1985. Many batches of vaccine were below the international standard. Some progress has now been achieved, as shown below:

PRODUCERS	BATCHES	PASSED 1985	PASSED 1986
B7	3	1/3	NT
K5	3	2/3	1/3
T4	3	1/3	3/3
D7	3	1/3	3/3
C6	3	0/3	NT
H10	3	0/3	2/3
H4	3	0/3	NT

The vaccine production laboratories of the region are government institutions. Due to lack of incentives, the staff do not have the real enthusiasm necessary for the promotion and accomplishment of high quality production. Under government management, it is difficult to produce good quality vaccines in sufficient quantity for the needs of the national campaigns and/or the Pan African Rinderpest Campaign (PARC). There are too many constraints (eg - lack of resources and foreign exchange, long bureaucratic procedures etc) which are not compatible with efficient vaccine production.

The trend toward regionalisation and/or the conversion into parastatal bodies may improve the situation. As the result of commercial pressures only the most competent laboratories will survive. The Economic Community of the Central African States has already taken steps in this direction. With the support of the FAO, EEC and other international donors, similar decisions must be taken in the near future in West Africa for the benefit of good vaccine producers and of animal health in general.

6. QUALITY CONTROL OF MODIFIED LIVING VIRAL VACCINES IN LIBYA, SOMALIA AND CZECHOSLOVAKIA

by

V Rozkosny

INTRODUCTION

Conventional vaccines constitute one of the most significant strategies for the prevention and control of infectious diseases, mainly in developing countries. Although the technologies for the production of many vaccines such as clostridial, anthrax, hemorrhagic septicaemia, contagious bovine pleuro-pneumonia, contagious caprine pleuropneumonia, rinderpest, sheep pox, lumpy skin disease as well as Newcastle disease, have been available for many years and most of them have been standardized, their quality in developing countries is still very variable.

The purpose of this paper is to summarize experiences in relation to quality control of modified living viral vaccines in small production laboratories in Somalia and Libya. A brief presentation of the quality control system for vaccines used in Czechoslovakia is also made.

Table 1 illustrates the system of production and quality control for some modified living viral vaccines, for example Parainfluenza-3 virus of cattle, as produced in Czechoslovakia. The process of vaccine production and control is divided into four independent institutions, each with full quality control responsibility. The first step is substrate control (kidney and growth serum). Both are obtained from bovine foetuses or postnatal calves originally from herds free of specific diseases (BVD-MD, Bovine Leucosis).

The virus strain for vaccine production is selected by a government advisory committee and the quality control (ie. purity, identity and viability) is under the responsibility of a special institution - the "Collection of Zoopathogenic microorganisms - Brno", where virus strains are stored and maintained.

Vaccine production itself is controlled in terms of quality by the producer according to accepted production norms, where all available tests for quality control are included. Production norms used are confirmed by a government advisory committee.

The highest level of quality control is undertaken at the Institute for Quality Control of all veterinary bioproducts in Czechoslovakia. This Institute has the status of an independent government organization. The production and control norms for all steps of vaccine quality control are regularly updated according to international standards issued by OIE, WHO or FAO.

Table 2 illustrates the quality control system applied to modified living viral embryonated egg vaccines, for example Newcastle Disease vaccine. The system of quality control is very similar to that mentioned above and is also divided into four independent steps each with its own quality control norms, which are regularly updated according to international standards.

Table 3 illustrates the system of production and quality control of rinderpest vaccine in operation in Somalia, where the Czechoslovak team worked from 1982-1986 under the FAO Project - SOM/82/004. More than four million doses of vaccine were produced for the local bovine population and one million doses were exported to Uganda.

Quality control was carried out according to the International norm for rinderpest (WHO. Geneva 1970, later revised FAO Rome 1985) and in line with the Czechoslovak control system. In the Independent Testing Programme (PARC FAO 1985) three samples submitted passed the tests for vacuum, sterility and purity. Two were consistently well above the minimum standard for potency thus being graded as "excellent" by one test centre, however, the third was consistently below the required potency standard when diluted for field use. Despite this, the vaccine, - which was produced in one of the smallest African laboratories, ranks among the four best produced in the Continent.

Table 4 illustrates the vaccine needs, vaccine importations and first stages of local vaccine production in Libya. It will be noted that Libya has imported more than 200 million doses of vaccines (mostly viral), per year. These are mainly for protection of poultry and the sheep population.

Attention has been focused on local production of viral vaccines such as Newcastle Disease vaccine and Gumboro vaccine for the poultry population and sheep pox vaccine for the population of local sheep. This programme has been in operation since 1989. Progress on the production of sheep pox vaccine has been good and over one million doses of vaccine have been produced and controlled for quality. The vaccine has been used in the field without adverse effects and to the satisfaction of the livestock owners.

The production of Newcastle Disease vaccine and Gumboro vaccine is going very well and more than 1 million doses of both vaccines have already been prepared and are being checked for quality. Large scale production of poultry vaccines will start next year.

CONCLUSIONS

Live viral vaccines, in general, offer significant advantages over other types of viral vaccines, namely induction of more effective cell mediated immunity and even long duration immunity.

However, such vaccines have, at present, some very important disadvantages:

- the possibility of an attenuated strain reverting to its original more pathogenic form
- some viruses may persist for lengthy periods in vaccinated hosts
- potential susceptibility of hosts other than the vaccinated population to the modified virus strain

contamination with other viral potential pathogens.

For these reasons, some modified viral vaccines have disappeared from the list of bioproducts of some European vaccine producers. In relation to other very effective vaccines such as rinderpest, Newcastle Disease, Gumboro and infectious bronchitis viral vaccine new, sophisticated and expensive methods have been introduced for their quality control. The application of these methods in small laboratories in developing countries is not easy since in addition to the high level technology needed, many freshly prepared diagnostic reagents and chemicals which are expensive, and the services of staff with professional qualifications and practical experience, are also required.

Table 1. Quality Control of Modified TC Parainfluenza-3 Living Virus Vaccine (Bovine Vaccines - Czechoslovakia)

A	B	C	D	E	F		G	
					FINAL PRODUCT		FINAL PRODUCT	
KIDNEY	GROWING SERUM	VIRUS STRAIN	SEED LOT	LIQUID VACCINE	BIOLOGICAL	TECHNICAL	BIOLOGICAL	TECHNICAL
1. BOVINE FOETUS 2. POSTNATAL ONE WEEK OLD CALF FROM HERD FREE OF SPECIFIC INFECTIONS BVD-MD BOVINE LEUCOSIS	1. CALF FOETAL SERUM 2. CALF PRE-COLOSTRAL SERUM 3. CALF POST-NATAL SERUM FROM HERD FREE OF SPEC. INFECTIONS BVD-MD BOVINE LEUCOSIS	SELECTED BY SPEC. GOV. COMMITTEE STERILITY IDENTITY MYCOPL. CONT.	STERILITY MYCOPL. CONT. VIRUS CONTENT SAFETY IDENTITY EXTRANEOUS AGENTS B/BOV. LEUCOSIS C/BVD	STERILITY MYC. CONT. VIRUS CONTENT	STERILITY MYCOPL. CONT. VIRUS CONTENT SAFETY IDENTITY EXTRANEOUS AGENTS STABILITY		STERILITY MYCOPL. CONTAM. VIRUS CONT. SAFETY IDENTITY EXTRANEOUS AGENTS STABILITY	RESIDUAL MOISTURE VACUUM

Table 2. Quality Control of Modified Living Newcastle Disease Virus Vaccine (Poultry Vaccines - Czechoslovakia)

A	B	C	D	E		F	
CHICKEN EMBRYO CHICKEN EMBRYO FIBROBLAST	GROWIN G CALF SERUM	VIRUS STRAIN	SEED LOTS	FINAL PRODUCT		FINAL PRODUCT	
				BIOLOGICAL	TECHNICAL	BIOLOGICAL	TECHNICAL
SPF EGGS (AS SPF STANDARD)		SELECTED BY GOVERNMENT COMMITTEE STORED AND MAINTAINED (CZECHOSLOVA K COLLECTION OF ZOOPATHOGENI C MICRO-ORGANISMS) (BRNO)	STERILITY MYCOPL. CONT. VIRUS CONTENT IDENTITY POTENCY STABILITY SAFETY USING CHICKEN EXTRANEOUS AGENTS USING EE AND TC	STERILITY MYCOPL.CONT. VIRUS CONTENT IDENTITY POTENCY STABILITY SAFETY USING CHICKEN EXTRANEOUS AGENTS USING EE AND TC	RESIDUAL MOISTURE VACUUM	STERILITY MYCOPL. CONTAM. VIRUS CONT. IDENTITY SAFETY USING CHICKEN EXTRANEOUS AGENTS USING EE AND TC POTENCY STABILITY	1. RESIDUAL MOISTURE 2. VACUUM

Table 3. Quality Control of Rinderpest TC Living Virus Vaccine (Somalia)

KIDNEY	GROWING SERUM	VIRUS STRAIN	SEED LOT	LIQUID VACCINE	FINAL PRODUCT
ONE WEEK OLD CALF GOVT. HERD FREE FROM INFECTIONS: BOV. LEUCOSIS FMD BVD-MD RINDERPEST LUMPY SKIN DISEASE CBPP BRUCELLOSIS S. DUBLIN TUBERCULOSIS	IMPORT CZECHOSLOVAKIA (CS NORM)	PIRBRIGHT RBOK	STERILITY MYCOPL. CONT. VIRUS CONTENT SAFETY IDENTITY EXTRANEOUS AGENTS A/LUMPY SKIN DISEASE B/BOV. LEUCOSIS C/BVD-MD	STERILITY MYC. CONT. VIRUS CONTENT	VACUUM STERILITY MYC.CONT. VIRUS CONTENT SAFETY IDENTITY EXTRANEOUS AGENTS A/LUMPY SKIN DISEASE B/BOVINE LEUCOSIS BVD-MD D/CHLAMYDIA

Table 4. Vaccines - Import. Local Production and Proposal for Production. (Libya - 1991)

IMPORT X1000	POULTRY/ANIMAL POPULATION X1000	VACCINES	IMPORT DOSES X1000	LOCAL VACCINE PRODUCTION DOSES X 1000		
				1991	1992	1993
FERTILE EGGS 40,000	BROILERS 70,000	NEWCASTLE	75,000	1000	16000	24000
		GUMBORO	75,000	800	16000	30000
		INF. BRONCHITIS	50,000			
1 DAY OLD CHICKEN 4000	PARENT STOCK 5000	FOWL POX	3,000			
16 WEEKS OLD HENS 2000	GRANDPARENT STOCK 20	MAREK	250			
		AVIAN ENCEPH.	750			
		TRIPOLE (NDV.IB.GUM) VACCINE (INACTIVATED)	750			
	SHEEP 7000	SHEEP POX	6,000	950	3000	3000
	CATTLE 40					

7. VACCINE PRODUCTION AND CONTROL IN SYRIA

by

G Khoury

It is well known that animal husbandry is the main source of income for a large proportion of the population in the developing countries. The methods of animal husbandry used in these countries varies from the labour intensive methods to modern industrial systems and therefore disease control may also be variable and difficult. The import of vaccines is sometimes impeded by lack of funds. The production of veterinary vaccines in the developing countries is therefore very important. As these conditions may be shared by many of the developing countries, it is important to consider various aspects of local vaccine production. These considerations are as follows:

1. It has often been shown that adequate vaccines are not obtainable immediately and easily when they are most needed, especially in the case of diseases with a rapid spread. This is due to the inability of some countries to obtain credit in time to buy and store an adequate supply of vaccines. For example, in Syria we faced this problem in 1982, when rinderpest had spread within the country. The losses were high because we could not provide vaccine at the proper time.

2. The execution of an adequate vaccination campaign requires a good stock of vaccines available at any time they are needed. The establishment of such a stock is often stopped or only partially implemented because of the above mentioned import problems.

3. The establishment of vaccine production in a developing country means much more than effective production work only. It also requires the development of isolation methods for pathogenic agents and their diagnosis. This provides opportunities for local veterinarians to understand and deal with pathogens in a proper manner, and to use the local strains for vaccine production. This can lead to a better and more efficient immunity against a wide range of bacterial diseases.

4. Finally, local vaccine production also means new job opportunities in places where not so many jobs are available. In consequence, it also helps to save needless expenditures by the elimination of repeated imports of vaccine which are often the only basis of vaccination campaigns in many developing countries.

Bearing in mind all of the above mentioned factors, the Veterinary Authorities in Syria have given special attention to the establishment and expansion of local vaccine production. They have provided technical staff, buildings and essential equipment in order to reach self sufficiency in this field. This input together with UNDP/FAO support has allowed us to achieve large scale vaccine production in the fields of both, viral and bacterial vaccines, with the exception of a few vaccines which will be implemented in the near future.

On behalf of the Syrian Veterinary Services appreciation is expressed to the Food and Agriculture Organization of the United Nations for the immense help in the establishment of the production of vaccines under the project SYR/86/008. This was mainly directed towards the production of virus vaccines and also some bacterial vaccines. Also the current project SYR/88/006 which concerns the extension of bacterial vaccine production by fermentation techniques. The latter project has now installed the fermenter units and has already produced some batches of Enterotoxaemia vaccines. On completion, this project will cover the need of the whole region for Enterotoxaemia, Brucellosis and sheep/cattle Pasteurellosis vaccines. In addition, it will be able to produce any other bacterial vaccine in large amounts; e.g E.coli vaccines.

The other subject which needs to be discussed, is the quality control of locally produced vaccines, and also imported ones.

There is no doubt that production and control activities have to be developed together, since production without good quality control can easily result in poor immunity and insufficient protection against dangerous diseases.

The Syrian Veterinary Services consider that the following requirements have to be available in order to reach an efficient level of quality control work:

1. The availability of well trained staff in the field of quality control work.

2. To keep updated with new technology concerning the methods of vaccine control and the related international standards.

3. The availability of modern and appropriate equipment necessary for this purpose.

For the fulfilment of these requirements it is suggested that the following are necessary:

1. Develop a programme to identify the factors most important to the establishment of new technologies in developing countries including methods for comparing the quality of products from different laboratories.

   The introduction of these methods will hopefully avoid the confusion created by different opinions and interpretations existing in this field.

2. Establishment and/or strengthening of international relations among different production and control centres in the developing countries. This programme should include the exchange of information and experience. This could be very important since it is known that contagious diseases can create not only local, regional and national problems but also international ones, as political borders do not stop the spread of diseases.

3. Plan and adopt a reliable system for the training of staff members concerned with production and control at both professional and technical levels. The training to be undertaken in the developed countries.

The FAO would be the best organisation to realise the above mentioned suggestions and to maximise the benefits and avoid obstacles that still exist in bilateral relations.

On the basis of all the above mentioned, the Syrian Veterinary Services wish to express their willingness in establishing co-operation with any organisation or group which might be interested in such relations. All interested parties will be welcome at the production and control centres. It is believed that the centres, both production and quality control are well equipped and organized and are ready to share knowledge with other centres. It is hoped that FAO will continue to help by providing experts and training facilities for our staff to improve vaccine production and quality control work. The Organization is also requested to help in providing facilities and knowledge in the field of multivalent vaccine production.

ASIA AND THE PACIFIC REGION

8. PRODUCTION AND QUALITY CONTROL SYSTEMS FOR VETERINARY BIOPRODUCTS IN CHINA

by

T Guiyun

INTRODUCTION

There are some 28 production units for the manufacture of veterinary bioproducts in China. Some of them were established for the production of anti-serum during the 1930's and 40's and many still function with old and outdated equipment from 30 or 40 years ago. These conditions obviously can not meet the requirements of Good Manufacturing Practice and therefore affect the quality of the products.

At the present time, the facilities have been improved in some manufactories, to meet the GMP requirements issued by the Ministry of Agriculture in 1988. The production conditions for bioproducts in these units have therefore been improved greatly.

In general, most factories are also making other products (antibiotics, pharmaceuticals, veterinary instruments etc).

In 1989, there were 78 types of vaccines involving a total output of 9.4 billion doses; poultry vaccines accounted for 8 billion doses; cattle vaccines 27.26 million doses; sheep and goat vaccines 120 million doses, and vaccines against zoonosis (eg Brucellosis ...) 200 million doses. In 1990 the comparable figures for 74 types of vaccine with a total out-put of 7.4 billion doses were: swine vaccines 1.1 billion doses; poultry vaccines 6.3 billion doses; cattle vaccines 28 million doses; sheep and goat vaccine 120 million doses; and vaccines for use against zoonosis 159 million doses.

The State has made unified quality standards for bioproducts. All producers have to meet these requirements accordingly. The quality control section of each factory is responsible for the inspection of raw materials and semi-products, the supervision of the whole production procedure and final tests. Products are not allowed to be released for use unless they have been checked by the Quality Control (Q.C.) section. The Q.C. section is responsible for submitting a report on the testing of products to the National Control Institute of Veterinary Bioproducts and Pharmaceuticals, monthly. Production units are given technical guidance by the Institute.

The National Control Institute of Veterinary Bioproducts and Pharmaceuticals (NCIVBP) set up by the Ministry of Agriculture is responsible for supervising, examining and appraising the quality of all veterinary bioproducts, having been entrusted by the Chinese Government according to the stipulations of "The Animal Drugs - Administration & Regulation".

The NCIVBP has 15 departments as follows: First Department of Bacteriology, Second Department of Bacteriology, Department of Virology, Department of Mycoplasmology, Department of Pharmaceuticals, Department of Biochemistry, Department of Culture Media Preparation, Breeding Unit for Laboratory Animals, Department of Equipment and Instruments, Office for Planning and Co-ordination, National Veterinary Culture Collection, Office of Veterinary Pharmacopoeia, Office of Review Committee of New Veterinary Products, Personnel Department and Administration Offices (logistics). The NCIVBP has a total of 263 staff including 172 technical staff of whom 34 are senior scientists, 65 assistant researchers and 50 junior scientists.

The main tasks of the Institute can be summarized as follows:

1. Preparation, appraising, storage and distribution of master seed cultures and standard or reference products for production and testing purposes, also for research use;

2. The provision of technical advice on quality control for 30 Provincial Control Institutes of veterinary bioproducts and pharmaceuticals and 28 Q.C. sections of veterinary bioproduct factories;

3. Sampling and retesting of veterinary bioproducts and pharmaceuticals;

4. Final arbitration in disputes on the quality of products;

5. Responsibility for conducting tests of new products (including vaccines, diagnostic reagents, drugs and feed additives) developed in China, and those registered in China by foreign enterprises;

6. Participating in the formulation of quality standards for veterinary bioproducts and pharmaceuticals;

7. Research on the development of new products, new technologies and techniques for production.

8. Training of technical personnel for factories.

Fig 1. System of Biobroducts Quality Control

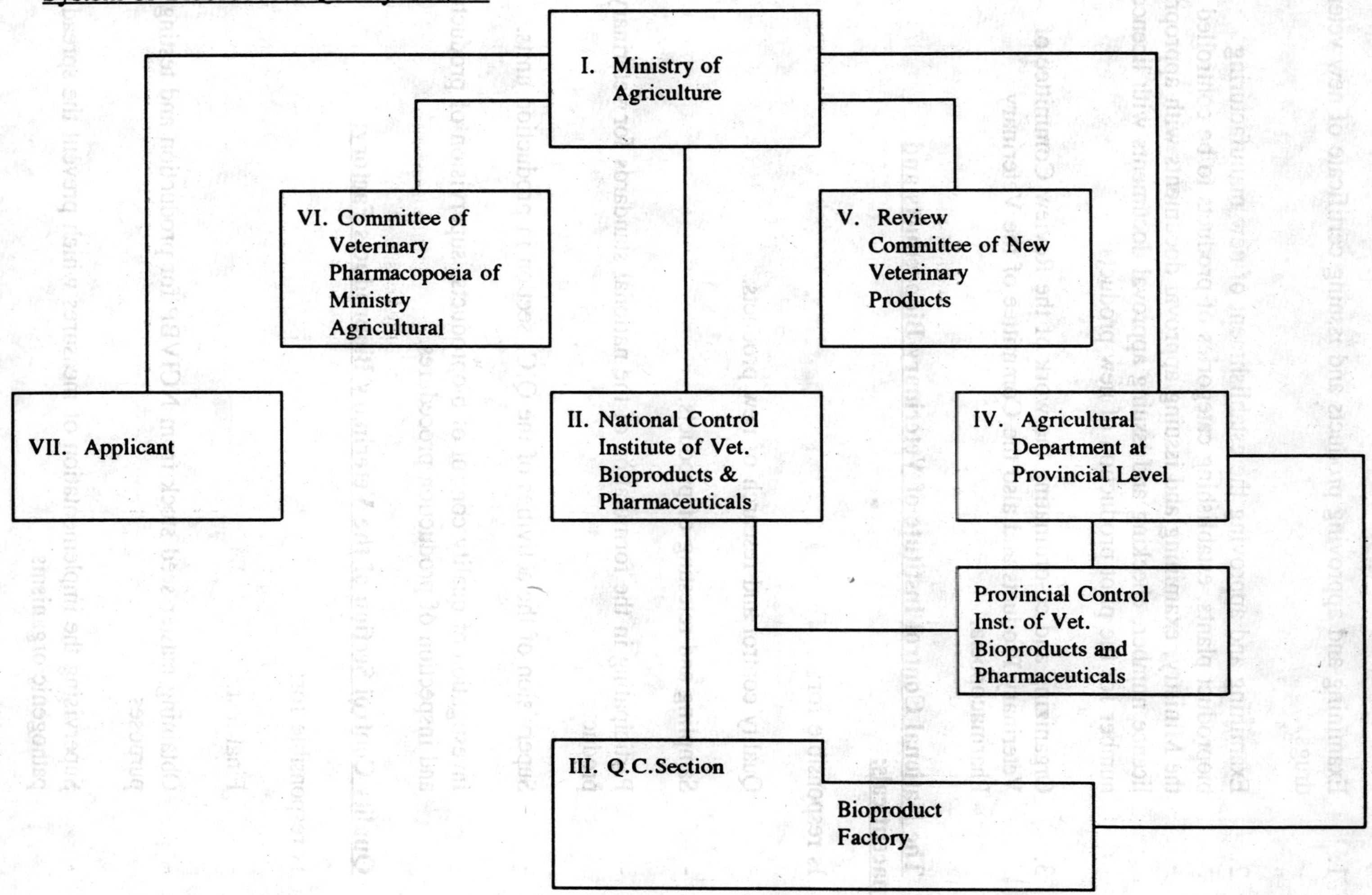

I. **Ministry of Agriculture:**

Has the following responsibilities:

1. Examining and approving products and issuing certificate of new veterinary drugs.

2. Examining and approving the establishment of new manufacturing bioproduct plants, establishing categories of products to be controlled by the Ministry, examining and issuing approval documents with appropriate licence number, checking and issuing approval documents with licence number for the pilot production of new products.

3. Organizing and co-ordinating the work of the Review Committee of Veterinary Products and also the Committee of the Veterinary Pharmacopoeia.

II. **The National Control Institute of Veterinary Bioproducts and Pharmaceuticals:**

Is responsible for:

- Quality control and research of new products.

- Sampling and retesting of products.

- Participating in the formulation of the national standards for veterinary products.

- Supervision of the activities of the Q.C. section in production units.

- Investigation of quality control of bioproducts, supervision of production, and inspection of production procedures.

III. **Quality Control Section of the Veterinary Bioproducts Factory:**

Is responsible for:

- Final test.

- Obtaining master seed stock from NCIVBP for production and testing purposes.

- Supervising the implementation of measures which prevent the spread of pathogenic organisms.

- Supervising the implementation of national standards throughout the whole production process.

Investigating the application and effectiveness of bioproducts in the field.

IV. Agricultural Departments at Provincial Level:

Are responsible for:

Examination and approval of veterinary bioproducts which already meet the national standard. Also rechecking and issuing of licence numbers for production.

V. Review Committee of Veterinary Bioproducts:

Is responsible for:

- Examining and reviewing new bioproducts application.
- Researching veterinary bioproducts under production.
- Reviewing and evaluation of veterinary bioproducts registered in China by foreign enterprises.

VI. The Committee for the Veterinary Pharmacopoeia of the Ministry of Agriculture:

- Formulates and revises the "Chinese Veterinary Pharmacopoeia" and quality standards.

VII. Application for a Product Licence:

Each application for the approval of a new product, requires that the following documents will be furnished to the Ministry of Agriculture:

- Official report
- Research report on the new bioproduct
- Report of the pilot production and field trial of the new product
- Quality standards for the new product
- Explanation of the drafting of the quality standards
- Instructions for use
- Feedback information from users.

Future Developments in the Production and Quality Control of Veterinary Bioproducts

Animal husbandry in China has developed rapidly for the past decade, especially in the intensive poultry raising industry, and there is therefore a need for high quality vaccines. Present production conditions do not meet the requirements of GMP. Technical improvements have been made at the existing factories in a planned programme. As an example, Nanjing Animal Drugs and Instruments Factory has set up a new building for production of bioproducts. This will be focused on the production of swine and poultry vaccines. The manufactured products will be directed towards use in the southern areas of the country. This establishment was financed by the Ministry of Agriculture. Other examples include: Hei Longjiang Veterinary Bioproduct Factory which has rebuilt its production units supported by local government. In Jiangxi Provincial Bioproduct Plant, a new production facility has been established. This is a joint venture co-operation with Sanofi - the French company.

The Ministry of Agriculture intends to set up a new biological production unit, designed according to the requirements of GMP, introducing advanced equipment and production techniques mainly to produce poultry vaccines which will be supplied to the northern areas of China. It is also planned to build a new production establishment for Foot-and-Mouth disease vaccine and other cattle and sheep and goat vaccines in the Lanzhou Bioproducts factory. These products will be mainly directed to the FMD immune zones of the border areas. Some small-sized factories in poor condition and incapable of technical improvement will turn to the manufacture of other products.

The first edition of the "Regulations for the Preparation and Testing of Veterinary Bioproducts" was issued in 1953 by the Ministry of Agriculture. It has been revised five times during the recent past years, and the sixth edition will be published in 1992 or 1993. International quality standards for veterinary bioproducts will be included and some methods of quality control developed by Chinese scientists will also form part of this edition.

The introduction of new regulations and implementation of new quality standards will be helpful in greatly improving the quality of veterinary bioproducts in China. This will bring the quality of bioproducts produced in China to levels very similar to those found internationa

9. VACCINE PRODUCTION AND QUALITY CONTROL IN INDIA

by

P N Bhat

INTRODUCTION

The organisation and function of veterinary vaccine production and quality control in India is governed by the Statutes of the Drugs and Cosmetics Act 1945. The country is self-sufficient in almost all the vaccines needed for livestock and poultry protection.

In India there are both State and Federal Administrations and agriculture comes under State Administration. Each State has its own biological production unit funded from the State budget, which produces vaccines for use in the State. Over the years some States have made great progress in this field, whilst others have lagged far behind and for economic reasons have given up vaccine production.

From the 1970's onwards multinational companies started production in India - the first of which was Hoechst with Foot and Mouth Disease vaccine. There are now 24 units in the Government sector producing biologicals and diagnostic reagents. These units have been established with aid of technology transferred from the Biological Production Division of the Indian Veterinary Research Institute (IVRI) which in turn has benefitted from technology brought in from abroad as the result of foreign aid programmes.

There are joint sector programmes in which the Government puts up the facilities with local funds and resources, and private sector companies provide the processes and management. In addition there are 2 major facilities totally owned by multi-national companies. There is a move in the country now towards increasing privatisation of production. This was not possible before, when the Government was both producer and purchaser of these products. The latter was for the benefit of the small marginal farmer who makes up some 65% of the total farming industry.

Legislation

The Drugs and Cosmetics Act defines the organisation for the control of biological production in the country. The principal authority for the licensing of vaccines and diagnostics is a joint panel of advisers drawn from the Ministry of Health and the Ministry of Agriculture. The licensing of production units is the responsibility of the appropriate State Drugs Controller. In addition there is a Federal Drugs Controller in the Ministry of Health who is advised on veterinary biologicals by the Director of the IVRI who is also one of the statutory authorities for the licensing of these products under the Act.

The Act is made up of a series of schedules based upon the Indian Pharmacopoiea and also the WHO, FAO and OIE guidelines. In formulating new standards, the Division of Standardisation of the IVRI is currently the National Standards Laboratory. Each

State-run biologicals production unit has to have an R and D section and there are regular inspections to ensure that quality control work is maintained after licensing.

It is now realised that the present organisation for control of biological products is less than ideal. In future it is intended that there should be a clear division between the controls for human and veterinary products. The intention is to establish a Central Veterinary Standardisation Laboratory supported by 4 Regional Laboratories. The Federal veterinarian in charge will be totally independent and act as a Statutory Authority located within the Ministry of Agriculture. He will take up his duties in 1992 after the necessary amendments to the Act have been made.

Future Developments

India has had no major problems in accessing the newer technologies. If a particular technology is not obtainable through bilateral aid programmes, the alternative is to purchase it. The major constraint to progress, as in most developing economies is lack of funds. In times of economic stress the first organisations to suffer are those connected with animal health and veterinary science. However progress is being made and the livestock industry is growing. In consequence there is now the possibility for the licensing of private companies to produce veterinary vaccines. It is anticipated that during the next 5 years a separate Act will be promulgated to control the products of recombinant DNA technology. The Department of Biotechnology of the Government of India has a major interest in developing a cadre of scientific manpower through training and research and development programmes. For this there is an investment programme of 400 million rupees. At present there are two P3 facilities in the country and there will shortly be a third at the new Institute under construction at Bhopal. There are also two P4 facilities for work with human viruses at Pune.

Normally, there is little need to import vaccines, however as a result of the large importation over the years of pedigree livestock or germ plasm, for livestock improvement, a number of extraneous agents have entered the country. This happened because there were no facilities for testing the imports at the time and reliance was placed upon the veterinary certificates from the exporting countries. In consequence there has been the appearance of Bluetongue disease and a number of poultry diseases for which vaccines have had to be imported.

India's programme for participation in the eradication of rinderpest from Asia is now underway and special arrangements for testing the vaccine for "Rinderpest Zero" have been put into effect. Efforts are being made to achieve batch standardisation. Quality control testing of every batch of other products is not normally undertaken, and maintenance of standards is on an 'honour' basis for each manufacturer. Four units will produce the vaccine using primary tissue cultures and every 5th batch will be sent to the Standards Laboratory for quality control tests. The batch will only be released after satisfactory results have been obtained.

10. THE ACTIVITIES OF THE VETERINARY DRUG ASSAY LABORATORY, GUNUNGSINDUR, BOGOR, INDONESIA

by

S B Siregar

INTRODUCTION

In order to ensure the quality of veterinary drugs distributed in Indonesia, the Government of the Republic of Indonesia established the Veterinary Drug Assay Laboratory (VDAL) in Bogor, West Java with financial aid from the Government of Japan. This project has been implemented under a technical co-operation program between the Government of the Republic of Indonesia and the Government of Japan. The executing agencies of both Governments are the Directorate General of Livestock Services, Department of Agriculture and the Japan International Co-operation Agency (JICA), respectively. This project was started in April 1984 for 5 years and extended until 1991.

The main functions of the laboratory are to examine the quality of veterinary drugs produced and imported, as well as to monitor the quality of veterinary drugs on the market.

Some information about the activities of the Veterinary Drug Assay Laboratory is given in this paper.

ORGANISATION AND FUNCTION OF THE VETERINARY DRUG ASSAY LABORATORY

1. Organisation

Veterinary Drug Assay Laboratory (VDAL) is one of the Technical Institutions concerned with animal health of the Directorate General of Livestock Services, Ministry of Agriculture, being charged with the quality control of veterinary drugs including vaccines, pharmaceuticals, premixes and other biologicals.

The Laboratory is organised into: Director's Office, three Major Sections, one Assay Group, six Sub Sections and five Assay Units. The three Major Sections are Administration, Sample Collection and Certification and Assay Facility.

The flow of assay activities is as follows: Samples of veterinary drugs are collected or received from the producers, importers, distributors, retailers etc by the sub section dealing with sample collection. The first tests to be made on the samples are concerned with sterility, vacuum level, moisture and preservative content etc. The samples are then distributed to the appropriate assay units for special tests of safety, potency, virus and bacteria content test etc. The assay results are collated by the staff of The Certification Sub Section.

2. Functions

The functions of the Laboratory are as follows:

(a) To examine the quality of veterinary drugs produced or imported before marketing, and issue quality certificates for the drugs.

(b) To monitor the quality of veterinary drugs on the market in order to ensure the use only of good quality veterinary drugs.

(c) To conduct training and provide technical guidance for veterinary drug inspectors.

(d) To promote the improvement of veterinary drugs and research on the development of assay methods.

(e) To assist the veterinary drug industry in improving drug quality.

ORGANISATION OF THE QUALITY CONTROL OF VACCINES AND BIOLOGICALS

The quality control of veterinary vaccines and biologicals is an integral part of veterinary drugs control in Indonesia.

At the national level, the control of the quality of vaccines and biologicals is conducted by the Veterinary Drug Assay Laboratory. Within the Directorate General of Livestock Services, the administration of vaccines and biologicals is performed by the Sub Directorate of Veterinary Drugs Control, under the Directorate of Animal Health.

The other institutions that are involved in some aspects of the quality control of veterinary vaccines and biologicals are as follows:

1. Veterinary Drug Commission

The function of the Veterinary Drug Commission is to make suggestions and advise the Minister of Agriculture and the Director General of Livestock Services on policies for the regulation of vaccines, biologicals and other veterinary drugs. Members of the veterinary drug commission are selected from the Directorate General of Livestock Services, Ministry of Agriculture, Universities, Ministry of Health and other related institutions. The Director of the Veterinary Drug Assay Laboratory is one of the members of the Commission and participates in the periodic meetings conducted by the Commission.

2. Veterinary Drug Assessment Committee

The function of the Veterinary Drug Assessment Committee is to assess veterinary drugs for registration. The producers or importers of vaccines and biologicals to be registered submit samples to the Veterinary Drug Assay Laboratory for testing of quality. This is one of the requirements to obtain a registration licence. The Director of the Veterinary Drug Assay Laboratory is a member of the Committee and attends the meetings conducted by the Committee. The members of the Committee are selected from the Directorate General of Livestock Services, Ministry of Agriculture, Ministry of Health and Directorate General of Fisheries.

3. Veterinary Drug Inspectors

Veterinary drug inspectors are veterinarians who have received special training in the technical and administration aspects of veterinary drug handling. They are assigned to every district and municipality throughout the country. The veterinary drug inspectors observe and inspect all aspects of vaccines and biologicals handling in the field. In particular, storage conditions of these materials at the retailers, packaging and transportation from the retailers to the farmer or user and any physical changes affecting the vaccines or biologicals.

In addition to retailers, the places of inspection also include manufacturers, importers, distributors and animal feed mills. Veterinary drug inspectors are also responsible for the administrative aspects of the use of vaccines and biologicals.

Hopefully by continuous inspections, abnormalities will be detected early preventing negative impacts on the livestock industry and also public health.

Continuous control of these activities in terms of supervision and information are therefore most important. There are about 300 veterinarians working as veterinary drug inspectors in every district and municipality throughout the provinces.

To improve the efficiency of inspectors in their tasks, training courses for veterinary drug inspectors have been conducted with the purpose:

1. To provide necessary knowledge and know-how on the regulation and scientific aspects of veterinary drugs.

2. To instruct and demonstrate laboratory technology of quality testing and inspections to be applied as part of the national quality control programmes.

3. To provide opportunities for observation and guidance at the points of manufacture, importation and distribution of veterinary drugs. Also efficient surveillance and control.

4. To exchange ideas and experience between participants under training.

The existence of a private organisation viz The Association of Veterinary Drug Businesses in Indonesia as a counterpart to the Government Sector, plays an important role in encouraging proper methods of veterinary drug handling.

The involvement of the Association is mainly is disseminating information and improving the technical abilities of member companies.

TECHNOLOGIES AND QUALITY CONTROL METHODS APPLIED TO DIFFERENT VACCINES AND BIOLOGICALS

1. Transfer of Technology

The methods of quality control of vaccines and biologicals at the Veterinary Drug Assay Laboratory have been introduced and developed through Technical Co-operation between the Government of Indonesia and the Government of Japan during the period of 1984 - 1991.

To facilitate the easy transfer of the technologies, the Government of Japan has provided equipment, materials, training of Indonesian counter parts in Japan and assignment of Japanese experts to the Veterinary Drug Assay Laboratory.

The basic technologies for laboratory tests and examinations was arranged at the beginning of the project and subsequently expanded to assay methods for each type of vaccine and biological. Although the range of vaccines and biologicals is very large, assay methods have been developed steadily and it has become feasible to introduce certification tests for official purposes. The guidelines for assay of veterinary drugs and biologicals were published in March 1989.

2. Types of Tests Undertaken

Tests can be classified according to their purpose as follows:

a. Preparatory Study Tests

Veterinary vaccines and biologicals which have not yet been licensed are subjected to preparatory study tests. These are concerned with a study of assay methodology and preparation of test materials and reference reagents. The types of vaccines and biologicals for preparatory study tests are selected taking into account the future plan of the Assay Program.

b. Trial Tests

Trial tests are applied to certain vaccines and biologicals for the purpose of assessing assay methods which will be introduced systematically as official assays. Samples are collected from producers or importers taken at the lot or batch level. Vaccines and biologicals to be subjected to Trial Tests are selected by consideration of the following factors:

i. Laboratory methods for quality assays of the said preparation are already established and applicable.

ii. Facilities, and materials including chemicals etc and trained staff needed for the test are already available.

iii. Economic and animal health importance of the preparation is appropriate.

iv. Other administrative and technical considerations.

Laboratory test procedures and interpretation of the results from Trial Tests are based upon procedures which can be introduced as the Official Assay Method in the near future. No certificate is issued after the Trial Tests, but the results are sent to the producer or importer concerned.

c. Certification Tests

Certification tests are applied to vaccines and biologicals whose methods of assay are already established. These tests are also used as an official test.

Samples of vaccines and biologicals for certification are collected from the following sources:

i. At the time of registration and renewing of registration.

ii. From the producer or importer concerned.

d. Tests for Monitoring

Samples of vaccines and biologicals collected from distributors, retailers, veterinary clinics and farmers, or samples received from other institutions including the commercial sector are tested for the purpose of monitoring. These tests are intended to evaluate the quality of vaccines and biologicals on the market or during field application.

APPLICATION OF NATIONAL AND INTERNATIONAL QUALITY CONTROL NORMS AND STANDARDS

conducting In the quality control of vaccines and biologicals, the Veterinary Drug Assay Laboratory uses national and international standards for viruses, bacteria, immune sera and other biologics. International standards are used for reference purposes and all national standards are callibrated against them.

In Indonesia, the collection, supply and standardization of viruses, bacteria and other biological materials for National Standards is carried out by the Research Institute for Veterinary Science (RIVS) located at Bogor. These materials are collected locally as field strains existing in the country and also obtained from foreign countries.

The Veterinary Drug Assay Laboratory also has close co-operation with the other institutions, agencies, universities, veterinary drug producers, importers etc in relation to the standards applied either in the country or in foreign countries.

QUALITY CONTROL OF IMPORTED VACCINES AND BIOLOGICALS

A number of vaccines and biological products are imported to be used for various animal health activities and improvement of livestock production in the country. Since 1986, there are 24 types of imported vaccines and biologicals, 200 samples or batches of which have been tested for certification at the Veterinary Drug Assay Laboratory.

The types of vaccines and biological products imported are as follows: poultry (67%), cattle (4%), swine (4%) and pet animals (25%). Three of the imported vaccines are combined vaccines.

There are no differences in the quality control methods, and assessment of results etc applied to the imported products, as compared to those produced in the country. Samples are collected at the time of registration and renewal of licensing. Depending on the nature of the imported products, the tests are grouped into preparatory study test, trial test and certification test. Tests are also conducted for monitoring of the quality of the imported products on the market.

11. VACCINE PRODUCTION AND QUALITY CONTROL IN MALAYSIA

by

A L Ibrahim and L H Seng

INTRODUCTION

Veterinary vaccines are an important tool in the control of animal disease. However, there is a growing concern on the hazards of low quality vaccines on animal productivity and health. On the other hand, development and production of high quality vaccines are expensive, especially in developing countries where the market size is small and production technology is limited. It may be difficult for a developing country to achieve high quality vaccine standards at low cost.

For these reasons, it is important that a national vaccine production and quality control institution plays a leading role to ensure vaccines in current use or in production conform to desired quality standards to bring maximum benefits to the animal industry.

This paper describes the experiences in Malaysia in areas of vaccine production as well as the establishment of national and regional vaccine quality control standards. It is hoped that this paper will stimulate further discussion on the formulation of effective quality control and vaccine production in the developing countries.

Vaccine Production - Current Situation

In Malaysia, the production and quality control of vaccines are under the care of government. There is no private veterinary vaccine manufacture in Malaysia. The Veterinary Research Institute (VRI), under the Department of Veterinary Services (DVS), Ministry of Agriculture, is the only Institution in Malaysia that produces vaccines as indicated in Table 1.

Table 1: Vaccine Production at the Veterinary Research Institute, Malaysia

Type of Vaccine	1990 Production In Million Doses
1. Newcastle disease 'S' vaccine	95
2. Newcastle disease 'F' vaccine	80
3. Fowl pox vaccine	80
4. Hog cholera vaccine	1.5
5. Contagious ecthyma vaccine	0.1

6.	H.Septicaemia oil adjuvant (Past.multocida) vaccine	0.25
7.	H. Septicaemia broth (Past.multocida) vaccine	0.03
8.	Combined Sal. dublin and Salmonella typhimurium vaccine	0.01
9.	Combined Past.multocida and Past.haemolytica vaccine	0.02
10.	Duck pasteurella vaccine (Past.multocida/Past.Anatifestifer)	0.70
	TOTAL DOSES	257.61

It is clear that Malaysia produces a limited number of vaccines because of the comparatively small animal population. Also the country is free from major diseases that might require the use of vaccine. Vaccine that cannot be economically produced is imported. There is a mechanism within the DVS for the approval of such importation.

Structure of Quality Control Organization

In vaccine production, the VRI follows a number of guidelines on good manufacturing practice (GMP). Briefly, the GMP carried out includes:

1. Establishment of good documentation and clear instructions for every production procedure. Results of operation and quality control tests are validated by trained personnel. Easily retrievable records are also kept to trace production batches after distribution.

   Poultry vaccine seeds are produced from certified SPF eggs. A seed lot system of production is instituted for every new vaccine.

2. Use of facilities that possess the following features:

   (a) Premises for production are situated in a separate area that presents minimal risk of contamination to materials and final products.

   (b) Facilities are designed, constructed and equipped for effective cleaning, disinfection and maintenance so as to avoid accumulation of dust and dirt as well as protect against entry of pests, animals and unauthorised persons.

(c) There is effective separation between the five major areas, viz: vaccine production, quality control laboratory, vaccine storage, experimental animal unit and ancillary areas such as reception rooms, washing and sterilisation room, workshop and toilets.

(d) Protected areas such as the vaccine production rooms are well-ventilated with positive filtered air. Entrance and exit points are equipped with an air-lock changing room.

3. An independent quality control department that carries out all defined and acceptable quality control tests in accordance with a national standard and ensures only safe and efficacious vaccine is produced.

<u>National Quality Control</u>

In carrying out quality control tests, the VRI follows its own national quality standards. The formulation and other modifications of these national standards were based on "in house" experience, expertise with the following documents as a guide:

(1) British pharmacopoeia.

(2) USDA Code of Federal Regulation. Title 9. Chapter 1, part 101-147.

(3) ASEAN Standards for Vaccines.

A document entitled "Minimum Vaccine Standards Requirements" was established as a national standard requirement. It consists of six clauses covering the following areas:

(a) Tests and methodology used in quality control.

(b) Specification of materials and substrates used for vaccine production and the quality control tests required thereof.

(c) Specification of vaccine strain, seed lot system in vaccine production and quality control required.

(d) Quality control required for production process and final products.

(e) Safety and potency test <u>in vivo</u>, including requirement of a field trial.

(f) Requirement of information to be given on the vaccine label.

One of the important quality control norms as stated in this national standard is the requirement of an <u>in vivo</u> safety test for each batch of vaccine in the ultimate host for which vaccine is intended. In addition, immunological tests in animals for the presence of adventitious organisms other than the vaccine itself are required following the safety test.

Application of National Quality Control Standards for Different Vaccines

In Malaysia, the Technical Advisory Committee on Biologics (TACB) in the Department of Veterinary Services (DVS) is responsible for the registration of important vaccines. Besides maintaining a list of registered vaccines approved for sale in the country, the TACB also appoints the VRI, if the need arises, to carry out the quality control tests for imported vaccines for the purpose of registration and certification. Hence, the VRI as a quality control institution, plays a role in such regulation.

Currently, TACB with the DVS of Malaysia tends to rely heavily on the data provided by reputable manufacturers for the registration of vaccines. Manufacturers must also provide documentary evidence that their vaccine production and quality control norms conform to a known international quality control standard. The actual quality control tests carried out by the VRI for imported vaccine is limited to a quantitative assay, since carrying out other quality control tests, especially a field trial on vaccine to test its efficacy under local conditions, is virtually impossible. In spite of these constraints, relying on the provisions of the "Minimum Vaccine Standards Requirements" as well as other administrative requirements as guidelines, the TACB has so far managed to evaluate and register 41 types of vaccine comprising 93 brands, manufactured by 22 different companies. However, there is no computerisation so far to establish a database of the results from these tests.

New Technologies

Research on vaccine development and production is being conducted at the Veterinary Research Institute Malaysia and the Faculty of Veterinary Medicine and Animal Science, Universiti Pertanian Malaysia. Research is underway at the Faculty of Veterinary Medicine and Animal Science to develop more effective vaccines through the application of biotechnology. The application of such technology in Malaysia is only at the beginning. Much more needs to be known about immunological mechanisms and the molecular biology of the infective agents before the potential of biotechnology is realised. The objective of the research project is to improve existing vaccines by standard vaccine methods and biotechnology. Targeted research efforts aimed at vaccine development have been identified for 4 important diseases viz: Newcastle disease, fowlpox, infectious bronchitis and contagious ecthyma. Such research involves:

(i) detailed study of the immunology of the disease and the molecular biology of the virus.

(ii) characterization and molecular cloning of vaccine virus.

(iii) formulation of vaccine for testing.

(iv) methods of presentation that will give greater convenience to users.

(v) the use of adjuvant and stabilizer to improve immunogenicity.

Many of these projects are collaborative undertakings between the University and Department of Veterinary Services. While the University concentrates on basic research, the VRI works on the process of scaleup for large volume vaccine production.

Constraints

One of the major constraints in vaccine quality control work in Malaysia is the shortage of skilled personnel and facilities. While all vaccines that are produced by the Institute are subjected to stringent quality control tests, the same tests are not applied to imported vaccines. Due to limited funds the Institute can not perform many of the quality tests. Certain tests are elaborate and costly to perform. Also special facilities, equipment and expertise are required for certain tests.

Strategies in Development and Application of a Quality Control Standard

For developing countries, the common strategy in developing a national quality control standard is to base its formulation on a known documented standard, taking into account each country's different needs, interests, resources and capability. It is important that in the application of a quality standard, there must be the concurrent development of an enforceable and adequate legislation to ensure its maintenance.

There is therefore a need to review and revise the existing regulations in developing countries pertaining to vaccine standards, such as those on certification by evaluation of laboratory tests, registration, distribution and other administrative procedures so that management of vaccine quality that affects livestock development can be assured.

Since it is costly to undertake laboratory quality tests for every type of vaccine, accredition of laboratories for testing a particular vaccine within countries will enable performance of recognised tests at lower cost in accordance with common vaccine standard requirements.

Developing countries have different needs for a variety of vaccines. But they must have easy access to veterinary vaccine production and quality control technology in order to make possible harmonisation of quality control standards. Establishment of training programmes on a bilateral basis or through the assistance of FAO, therefore, will expedite the harmonisation and improvement of veterinary vaccine quality control standards in developing countries.

Discussion

The production of potent and effective vaccines is very difficult and may not be achieved by all laboratories. The ability to produce potent, pure and safe vaccines depends primarily on the establishment of a seed virus bank that has been well characterised so that its properties are known and its freedom from entraneous agents is well established. This is very important especially in the production of viral vaccines. If there are contaminants, no amount of testing and retesting of the final product will help. The source of contamination may be: i) the cells or eggs in which the virus is grown ii) media and additives used in virus culture and iii) the environment in which the virus is being prepared.

The use of characterised seed virus is a basic requirement in vaccine production. The second requirement is the development of simple, sensitive standardised procedures for evaluating potency, purity and safety. There is a need to standardise serological methods and techniques within and between laboratories. The third requirement for the production of good vaccine is the availability of a suitable manufacturing process. Finally the availability of trained manpower who are familiar with good laboratory practices is a prerequisite to good vaccine production.

LATIN AMERICA

12. FOOT-AND-MOUTH DISEASE VIRUS PRODUCTION AND CONTROL OF VACCINES IN SOUTH AMERICA

by

R A Casas-Olascoaga

Overview of Foot-and-Mouth Vaccines in South America

Vaccines currently used in FMD immunophrophylaxis are of the inactivated type.

During the 1960's, several countries dedicated considerable research to developing vaccines of the attenuated live-virus type; expectations were high and the use of this virus was indicated for some countries. In South America, the attenuated live-virus FMD vaccine was extensively administered in Venezuela until its manufacture and use were banned in August of 1990.

Inactivated vaccines produced in South America are of the following types: aluminum saponin-hydroxide vaccine, oil-adjuvanted water-in-oil emulsion, and a mixture of aluminum hydroxide and oil-adjuvanted. Vaccines using the synthetic amino-lipoidal adjuvant AVRIDINE (N,N-dioctadecy1-N', N'-bis (2-hydroxyethy1) propanodiamine) have been registered in Brazil.

Total production of FMD vaccine for the region in 1990 was 407.4 million polyvalent doses (types O, AC and OA), some 12 million more than for 1989.

In comparison to 1989, the production of oil-adjuvanted vaccine in 1990 increased 87% while output of saponin-hydroxide vaccine fell by 11%. A total of 457.1 million polyvalent doses was recorded (included those left over from 1989), of which 303.1 million corresponded to saponin-hydroxide vaccine and 154.0 million to oil-adjuvanted vaccine. Tables I and II show vaccine production and control in South America for 1986-1990.

Between 1986 and 1990, more than 2 billion doses of polyvalent FMD vaccine were manufactured in South America.

In Argentina, Paraguay and Uruguay all FMD vaccine is made by private laboratories (10, 2 and 5, respectively). In Brazil, production involves 7 private and 2 government laboratories; in Colombia there is one semi-official laboratory (a collaboration between the Ministry of Agriculture and rural-production associations) and one private laboratory.

In Ecuador and Peru, production is handled by the government through their Ministries of Health. Venezuela has one private laboratory that turns out limited amounts of vaccine. The Ministry of Agriculture and Livestock Breeding (MAC) is building a plant with a production capacity of 20 million bivalent doses. The MAC has recently decided to study the privatizing of this plant as it now stands (90% completed) and all available equipment acquired so far through international bidding. In the meantime, Venezuela has chosen to import most of its FMD vaccine from Brazil and other countries.

Bolivia has no production laboratories but instead imports FMD vaccine from neighbouring countries - Argentina, Paraguay and Brazil. One may generally conclude that South America has an installed industrial capacity larger than its needs and the demand for vaccine, especially in the case of Argentina, Brazil, Colombia, Paraguay and Uruguay. On the other hand, production is low and insufficient for Ecuador and Peru, which are facing difficulties in obtaining supplies of raw materials needed to sustain effective output.

Most countries have well-equipped manufacturing plants, with modern technology and skilled personnel adequately trained to turn out efficacious, stable and innocuous vaccines. With few exceptions, laboratories in South America lack a strong research sector, which in the medium run will limit technological development. This situation will most likely worsen as production by European laboratories declines owing to fewer investigators working in FMD-related R & D, thereby slowing down scientific progress in this area.

Foot-and-Mouth Disease Virus Strains Used to Produce and Control Vaccines in South America

The following are the strains most used in South America: 0_1 Campos, A_{24} Cruzeiro, C_3 Indaial and C_3 Resende. These strains provide effective coverage against most field-occurring viruses. Certain countries, however, have begun producing other strains that have shown significant antigenic and immunogenic variations relative to the ones above. For example, in Brazil Valencia A has been supplemented by A Venceslau; in Argentina by the A_{79}, both strains of the A_{24} group, and in Colombia by the A_{85} Sabana, during the epidemic caused by this virus.

The Pan American FMD Center has a bank of serum from animals primary-vaccinated and revaccinated with vaccine strains, which makes it possible to constantly monitor relevant strains appearing in South American countries.

It also has a battery of monoclonal antibodies that is extremely valuable for studying vaccine strains used by private and government laboratories for both vaccine production and control. By monitoring with these monoclonal antibodies, the occurrence of changes or variations in strains used in antigen production as well as challenges in vaccine efficacy-control testing, can be determined.

Antigen Production

In South America, most antigens are produced in BHK21 Clone 13 cell cultures, in tanks with deep suspended culture, and at a considerably reduced scale in cell multilayers in roller flasks. The Frenkel method, which uses explants of tongue epithelium kept alive in special media, continues to be frequently used by three laboratories in Argentina, one in Paraguay, one in Ecuador, and two in Uruguay. Although this method makes it possible to obtain highly immunogenic antigens, its production is falling off due to a limited supply of tongue epithelium, which depends on abattoirs and slaughterhouses. The availability of a stable line of kidney fibroblast cells from newborn hamsters (MacPherson & Stoker, 1962), along with proof of their susceptibility to FMD virus (Mowat & Chapman, 1962), has created an extraordinary source for replicating the virus on an industrial scale. Growing the culture in monolayers using static flasks, in cell multilayers using roller flasks - developed on an industrial scale (Ubertini et al.) - and its adaptation to multiplication in deep suspended culture (Capstick, 1963) has resulted in a widespread global increase in the production of FMD virus using antigens prepared in cell cultures.

In Europe, particularly in Spain, the production of vaccines for pigs has used the pig kidney cell line IBRS2, developed in Brazil by Pereira de Castro (1970).

The predominant method currently used in Latin America involves producing suspended cultures in large stainless-steel in-line tanks, with automatic controls for pH, temperature, aeration, etc, needed to optimize the output of cells and viral replication.

Although it is possible to obtain highly concentrated immunogenic antigens in cell cultures using rotating flasks, this method is limited to a few laboratories with low production capacity - two in Brazil, one in Peru and one in Uruguay.

A number of purification and concentration methods are used to manufacture antigens in laboratories in Argentina, Brazil, Colombia, Paraguay and Uruguay: ultrafiltration, ultracentrifugation, treatment with polyethylene glycol (PEG), trichlorotrifluroethane, and chloroform, among others.

Nowadays, there are alternative methods for high-density cell cultures. These include perfused microcarriers (glass beads, gelatin, biosilon, polyacrylamide, cytodex I, II or III), ceramic matrix, microencapsulation, hollow fibers, collagen sponges, etc, by which concentrations ranging from 10^7 to 10^8 cells per milliliter can be obtained. In South America, considerable efforts are being made to develop certain of these methods; as of now, however, no country is using them to produce FMD vaccine.

Inactivation

Antigen inactivation is extremely important since it allows for the destruction of the virus's capacity to replicate while maintaining its immunogenic properties.

For several decades formalin was the inactivant most often used to inactivate FMD virus. It is nevertheless slow-acting and its kinetics non-linear, thus making it impossible to determine if the virus ha been totally inactivated. Owing to the "tail effect" in the inactivation curve it is not always possible to be certain that complete inactivation has taken place.

The development of a first-order inactivant with constant kinetics rendered antigen inactivation safer, consequently increasing the safety and immunizing potency of FMD vaccines. It acts rapidly to destroy the infectiousness of the virus with constant linear kinetics throughout the process while preserving the antigenicity and immunogenicity of the antigen.

In South America, n-acetylethylenimine (AEI) (Brown et al., 1963) was first used, followed by glycylaldehyde (GDA) (Martinsen, 1964), and especially bromoethylenimine, or binary ethylenimine (BEI) (Bahnemann, developed at PAFMDC in 1974).

Some years ago, the South American Commission for the Control of FMD (COSALFA) recommended that South American countries replaçe formalin with first-order inactivants. Colombia and Brazil were the first countries to use them exclusively in making FMD vaccines. Other countries later accepted the recommendation, and in 1990 Argentina, Paraguay and Uruguay also made the use of first-order inactivants obligatory. The great majority of South American laboratories use BEI for inactivating antigens intended for producing vaccines.

BEI offers a number of advantages: It can be more safely and easily handled, and its chemical components are less expensive.

The virus suspension should be checked to determine that it is at the desired temperature and at a pH of -7.4 before the inactivant is added. It is also advisable to control the osmolarity of the virus suspension, which for cell-culture-produced-FMD virus is approximately 320-340m0sm.

The pH and osmolarity of the virus suspension affect the rate of inactivation. Increasing alkalinity reduces the inactivation rate. This is in contrast to formalin inactivation where the velocity of inactivation was found to increase with increasing alkalinity. Increasing osmolarity also slows down the inactivation rate. The pH and osmolarity effects on the inactivation rate are perhaps due to conformational changes in the viral capsid proteins that affect the permeability of the inactivant.

A computer program has been written to assist with the calculations needed for controlled inactivation of viruses with BEI or any other first-order inactivant. The program runs on DOS and is available in English (vine.exe) or in Spanish (vins.exe). Copies of either program can be obtained by sending a formatted double-density/double-sided 5.25" diskette. Requests should be sent to the Centro Panamericano de Febre Aftosa, Caixa Postal 589, 20001, Rio de Janeiro, Brazil.

Owing to their toxicity, the handling of inactivants requires vigorous safety measures to avoid risks to health.

The inactivating method developed by Scodeller et al. in Argentina is worthy of note: It involves the endonuclease of the virus obtained by incubating integral virus suspensions or viruses purified at a temperature of 37 °C in the presence of high concentrations of monovalent cations such as K^+, C_s^{+2}, and NH_4 at pH 8.5. Inactivation kinetics are first-order, quick and with no toxicity.

Antigen quality control during preparation is based on controls that include the infectivity titer, the complement fixation capacity, antigenicity evaluated using monoclonal antibodies, assay of antigenic mass (particle 140S) by density gradient centrifugation, the integrity of the viral polypeptides, especially VP1, by SDS-polyacrylamide gel electrophoresis (PAGE), and innocuity testing in cell cultures and animals. These are some of the techniques that allow for a reliable evaluation of the quality of the antigen.

Adjuvants

In South America, laboratories that manufacture saponin-hydroxide type FMD vaccine use aluminum hydroxide with a saponin aggregate so as to boost the immunogenic effect of vaccines. Aluminum hydroxide acts on the viral suspension by adsorption as well as making it possible to concentrate the antigen by eliminating the supernatant when the aluminum hydroxide-antigen complex settles out.

Current methods for preparing aluminum hydroxide are very efficacious, with uniform output and a high adsorption capacity. The use of saponin in conjunction with aluminum hydroxide provides excellent coadjuvanting action. Extreme care must be taken in selecting the saponin due to the large variety of commercial products, as well as the differences that may exist among different batches of the same product.

When Quill A, an active adjuvanting substance with lower inflammatory effect is administered at 1 mg per dose, its adjuvanting effect is very satisfactory and it causes less tissue reaction at the inoculation site. Quill A is also used in ISCOMS (immunostimulant complexes). When Quill A has been combined with SGP (Schering), a direct effect on B cells has been demonstrated.

During recent years in South America, there has been a considerable increase in the production of oil-adjuvanted FMD vaccine. Vaccines are made with an incomplete oil adjuvant (Freund) wherein the (aqueous) virus suspension is emulsified in equal parts in 10% emulsifier (a mannitol oleate) and 90% light mineral oil. With constant agitation an emulsion of the water-in-oil type (primary emulsion) is formed.

Mineral oils for medicinal use are described in the U.S. Pharmacopoeia, which contains detailed specifications regarding their characteristics and properties.

The current commercial availability of highly efficient emulsifiers has led to the preparation of oil-adjuvanted vaccines on an industrial scale. These vaccines exhibit very low viscosity and a very high fluidity characteristics which makes possible their widespread use in the field.

A number of private laboratories in Argentina, Brazil, Paraguay and Uruguay produce vaccines that combine aluminum hydroxide at low concentrations - to absorb and concentrate the antigen - and the oil adjuvant. These vaccines generally tend to produce a higher reactivity at the inoculation site in vaccinated animals.

Vaccines administered to pigs in South America are of the double emulsion type (water in oil-in-water), which provide adequate protection for these animals. It should nevertheless be pointed out that pigs are vaccinated only as a strategic measure when risks arise, rather than being done systematically.

The Pan American Foot-and-Mouth Disease Center constantly transfers oil-adjuvanted vaccine technology to both government and private laboratories. PAFMDC also co-ordinates and carries out demonstration-area projects in South American countries affected by endemic FMD, with constant evaluation of results. More than one million animals have been vaccinated in these areas, which reflect differing geographical conditions, climates, breeds of cattle and handling methods, as well as different epidemiological characteristics of the disease.

The results of these projects have been highly satisfactory, opening the way for the massive production of oil-adjuvanted vaccine.

In view of the conditions in South America, oil-adjuvanted FMD vaccines have been proven to confer a longer period of immunity in cattle, which allows for longer intervals between vaccinations. They are efficient in immunizing swine, and particularly so in young cattle.

One drawback of oil-adjuvanted vaccines is that they leave a residue in the tissues of vaccinated animals.

Among other adjuvants, two are of special interest: dimethyldioetadylamine (DDA Eastman) and N,N-dioctadecy1-N'-N'-bis(2-hydroxyethy1) propanodiamine (AVRIDINE - Pfizer). These substances have been shown to have very good adjuvanting activity for various viruses.

Vaccines made with AVRIDINE have been registered and approved in Brazil. At the admission test they show a long-lasting antibodies profile and complete protection for primary vaccinated cattle challenged at 90 days postinoculation.

In addition to the adjuvants referred to above, other mechanisms are being developed that allow for a regular, delayed release of the antigen, such as multilaminate liposomes, biodegradable capsules and microspheres. These antigen-release systems allow T and B cell growth factors to be incorporated.

New Vaccine Developments

Current advances in recombinant DNA techniques, and vectors, sequencing techniques, peptide chemistry development and monoclonal antibodies coupled with advances in immunology provide a powerful means of aiding the development of new vaccines provided that the identification of critical antigenic determinants, genetic determinants of attenuation and targets of humoral and cell-mediated immunity and their role in protection are elucidated.

Great interest is now being focused on the optimal conditions for introducing antigens to the immune system. The development of new FMD vaccines is desirable to avoid in the future the biological risks caused by handling large volumes of infectious virus, incomplete inactivation, and also alterations of the antigenic structures due to inactivation and other procedures during vaccine production. There is also the need to refrigerate conventional vaccines during storage and distribution, especially in tropical countries.

Nevertheless there appears to be little possibility of substantial improvements in FMD vaccines developed through new synthetic or genetic procedures in the short term.

It has to be appreciated that insufficient results from current immunoprophylaxis programs are mainly due to the difficulties in gaining quick and effective access to herds under certain forms of livestock production. In most cases, this is not due to problems involving the quality or efficacy of available vaccines. The factors mentioned above - the risks of viral manipulation and the potential these modern techniques have to generate products that can simultaneously immunize against a range of diseases - will make vigorous research to develop such vaccines rewardable.

FMD Vaccine Quality Control

Standardized quality control of FMD vaccines is of utmost importance for the success of FMD control and eradication programs in South America.

In Argentina, Brazil, Colombia, Paraguay and Uruguay official control units systematically test all vaccine lots produced. This accomplishment has been reached gradually, demanding time and the solution of technical and logistic problems.

The Pan American Foot-and-Mouth Disease Center is actively collaborating with governments to improve their vaccine control services through workshops, seminars, courses or in-service training of national professionals. The Center also provides standard reagents, reference FMD strains, consultancy, transfer of technology and guidelines on quality-control standards and techniques.

The most important aspects of quality control regarding the final product are the innocuity and efficacy that are tested at the laboratory level.

It is very important to have a surveillance system to follow up the behaviour of the vaccine in the field, especially in relation to stability, antibody responses in herds, and local tissue reactions. This also includes local and general hypersensitivity (allergenic and anaphylactic reactions) occurring in individual animals or in particular herds. Vaccine innocuity is tested in cell cultures and in cattle. Efficacy control should be assessed, preferably in the host for which the vaccine will be used. In the standard efficacy test, the challenge virus will be homologous with the strain used for vaccine production. Control in guinea pigs should be used only for screening control of vaccine but not for official decision making for approval or rejection.

In Argentina and Brazil, the systematic control of all vaccine batches produced between 1979 and 1987 utilized the DPB50 method as recommended by the European Pharmacopoeia, which sets 3DPB50 as a minimum for vaccine approval. Following correlation studies and combining results from 2 countries in a total of 658 vaccine batches involving more than 9,000 animals, it was shown that there was no concordance with the dose response in 22% of vaccines tested. As of then, Argentina, Brazil and Colombia began employing the footpad generalization protection test (FGP), which utilizes 16 cattle vaccinated with undiluted vaccine and 75% minimum protection 21-28 days postvaccination. This test has proven to be more reliable and allows for complementary antibody testing of all virus types present in the vaccine under assay. In this respect, the Center and the countries have wide experience and information correlating challenge results with antibody titer measurements by neutralization and mouse protection tests. In FGP reproducibility testing carried out in Brazil using commercial vaccines with some 65 repetitions, the method was shown to be rather more reliable. In addition to the FGP method, Paraguay, Uruguay and Venezuela use serological methods such as mouse-protection and seroneutralization for vaccine control.

In Argentina, efficacy control procedures have been modified so as to assess vaccines with a longer lasting immunity. This involves administering the viral challenge 90 days post-primary vaccination in 16 animals for each valency. Brazil and Uruguay have adopted the same criteria.

The PAFMDC has developed and has been using for several years the Expected Percentage of Protection (EPP) as an internal control of vaccines produced at its plant. This method consists of taking individual mouse-protection rates obtained from at least 16 vaccinated cattle and using probits to convert them to percentages. In averaging the EPPs, consideration is given to the standard error (SE) and the lower limit of reliability (0.95). EPPs may be calculated for the 3 vaccine valencies using the same number of vaccinated cattle. Comparative studies of FGP and EPP have shown a high correlation - Table III.

The European Community has recently signed an agreement with the PAHO regarding a project to correlate direct and indirect testing of efficacy control of FMD vaccines. The project will be carried out under a Technical Co-operation Agreement signed by Argentina, Brazil, Uruguay and Paraguay, which joined up in 1991, and the PAHO, through the PAFMDC. The EC has given a grant of US$ 450,000. This project will also aim at standardizing production strains and vaccine control in the 4 countries so as to facilitate integration of this subject into Mercosul.

Biosafety and Environmental Protection

Based on the current status of FMD prevention, control and eradication programs in South America, it is essential that environmental-protection and biosafety systems be adopted in laboratories that handle FMD viruses.

Modern methods for identifying and characterizing viruses (fingerprinting, sequencing, monoclonal antibodies) often make it possible to identify the origin of virus strains that cause outbreaks in the field. Various mechanisms have been used to verify virus escapes from laboratories that have led to FMD outbreaks in the field in Central Europe and South America. They demonstrate the need to develop systems and methods for biosafety and environmental protection.

CONCLUSION

During the 1980's, most South American countries recorded substantial and continuous improvement in general vaccine quality, mainly in innocuity and potency.

There is a well established quality-control system among producers and efficient government control in those countries with the largest vaccine production. Major efforts must still be exerted to improve biosafety and protection if escapes of virus from laboratories to the field and livestock are to be avoided.

Table I. Production and control of FMDV aluminum hydroxide vaccine in South America (1986-1990)

		1986	1987	1988	1989	1990
Argentina	PROD.	149.566.550	196.151.500	115.402.000	129.833.600	127.568.500
	APROV	142.191.935	188.349.570	109.452.000	110.199.400	120.380.100
Bolivia		-	-	-	-	-
Brazil	PROD.	219.492.570	214.175.030	246.739.000	158.730.500	147.028.900
	APROV	196.229.730	159.772.010	198.767.800	154.057.000	136.497.200
Colombia	PROD.	29.619.378	24.429.650	23.375.500	13.260.200	-
	APROV	29.500.000	20.722.620	21.447.100	16.405.200*	1.829.600
Chile		-	-	-	-	-
Ecuador	PROD.	941.000	600.000	420.000	463.500	317.400
	APROV	941.000	600.000	420.000	463.500	317.400
Paraguay	PROD.	9.609.750	8.817.210	11.201.500	7.835.700	7.756.100
	APROV	9.609.750	8.817.210	11.201.500	7.835.700	7.756.100
Peru	PROD.	1.140.240	520.000	-	120.000	-
	APROV	768.440	520.000	-	0.0	-
Uruguay	PROD.	33.076.060	49.829.125	45.088.900	25.163.900	18.243.500
	APROV	28.218.250	53.460.980*	36.588.100	29.431.200*	20.416.300*
Venezuela	PROD.	7.644.950**	7.174.500	6.354.900	3.190.000	568.600
	APROV	7.644.950	7.174.500	6.354.900	3.190.000	568.600

* Include vaccines produced in the past year
** Modified live virus vaccines

PROD. Produced
APROV Approved

Table II. Production and control of FMDV oil vaccine in South America (1986-1990)

		1986	1987	1988	1989	1990
Argentina	PROD.	-	-	9.816.000	7.201.600	23.365.000
	APROV	-	-	7.551.000	6.106.600	21.472.500
Bolivia		-	-	-	-	-
Brazil	PROD.	16.944.230	17.340.070	35.066.900	36.980.700	40.974.900
	APROV	12.095.515	10.731.650	30.658.300	35.502.500	35.542.100
Colombia	PROD.	910.360	1.664.555	2.446.500	9.170.500	23.048.800*
	APROV	762.900	1.294.654	1.680.700	7.428.300	15.925.600
Chile		-	-	-	-	-
Ecuador		-	-	-	-	-
Paraguay	PROD.	120.000	283.460	1.229.000	1.219.800	5.121.600*
	APROV	120.000	283.460	1.229.000	1.219.800	3.758.200
Peru	PROD.	-	260.000	-	192.100	113.800
	APROV	-	260.000	-	192.100	113.800
Uruguay	PROD.	-	-	-	-	9.318.100
	APROV	-	-	-	-	9.084.100
Venezuela	PROD.	-	-	1.244.000	2.000.000	4.000.000
	APROV	-	-	244.000**	2.000.000	4.000.000

* Exceeds doses controlled in 1991
** Approved doses for pigs

PROD. Produced
APROV Approved

Table III. Results of FGP and EPP of an oil adjuvanted vaccine OL 333, produced by PAFMDC, challenged against 0_1 and A24 FMD viruses.

	0_1 Virus				A_{24} Virus		
Bovine n^0	MPI[1]	EPP	FGP		MPI	EPP	FGP
01	2.85	95	P*		3.91	99	P
02	2.85	95	P		3.91	99	P
03	5.60	99	P		5.40	99	P
04	5.32	99	P		0.65	41	3F
05	3.20	97	P		3.40	98	1F
06	3.82	99	P		4.47	99	P
07	5.60	99	P		4.51	99	P
08	2.60	92	1F**		3.40	98	P
09	5.60	99	P		4.40	99	P
10	5.20	99	P		1.90	79	P
11	2.20	86	P		5.15	99	P
12	2.85	95	P		3.90	99	P
13	4.60	99	P		5.05	99	P
14	2.20	86	P		5.40	99	P
15	1.10	55	2F		5.40	99	P
16	4.35	99	P		2.90	95	P

	0_1 Virus	A_{24} Virus
XEPP=	93.30	93.30
SD=	11.10	14.90
ASE=	2.80	3.70
LLC=	88.40	87.30
FGP=	14/16= 87.50	14/16= 87.50

[1] mouse protection index
P = protected
1F= generalization 1 foot
SD= standard deviation
ASE= average standard error
LLC= low limit of confidence

REFERENCES

Abaracón, D., Casas Olascoaga, R. (1984) Vacinas contra a febre aftosa. A Hora Veterinária, **17**:45-52, Janeiro/Fevereiro.

Alonso, A., Casas Olascoaga, R., Astudillo, V.M., Söndahl, M.S., Gomes, I., Vianna Filho, Y.L. (1987) Updating of foot-and-mouth disease virus strains of epidemiological importance in South America. Bol. Centr. Panam. Fiebre Aftosa **53**:11-18.

Alonso, F., Gomes, I., Bahnemann, H.G. (1988) La inducción de anticuerpos anti-VIAA en bovinos vacunados y revacundos con vacuna inactivada antiaftosa. Bol. Centr. Panam. Fiebre Aftosa **54**:51-52.

Alonso, A., Gomes, M.P.D., Martins, M.A. and Söndahl, M.S. (1990) Detection of foot-and-mouth disease virus infection-associated antigen antibodies: Comparison of the enzyme-linked immunosorbent assay and agar gel immunodiffusion tests. Preventive Veterinary Medicine, **9**:233-240.

Augé de Mello, P. (1979) Reflections on the prevention of foot-and-mouth disease in swine. Boletin del Centro Panamericano de Fiebre Aftosa, **35-36**:59-61.

Augé de Mello, P. and Gomes I. (1978) Foot-and-mouth disease oil adjuvanted vaccines for pigs. Boletin del Centro Panamericano de Fiebre Aftosa, **31-32**:7-12.

Bahnemann, H.G. (1975) Binary ethylenimine as an inactivant for foot-and-mouth disease virus and its application for vaccine production. Arch. Virol. **47**:45-56.

Bahnemann, H.G. Inactivation of viral antigens for vaccine preparation with particular reference to the application of binary ethylenimine. Vaccine, vol. **8**, August 1990, 299.

Casas Olascoaga, R., Sutmöller, P., Alonso Fernández, A., Abaracón, D. Foot-and-mouth disease virus production and control of vaccines in South America. Proceedings of XVI Conference of Foot-and-Mouth Disease Commission, Office International des Epizooties, Paris, 14-17 September, 1982, Vol. **1**:139-152.

Casas Olascoaga, R., Augé de Mello, P., Bergmann, I. Prospects for new vaccines in Latin American and Caribbean Countries. Bol. Centr. Panam. Fiebre Aftosa **54**:21-33, 1988. Presented at the Meeting sponsored by FAO, "Expert Consulation of the Application of Biotechnology in Livestock Production and Health in Developing Countries", La Habana, Cuba 7-10 September, 1988.

Casas Olascoaga, Raúl. Foot-and-mouth control in the Americas. Continental Strategy. XXIV World Veterinary Congress, Rio de Janeiro, Brazil, August 18-23, 1991.

Dalsgaard, K., Jensen, M.H. and Sorensen, K.J. (1977) Saponin Adjuvants. IV. Evaluation of the adjuvant Quil A in the vaccination of cattle against foot-and-mouth disease. Acta. Vet. Scand. **18**:349-360.

Ebbesen, P., Dalsgaard, K. and Hour-Madsen, M. (1976) Prolonged survival by AKR mice treated with saponin adjuvant Quil A. Act. Path. Microbiol. Scan. Sect. A., **84**:358-360.

Flebbe, L.M. and Braley-Mullen, H. (1986) Immunopotentiating effects of the adjuvants SGP and Quil A. I. Antibody responses to T-dependent and T-independent antigens. Cell Immunol. **99**:128-139.

Mesquita, J.A., Sutmöller, P., Casas Olascoaga, R. Control of the production of foot-and-mouth disease vaccines under good manufacturing practices (GMP). XXIV World Veterinary Congress, Rio de Janeiro, Brazil, August 18-23, 1991.

Morein, B. et al. (1984) ISCOM, a novel structure for antigenic presentation of membrane proteins from enveloped viruses. Nature, **308**:457-460.

Neitzert, Erika, Ewald Beck, Paulo Augé de Mello, Ivo Gomes and Ingrid E. Bergmann. (1991) Expression of the aphtovirus RNA polymerase gene in Escherichia coli and its use together with other bioengineered nonstructural antigens in detection of late persistent infections. Virology **184**:799-804.

Pan American Foot-and-Mouth Disease Center. Situation of the Foot-and-Mouth Disease Control Programs in South America, 1990. March 1991.

Pan American Foot-and-Mouth Disease Center/Regional Support Laboratory for Animal Health. Production and control of oil adjuvant foot-and-mouth disease vaccines at the Pan American Foot-and-Mouth Disease Center and the Regional Support Laboratory for Animal Health of the Ministry of Agriculture and Agrarian Reform, Brazil. Bol. Centr. Panam. Fiebre Aftosa. No. 56, 1990. In press.

Pinto, A.A., Garland, A.J.M. (1979) Immune response to virus-infection-associated (VIA) antigen in cattle repeatedly vaccinated with foot-and-mouth disease virus inactivated by formalin or acetylethyleneimine. J. Hyg., Camb., **82**:41-50.

Rweyemamu, M.M., Umehara, O., Medeiros Neto, R.R., Schiappacassi, C.A. AVRIDINE: a new synthetic adjuvant for veterinary vaccines. Proceedings of the X Pan American Veterinary and Zootechnic Congress. Buenos Aires, 23-27 September, 1985 paper no. 384.

Scodeller, E.A., Rebendiker, M.A., Dubra, M.S., Basarab, O., La Torre, J.L., Vasquez, C. An inactivation process for FMDV based on activation of virus-associated endonuclease. Proc. of 16th Conference of the FMD Commission Office international des Epizooties, 43-50, 1982.

Viana Filho, L. Ydérzio, Gomes, I., Fernandez, Graciela, Ravison, A., Fernández Alonso, A. Correlation between 50% bovine protective dose (BPD50) and percentage protection against foot generalization (PG) in FMD vaccine potency. Report of the Ses. Res. Group of the St. Tech, Comm, of the European Commission for the Control of FMD. Manuscrito em preparaçao.

Ydérzio L. Vianna Filho, Vicente Astudillo, Ivo Gomes, César E.E. Rozas, José A. Ravison, A. Alonso. Reprodutibilidade do teste de proteçao a generalizaçao podal (PGP) e estabilidade imunogênica de vacinas comerciais hidróxido-saponinadas e com adjuvante oleoso. Manuscrito em preparaçao.

EUROPE

13. VACCINE CONTROL IN ITALY

by

M Tollis

The Istituto Superiore di Sanita (ISS) is the main national Italian authority in charge of quality control work on vaccines both human and veterinary. The Department of Veterinary Medicine supervises the control of two categories of veterinary vaccines viz:

(a) Batch to batch control of vaccines used for compulsory State immunisation programmes eg FMD, Classical Swine Fever, Rabies, Brucellosis etc.

(b) Quality assessment of other veterinary vaccines prior to their being given a product licence. In the case of these products they are controlled officially only once during the commercial life of the product, except perhaps occasionally when it is decided to assess vaccine as used under field conditions.

Italy is not a big producer of veterinary vaccines and most of the control work is related to assessment of imported products.

The philosophy of the quality control procedures used, is to apply standards which are either national or are from the European Pharmacopoeia. If there are no recognised standards for some vaccines, specific tests which have been agreed between the authorities and the manufacturers are carried out. In this case the costs involved are borne by the manufacturer. Subsequently, application is made for a product licence and this is considered by an expert committee made up of representatives from the ISS, the Universities, the Ministry of Agriculture and members of the Pharmaceutical Association. This committee gives a final opinion of the product and recommends licensing or otherwise.

The ISS is also responsible for standardisation of technical procedures to be used in production units thus promoting Good Manufacturing Practice. The ISS does not produce vaccines as such, but in the appropriate cases will be responsible for the development and distribution of important vaccines strains to Government production laboratories.

14. VACCINE PRODUCTION AND CONTROL IN FRANCE

by

R M Lombard

Being members of the EEC, both France and Italy follow the same quality control procedures for veterinary vaccines.

In France there are two principal producers of these vaccines:

(a) Virbac, which is concerned with vaccines for companion animals, poultry and also the oral immunisation of wildlife against rabies, and

(b) Rhone Merieux which produces a wider range of vaccines for domesticated livestock ie cattle, pigs, small ruminants, rabbits, poultry and companion animals.

There are some eight laboratories located throughout the country for official quality control work. These are all State laboratories and each of them concentrates their activities on work with one particular animal species. As in Italy, all vaccines used in the field must have a product licence and this applies to both locally produced and imported products.

For vaccines used in compulsory vaccination campaigns instigated by the State, all batches must be tested and the legislation is such that the manufacturer and the quality control laboratory can be sued if adverse reactions follow the use of a particular batch of vaccine.

Other veterinary vaccines must be produced according to the requirements of the European Pharmacopoiea and the OIE norms or according to specific conditions required of the manufacturer by the State authorities as defined in the product licence.

15. VACCINE PRODUCTION AND QUALITY CONTROL IN POLAND

by

Z Pejsak and J Gorski

INTRODUCTION

Thirty-seven vaccines against bacterial infections, 19 viral vaccines and 2 vaccines against mycosis are produced at present in Poland. These biologicals are made by three manufacturers.

These vaccines include monovalent preparations, polyvalent preparations (containing several serotypes of the same micro-organism, eg Leptospira and Pasteurella vaccines) and combined vaccines (eg distemper and Rubarth disease vaccine, and atrophic rhinitis vaccine). There are inactivated preparations (37 vaccines) and live ones (21); most of them are lyophilised. These vaccines are used for the immunisation of 10 different species of animals.

ORGANISATION OF QUALITY CONTROL OF VETERINARY VACCINES IN POLAND

Each vaccine is subjected to a 4-stage control system.

1. Control of seed lots of viruses and bacteria - performed by the National Veterinary Research Institute (NVRI).

2. In-process control of biologicals, performed by the manufacturer.

3. Batch control performed by the manufacturer.

4. State control of biologicals performed by NVRI.

METHODS APPLIED

Stage 1. Checking of production strains (seed management)

This is performed by the NVRI before delivering a viral or bacterial production strain from the NVRI bank to the vaccine producer. Seed lots of virus and or any continuous cell line used for virus growth shall be free from bacteria, fungi and mycoplasmas, and those pathogenic viruses and other pathogens which can be transmitted from the species of origin to the species to be vaccinated. Seed lots of bacteria shall be free of other bacteria as well as fungi and mycoplasmas. The following other features are also checked: taxonomic properties of the strain (biochemical and/or serological identification); antigenic properties; biological properties; reversion; vertical and horizontal transmissions; immunosuppressive properties (absence of contaminations), genetic stability and homogenicity (eg size of plaque).

Stage 2. In-process control in producer's laboratory

The aim of this work is:

(a) control of contamination in nutrient media; primary and continuous cell lines; semi-finished product; inactivation substances, adjuvants; enzymes and other necessary reagents.

(b) determination of the titre of a propagated micro-organism in living vaccines and its titre or density in inactivated products.

<u>Stage 3. Testing of each batch of vaccine in the manufacturer's laboratory</u>

To include:

tests for sterility and freedom from contamination:

<u>Living viral vaccines</u> - are tested for sterility according to the General Requirements for Sterility of Biological Substances (Requirements for Biological Substances No. 6) of the WHO. Each batch of vaccine shall pass tests to prove that the vaccine is free from extraneous viruses (tests in cell cultures susceptible to viruses of the species to be vaccinated, tests in embryonated eggs, and, where necessary, tests in animals);

<u>Inactivated viral vaccines</u> - are tested for efficiency of inactivation of the vaccine virus;

<u>Live bacterial vaccines</u> - are tested for sterility carried out using solid media and ignoring the growth of the vaccine bacterium;

<u>Inactivated bacterial vaccines</u> - are tested for inactivation of the vaccine bacterium.

Each batch of vaccine is also tested for: toxicity for laboratory animals; residual moisture (in lyophilized biologicals); concentration of inactivating substances; amount of adjuvant; lack of contamination and stability of an oil emulsion.

<u>Stage 4. State Quality Control</u>

The NVRI is the only institution authorized for performance of the state control of veterinary biologicals permitted for use in Poland. The state control always includes tests for viability and bacterial titre in live vaccines and efficiency of inactivation in inactivated preparations; tests for absence of contamination (microbiological sterility is rigorously required); evaluation of vaccine safety for laboratory animals (mice, guinea pigs, rabbits, pigeons etc). In the majority of cases the state control also includes:

(a) tests of safety for the specific species for which the vaccine is intended, given at normal dosage and 2 to 100 times larger doses. Most vaccines are compulsorily tested for safety in the specific species of animals. These include the vaccines against foot-and-mouth disease (FMD), classical swine fever (CSF), distemper, infectious canine hepatitis and all vaccines for poultry;

(b) evaluation of potency of lyophilised viral vaccines is carried out by estimating its titre as determined by means of the appropriate laboratory test (eg - CPE, HA, CF, ELISA, IF and NPLA) - or on laboratory animals (LD_{50}) and hen eggs (EID_{50}).

(c) evaluation of immunogenicity is performed by testing immunity against challenge infection eg - CSF, erysipelas, distemper, etc. or by evaluation of sero-conversion 7 to 21 days after vaccine administration eg canine parvovirus and leptospirosis. The kinetics of sero-conversion is determined in specifically sensitive animals of the species to be protected or, if it is possible and economically justifiable, on laboratory animals.

Vaccines against diseases mentioned in list A of the O.I.E.

In Poland only vaccines against CSF are subjected to more precise and rigorous tests. Each batch of modified live CSF virus vaccine (lapinized or cell culture) must be prepared according to the production protocol (accepted by NVRI) and under the conditions laid down for the registration of the final product.

In process and batch control includes

(a) identity; the vaccine must induce neutralizing antibodies against a virulent strain of CSF virus.

(b) sterility.

(c) safety - 10 pigs are vaccinated with 10 vaccine doses each. During 21 days after vaccination no pig should die or show signs of disease attributable to the vaccine, and the average of daily body temperature must not reach 40.5° C or more.

(d) purity - 3 pigs are inoculated i.m. with 10 vaccine doses of "cell culture" vaccine. Serum samples are collected at the time of inoculation and 5 weeks later. Collected samples are tested for antibodies for BVDV and PPV. All 3 pigs must remain free from such antibodies.

(e) 1 dose of vaccine should contain at least 100 PD_{50}.

QUALITY CONTROL OF IMPORTED VACCINES

Several vaccines imported from Western Europe and the USA are used in Poland. Many of them are used in parallel with Polish biopreparations. Other biologicals (eg FMD vaccine) are imported when necessary since they are no longer produced in Poland.

According to legal mandatory regulations veterinary biologicals and drugs may be introduced for sale and general use only on the basis of a licence granted by the Veterinary Department and authorized by the Minister of Agriculture. Such a licence is issued after examination and acceptance by the State Drug Commission. The Commission gives its opinion after detailed investigation of the technology of production and control methods presented by the manufacturer. The Commission also takes into consideration the results of tests for sterility, safety, immunogenicity and potency carried out by the NVRI. The documentation presented by the manufacturer, who wishes to register his product, should contain the following information: origin and description of physico-chemical properties of a production strain; results of tests for vertical and horizontal transmission (for living vaccines); reliability of inactivation (for inactivated vaccines); stability of the vaccine at 4° C and under unfavourable conditions (accelerated stability test 37° C) during 7-14 days; safety for specific animals and closely related species and data on dynamics of sero-conversion and persistence of antibodies.

Tests carried out in the NVRI always include the verification of declared physical features, absence of extraneous contamination and safety for laboratory animals and species for which the biological is intended. A control inoculation (challenge) is performed with micro-organisms isolated in the country or with international standard challenge strains (eg Snyder Hill - CVS, Pseudorabies - NIA-3). Kinetics of sero-conversion is also determined. After preliminary laboratory examinations the protective value of the vaccine is always tested under field conditions by two or more different reference veterinary clinics. After obtaining positive results of laboratory examinations and field observations the NVRI sends its findings to the State Drug Commission. All batches of imported veterinary biologicals, destined for control of diseases from list A of the O.I.E., are subjected to State quality control tests according to the "Manual of Recommended Diagnostic Techniques and Requirements for Biological Products for Lists A & B Diseases" edited by OIE (1990).

Summarizing

It may be stated that permission for use and sale of new veterinary biopreparations imported or produced in Poland is based on substantial legal principles. Permission is always preceded by laboratory control and the results are evaluated by independent, highly qualified experts. Vaccines already registered, before introduction for sale are subjected to a preliminary quality evaluation in the NVRI.

The procedures described have proved to be very satisfactory and have effectively protected the country against the use of veterinary biopreparations of low value or capable of causing epizootiological hazards.

APPLICATION OF INTERNATIONAL NORMS

International norms are used for the quality control of all biologicals destined for control of diseases mentioned in list A & B of the OIE.

ACCESS TO NEW TECHNOLOGIES ON VACCINE PRODUCTION/QUALITY CONTROL

Many bacterial and viral vaccines are produced in a closed cycle system using cell suspensions in fermentors, cell lines and primary cell cultures for the propagation of viral strains for vaccine production. Studies for the development of new bio-engineered vaccines eg a deleted TK , gI pseudorabies vaccine for swine have been recently undertaken.

LEVEL OF COMPUTERIZATION

Up to now, no computer systems have been used for the control of production and quality assurance of veterinary biologicals.

MAJOR CONSTRAINTS

Biological manufacturers are not adequately equipped, and they do not yet use modern technologies of production for some biologicals. As an example, they rarely produce antigen for vaccines in fermentors. Not all biologicals produced in Poland meet the requirements recommended by the Standards Commission of the OIE.

DEVELOPING STRATEGIES

It is intended that the following be promoted:

The application of inactivated vaccines in place of live ones;

The introduction of modern methods (restriction enzyme analysis) of strain selection for vaccine production;

The improvement and use of modern adjuvants in inactivated vaccines;

The production of polyvalent and subunit vaccines.

RECOMMENDATIONS/COMMENTS

It is considered that it would be of great value to introduce universally applicable principles for the control and registration of all vaccines and that adherence to these principles would be mandatory both for producers and the control institution.

16. VACCINE PRODUCTION AND CONTROL IN HUNGARY

by

V Palya

Until recently, Phylaxia Biologicals which was set up in 1912, was the only vaccine producer in the country. A few years ago a second production unit started up. Phlyaxia have produced a wide range of immunobiologicals covering almost 50 viral and 30 bacterial diseases in addition to pharmaceutical products and antibiotics.

The policy in Hungary requires that before a biological product can be used in the field, a product licence must be obtained from the Ministry of Agriculture. This will only be granted after the National Institute for Quality Control has examined a very comprehensive dossier of data on the origins of the seed strains used and the provenance of the raw materials used in manufacture together with details of development work and the manufacturers 'in house' testing. Samples of the new product are submitted to further testing by the State organisation following standards obtained from the British or European Pharmocopieas.

Until recently, licensing of imported vaccines was not a requirement for their use in Hungary. Some vaccines were tested for safety, but potency assessments were not undertaken. This has now changed and all imported vaccines have to be licensed. This requires tests by the National Quality Control Institute followed by approval of the Ministry of Agriculture and finally by the Ministry of Health who is the final arbiter.

Discussion

Dr Sylla commented very favourably on the work of the PAFMDC in Rio and thought its activities provided a very useful model for the needs of other regions - particularly Africa. In his opinion the assistance of FAO and similar organisations was urgently needed to establish a co-ordinated system of quality control for vaccine work along the lines of that in Latin America which has proved to be so effective. Dr Sylla thought that a strong recommendation from the consultation on this matter would be a helpful first step.

Dr Nagy put a question to Dr Mannathoko about the policy of the Botswana Vaccine Institute on product development and marketing. Dr Nagy thought that the statement that there were no other vaccines (besides FMD vaccine) worthy of production and sale in the SADAC region, very disappointing. He quoted the example of Kenya which produces 14 vaccines which were available for export.

Dr Mannathoko in reply stated that the Institute had looked very carefully at the possibility of marketing other viral vaccines but had come to the conclusion that the prospects for success were not good. The political climate of the region was not conducive to such a venture. Another factor of importance was that South Africa was already in the market as a large producer of high quality veterinary immuno-biologicals and the BVI would not want to duplicate the activities of Onderstepoort.

Dr Chema in reply to the comment on vaccine production in Kenya, pointed out that the basic market for these products was the home one. If export sales fell significantly, then the home market was sufficiently strong to maintain the viability of the producing organisation. Other producers might be more vulnerable to the effects of fluctuations in the export markets.

Dr Mannathoko illustrated the problems associated with a fluctuating market from his experience with producing FMD vaccine at the BVI. Botswana and Zimbabwe are the main customers for this vaccine. Both countries export beef to the European Community - who will not accept meat from vaccinated cattle. When the incidence of FMD falls in these countries as a result of the vaccination campaigns, the sale of vaccines also falls and vaccination is confined to the high risk areas. In consequence the BVI is in danger of operating at a loss. However, the low incidence of FMD promotes the sale of meat to Europe and to compensate the BVI for its reduced income, the Botswana Meat Commission provides it with a financial subsidy.

Dr Rweyemamu thought that the following points which had arisen during the presentation of reports needed emphasis:

Vaccine manufacturers must maintain their own quality control unit. Under no circumstances should a national quality control agency be regarded as a substitute for the producers own 'in house' quality control organisation.

The new adjuvant AVRIDINE was mentioned in one of the contributions and since it shows considerable promise of improvement for some vaccines, Dr Rweyemamu would like to see it tested widely and not be allowed to become the subject of a monopoly.

Thirdly, and most importantly, he much regretted the reducing interests of the bioproducts industries of the developed countries, to undertake research and development work for the benefit of the less developed countries. He asked how can the small, inefficient and under supported producer in these countries be expected to be self supporting without considerable technical help to become so. There is a real need for technology and process and product development work. He suggested that this Consultation should give advice on how best to involve the appropriate organisations in the developed countries to take up this very necessary task.

Dr Chema also expressed his concern on this matter. From his experience of research project funding in Africa he quoted that there was money for research, but for some reason projects based on livestock were not being supported.

Dr Pejsak thought there was a lesson from past experience in Poland to be learnt in the developing countries. Previously due to lack of registration requirements, producers were protected from investigation of the quality of their products, and that resulted in many small companies trying to take advantage of the situation there. Now with official registration the situation has been considerably improved. Dr Pejsak thought that if such a situation should arise in the developing countries the use of immunising agents could fall into disrepute - and he quoted one area where local farmers thought vaccination against Swine

Fever not worthwhile because the vaccine was ineffective. However the real reason was that the particular batch of vaccine used, was not potent. Dr Pejsak emphasised that potency of vaccine must be checked after official registration.

Dr Lombard made the point that in some developed countries the requirements of the export licence related only to safety, and ensuring that products were potent was the responsibility of the importing country.

Dr Ozawa of the Office International des Epizooties gave a very brief history of the efforts of the main international agencies to promote the establishment of universally accepted standards for some of the most important vaccines in widespread use. In the 1970's, WHO was responsible for promoting quality control of veterinary vaccines and tried to establish norms for Newcastle Disease and other vaccines. FAO and the WHO experienced difficulties in inaugurating standards for rinderpest vaccine. Eventually, FAO had difficulties in continuing this this vaccine.

Recently, OIE have taken the decision to publish internationally accepted standards for vaccines for all domesticated livestock including poultry and fish. Dr Ozawa brought to the attention of the Consultation the proposed OIE Manual which will be a sister publication to the OIE International Animal Health Codes. The Manual will contain details of diagnostic methods and recommended standards for the appropriate biological products for control purposes. This information will relate to all the diseases in the OIE lists A and B. Dr Ozawa admitted that so far there are not many vaccine standards that have been universally accepted by member countries of the OIE. However, OIE's task is to promote acceptance of standards by member countries and hopefully the other international agencies will contribute to this work. Dr Ozawa emphasised that at present the Manual is simply a book of recommendations, but perhaps it should eventually become the central source for the establishment of mandatory requirements. However, who should take the lead in bringing this about? Recommendations given in the Manual have been accepted already by some member countries and Dr Ozawa hoped that it would be taken up widely in the near future. He pointed out that it was intended to revise and update the Manual on a regular basis.

Dr Nagy questioned the value of attempts to assess the efficacy of vaccines when used under field conditions. Dr Pejsak in response, thought that in certain situations, such as obtained with large herds of housed pigs, that it was perfectly possible to plan sampling regimes which would give useful results. Dr Jeggo again emphasised the need to prove the efficacy of vaccines, particularly in the developing countries - since poor performance would result in 'consumer resistance' and apathy, leading to a resurgence of disease. In extreme situations the very survival of veterinary services in some countries might be in doubt.

Dr Doel pointed out that the potency tests of some vaccines are very expensive to perform and quoted FMD as an example. Groups of susceptible cattle are needed for an end-point of immunity assessment, and this was indeed very expensive. For vaccines in this category there was much to be said for the establishment of a vaccine co-ordinating institute as was now being developed for the benefit of the members of the European Economic Community. This Laboratory will in future be responsible for checking on a random basis vaccines produced for inclusion in the European Vaccine Bank.

Dr Sylla thought that more and more, the smaller vaccine producing laboratories - particularly in Africa - could not hope to make vaccines of high quality - due to the lack of funds and staff etc. He thought that regionalisation of biologicals production appears to be the answer and the idea has already been put to a meeting of Heads of Laboratories held in Nairobi in September 1990. The concept was accepted and is being further considered by Directors of Veterinary Services before advising their Governments. Dr Sylla recommended that the Consultation should also accept this idea and should take steps to promote it. He strongly advised that small producing laboratories should be encouraged to close and regionalisation of vaccine production established.

Dr Cheneau stated that this problem was not confined to Africa but was global. He had the impression that laboratory directors thought that "the next laboratory to close will not be mine"! This led to complacency and poor products. The farming community needs good and safe products and Donors will require reassurance of quality before investing in this type of aid work. Perhaps there are socio-economic factors involved in the maintenance of large numbers of inefficient laboratories - however the main objective is to control, if not eliminate, disease.

Experience with PANVAC has shown the benefits of payment only for quality products. It would appear that some producers are not making proper estimates of the real cost of production. It seems likely that in future Donors will only support laboratories that are seen to be well managed and not wasteful. Experience has shown that the statal or parastatal organisation soon runs into financial problems and not having financial autonomy has to fall back on central government for support for basic functions such as the cost of power or staff salaries.

Donors will be more critical and expect better management of both laboratory and finances in future. Such organisations if they are to survive will have to be self sustaining. In many African countries such laboratories will not be able to afford their own quality control units and in such situations the virtues of having a fully functional Regional Institute eg PANVAC - becomes obvious.

Some Technical Aspects of Vaccine Production and Quality Control

LIVE VIRAL VACCINES

by

L E Carmichael

INTRODUCTION

The history of live viral vaccines reveals similarities in the nature of problems faced by those who seek to control or eradicate infectious diseases through the use of vaccination, whether produced by crude or by 'modern' methods (11, 22, 26). Vaccination as a conscious endeavour to protect man and animals against serious diseases commenced some 2000 years ago in Asia with the practice of 'variolation'. The unrefined methods used then not infrequently provoked serious reactions, even death - events that still occur today, especially when procedures and precautions learned over the past 25 - 30 years have not been rigorously followed.

Jenner (1798) recorded the first scientific attempt to control an infectious disease, variola, by deliberate inoculation of individuals with a living agent - "cowpox". It might be noted that vaccinia, the name given to the agent for Jennerian vaccination, is somewhat distinct from true cowpox, although its origin and the mechanism of its evolution are uncertain (17). It is interesting to note that 13 years earlier a cattle farmer, Benjamin Jesty, purposefully inoculated his wife with cowpox in the face of a smallpox epidemic - an experiment acknowledged by Jenner and often ignored by medical historians, but engraved boldly on Jesty's tombstone!

Jenner is considered "the father of immunization", however Pasteur was it's midwife. Pasteur's first living 'vaccine' was fowl cholera, a bacterial disease(P. multocida) - and later rabies (infected animal tissue) - but experience with those diseases and, later, yellow fever, laid the foundation for the development and scientific testing of vaccines against several human and animal diseases, with safety and efficacy as the causa sine qua non - requirements that, even today, are not always satisfied with many veterinary vaccines.

The modern era of 'vaccinology' began about 1950 when cell culture methods had improved. Techniques for dispersion of cells were developed in 1950 and, shortly thereafter, applied to large-scale propagation of viruses such as polio (early 1950's), measles (1960) and several veterinary vaccines. Originally, live virus vaccines were the focus of research because only this kind of vaccine was able to be produced. Later, when methods were developed for the plentiful growth of viruses in cell culture, there was renewed interest in inactivated vaccines, which continues today because of more effective methods of inactivation (eg, BPL, BEI). However, since killed vaccines have been found to produce relatively poor local (mucosal) immunity, live vaccines are considered to be superior for many diseases, especially those of the respiratory and enteric systems. Clearly, inactivated vaccines provide greater safety, but the usefulness of a killed vaccine depends on whether it can engender adequate immunity, especially when the goal is control or eradication of a disease in a population. Norrby (18) points out that inactivated vaccines may provide efficient immunity in situations where viraemia is an essential part of the pathogenetic process, such as in poliomyelitis and hepatitis. In some instances, however, inactivated vaccines protect animals from disease only, but not from infection. In such cases, transmission of virulent virus is not interrupted (8). The choice of different types of vaccines is not within the scope of this review.

GENERAL ASPECTS OF LIVE VIRAL VACCINES

"Classic" living viral vaccines, the ones most commonly used in veterinary medicine, are mutants of wild type viruses that emerge attenuated to varying degrees following the empirical process of passage in some unnatural host eg: embryonating eggs, cell cultures or animals. If a virus responsible for serious disease can be purified (cloned) and propagated to acceptable titer in the laboratory, and proved safe (attenuated), it may be the vaccine of choice since most live vaccines provoke immune responses that closely simulate those which attend natural infections. Historical aspects of the evolution of vaccinology are dealt with by several authors (11, 12, 17, 22, 26). A list of the common live-virus veterinary vaccines is given in Table 1. Several of the vaccines listed also are available in inactivated form.

TABLE 1 Commonly Used Live Viral Veterinary Vaccines (refs. 1, 2, 23)

A. NORTH AMERICA

Species	Vaccine
Canine	Distemper
	Infectious hepatitis (canine adenovirus 1,2)
	Canine parainfluenza virus (Type 2)
	Canine parovirus - type 2
	Rabies[1]
Feline	Feline parvovirus (panleukopenia)
	Feline herpesvirus - 1 (rhinotracheitis)
	Calicivirus
Porcine	Hog cholera (swine fever)
	Rotavirus (porcine)
	Pseudorabies (Aujesky's disease)[2]
	Coronavirus (transmissible enteritis)[3]
	Porcine enterovirus (some strains)
Equine	Equine herpesvirus (rhinopneumonitis)
	Equine viral arteritis
	Venezuelan equine encephalomyelitis
Ovine/Caprine	Ovine contagious ecthyma ('Orf')
	Bluetongue (various types)

[1]Inactivated rabies vaccines are now recommended in many countries.

[2]Some vaccinal strains have been genetically altered.

[3]Both attenuated and fully virulent virus is used.

Bovine	Bovine-herpes-1 (infectious bovine rhinotracheitis)
	Rotavirus (bovine)
	Bovine coronavirus
	Bovine parainfluenza - 3
	Bovine respiratory syncitial virus
Avian	Avian encephalomyelitis
	Infectious bursal disease ('Gumboro')
	Duck viral enteritis (duck plague)
	Duck viral hepatitis
	Fowlpox
	Newcastle disease
	Infectious bronchitis
	Avian arthritis (tenosynovitis)
	Marek's disease

B. OTHER COUNTRIES (eg AFRICA, ASIA)

Species	Vaccine
Dogs and Cats	As above (variably available)
Porcine	Hog cholera (swine fever)
	African swine fever (experimental)
	Teschen disease
Equine	African horse sickness
Ovine/Caprine	Bluetongue
	Sheep and goat pox
	Contagious ecthyma ('Orf')
	Rift Valley Fever
	Nairobi sheep disease (experimental)
	Peste de petit ruminants (rinderpest vaccine)
Bovine	Rinderpest
	Foot and mouth disease
	Rift Valley Fever
	Lumpy skin disease
Avian	Newcastle disease
	Infectious bronchitis (some countries)
	Fowl pox
	Avian laryngotracheitis
	Infectious bursal disease ('Gumboro')
	Marek's disease (some countries)

It should be recognised that 'attenuated' is an ambiguous term that means, literally, a virus which is less likely to cause disease than is the wild-type parental strain. Most attenuated viruses undergo limited replication in the vaccinated animal. Attenuated vaccines are, essentially, the product of a process of 'genetic roulette' with the desired properties of reduced virulence and retained immunogenicity (17). It should be recognized that there is very little knowledge concerning the mechanism of attenuation with most viruses. Changes in less than 1% of the genome, sometimes only 1 - 10 codons, have been associated with reduced virulence in several instances. It should be recognised that a virus passaged many times in an alien host may accumulate several mutations in critical sites, ones that render it incapable of replicating in the target host and thus fail to engender immunity. This phenomenon has been a problem on several occasions with canine parvovirus vaccine production (8).

Various conditions have been imposed to favour the development of mutants (9, 12, 17, 19). These include: passage under unnatural temperature conditions (cold-adapted and ts mutants), deliberately mutagenized or reassorted genomes and, more recently, by way of DNA modifications obtained by techniques of genetic engineering. Examples of deletions associated with reduced virulence include the deletions in human (alpha 22), or suid herpesvirus TK or glycoprotein genes (14). Some viruses can be distinguished from their wild-type parents by characteristics other than pathogenicity for the natural host; for example, temperature-sensitivity, plaque characteristics in cell cultures, antigenicity -reactivity with monoclonal antibodies, or nucleotide sequence differences.

Vaccine strategies differ, but all successful ones take into account the pathogenesis of the disease, the elements of the immune response repertoire that are stimulated to produce antibodies or cell-immune components - and the recipient. In animals, breed, age (susceptibility of the very young; presence of maternal antibodies), and whether the intended recipient of a vaccine is immunocompromised, are important determinants of successful immunization. Interference between viruses in multiple vaccines is well documented for polio vaccines, but this phenomenon is not regarded as a problem with licensed veterinary vaccines. The presence of one or more viruses in a multiple vaccine may, however, engender some degree of immunosuppression (21, 25). 'Reactivation' of virulent virus has been recorded with live, attenuated polio strains, and with some experimental encephalitis vaccines, but it has not been a recognized problem with veterinary biologics.

THE "IDEAL VACCINE" SHOULD BE SAFE AS WELL AS EFFECTIVE

Ideally, a vaccine should have the following characteristics:

- It should be completely <u>safe</u>; ie, it should cause no illness to the recipient, or to contact animals, if transmissible. It should not cause foetal infection or affect reproduction.

- It should be highly <u>protective</u>. Protective antibodies or cell-mediated immune responses should be generated quickly and immunity should be <u>durable</u>, ie, sustained for a reasonable period (1 year).

- It should <u>prevent infection</u>, or establishment of latency by wild virus (eg, herpesviruses; retroviruses).

- The ideal vaccine should <u>interrupt transmission</u> of wild-type viruses, especially those which are highly contagious such as distemper, rinderpest, or canine parvovirus. With such diseases, control in populations depends upon establishing 'immune barriers'.

- If the vaccine does not prevent infection, but only suppresses disease, the virus load should be reduced >99% in vaccinated hosts so that host immune responses may cope with the remainder. <u>Prevention of disease</u> in successfully vaccinated individuals, but <u>not transmission of virulent virus</u>, is common with <u>inactivated</u> products.

- With <u>enveloped viruses</u>, especially, vaccine should generate specific <u>CMI responses</u> (Class I, MHC-restrict T-cells), which are important in clearing infections.

- Vaccine should immunize at an age when an animal becomes susceptible to infection, ie, prior to the decline of maternal antibodies below protective levels, an uncommon attribute with canine parvovirus or infectious hepatitis.

- The vaccinal virus should be <u>genetically stable</u> during laboratory propagation and not generate non-immunizing variants during scale-up to production lots.

- Vaccine should be relatively <u>inexpensive</u> to produce.

- Vaccine should be <u>stable</u> during lyophilization so as not to lose potency (titer). In tropical countries the vaccine should have <u>thermo-protective stabilizers</u> to prevent inactivation during delay in storage or administration, eg, measles, distemper, rinderpest vaccines.

<u>SOME PROBLEMS WITH LIVE VIRUS VACCINES</u> (2,6,13,17,18,25)

- <u>Back-mutation</u> to virulence (eg, polio-3).

- <u>Interference</u> by endemic enteroviruses (eg, polio).

- <u>Inadequate attenuation</u> ('residual virulence'), leading to disease may be a consequence of the nature of the virus or result from insufficient or faulty research. There are numerous examples (25). A partial list includes: <u>Equine herpesvirus-1</u> (rhinopneumonitis) - paralysis; <u>rabies</u> - encephalitis; <u>canine distemper</u> (some strains) - encephalitis, especially in young animals; <u>bovine herpesvirus-1</u> and <u>bovine virus diarrhoea virus</u> (BVD) - immunosuppression and abortions; <u>infectious canine hepatitis (CAV-1)</u> - 'blue eyes' (type II hypersensitivity); <u>feline panleukopenia</u> (parvovirus) and <u>bluetongue virus</u> - arrest of brain development; <u>human measles</u> - 'measles', encephalitis, SSPE; disease in <u>exotic animals</u> - distemper in grey, foxes, lesser pandas and kinkajous; BVD - persistent fetal infections, sometimes with anomalies; canine coronavirus vaccine - meningitis, encephalitis, pancreatitis.

Contamination of live vaccines has been a recurrent problem, not only in developing countries. Examples include: frequent contamination of several bovine vaccines with BVD virus - commonly present in commercial sera; reticuloendotheliosis virus in vaccine (turkey herpesvirus) for Marek's disease; pestivirus (BVD/Border Disease?) contamination of pseudorabies vaccine. Mycoplasmas commonly contaminate vaccines, but their significance is uncertain.

- Thermolability - rinderpest and other live vaccines used in the tropics. There is a great need for development of lyophilizing processes that would reduce the need for emphasis on the "cold chain" (16).

TABLE 2 Live Versus Inactivated Vaccines - Some Comparisons

Attribute	Live Virus Vaccine	Inactivated Vaccine
1. Duration of immunity	Lengthy	Months (exceptions)
2. Safety	Variable (see above)	High (local reactions)
3. No. doses required	Single (usually)	Multiple (2 or more)
4. Mucosal immunity	Usually good	None, or limited
5. Antibody responses	Early onset; IgG	Delayed (1° IgM → 2° IgG)
6. CMI responses	Good	Weak, variable
7. Interference	Rare (vet. vaccines)	No
8. Adjuvant required	No	Usually
9. Thermolability	Yes ($\propto$ stabilizer,etc)	No
10. Cost	Low	*Relatively high
11. Amount of antigen to provoke immunity	Small	Large

DEVELOPMENT AND EVALUATION OF A LIVE VIRUS VACCINE

Several strategies have been employed to develop attenuated live viral vaccines, however, the approach currently used for most veterinary vaccines follows a 'classical' protocol. The most important prerequisite is the need for good methods of propagating virus in the laboratory, eg, in cell cultures or embryonating eggs. In some instances the 'Jennerian Approach' (17, 19) has been used. This involves the use of a virus of one animal species to immunize against an antigenically related virus of a different species. Such empirical vaccines include vaccinia (cowpox?) for humans; heterotypic parainfluenza viruses for dogs, cattle or primates; mammalian rotaviruses for humans; alien influenza viruses for heterologous species; human measles for dogs; bovine diarrhea virus for swine fever; and a turkey herpesvirus for prevention of Marek's disease.

In the future, new strategies are envisioned for making live virus vaccines (2,9,12,17,19). These are not discussed here, but they involve vaccines constructed through genetic engineering or other methods of molecular biology. These include recombinant viruses, with vaccinia or other viruses with redundant genes as vectors, and the creation of deletion or insertion mutants by DNA modification.

VACCINE FAILURES

Although there are special requirements for each vaccine, the *conditio sine qua non* is acceptable potency (confirmed by efficacy tests) and safety. Other attributes, such as rapidity of onset of immunity, are important, though less so. Vaccines occasionally fail because of low standards - failure to control potency, emergence of non-immunizing mutants in vaccine lots during expansion from working seed (not an uncommon event with canine parvovirus) or the presence of contaminating agents. In many developing countries, it is not possible to monitor the quality of vaccines on a regional basis, even ones of great economic significance. In Africa this critical need is now being addressed through 'PANVAC', a regional project of FAO/UNDP to upgrade vaccine production and quality control of priority vaccines (20). Additional problems concern modes of vaccine storage, transportation and administration.

Vaccines which have been manufactured according to high standards ('Good Manufacturing Practices') also have failed in the field. Documented reasons include: use of out-dated vaccines; inactivation of viruses by residual disinfectant in needles/syringes used for vaccination; 'dose-splitting' (using smaller doses for smaller animals, etc); heat-inactivation of thermolabile vaccines such as measles or rinderpest. Improper use of vaccines in pregnant dams, very young animals or in non-intended species has also caused 'vaccine failures'.

Steps in the development of commercial vaccines follow the general scheme presented in Table 3. Regardless of the protocol followed to achieve the selection of a less-virulent virus population from wild-type stock, each requires satisfying the fundamental requisites of safety and immunogenicity ('potency').

TABLE 3 Steps in the Development of a Commercial Vaccine[1]
(Modified from Baker and Robson, 1978, ref.3)

Wild-type or Virulent virus
Produces illness and productivity loss in natural host

↓

Serial passage in alien host
Test for pathogenicity in susceptible animals at approximately each 10th passage. Use standard host (age, breed); viral dose

↓

'Attenuated Virus'
Stop passage when diminished pathogenicity observed in preliminary tests, ie, produces no signs of typical illness, or modified, acceptable signs of illness

[1] It is assumed that virus has been isolated and propagated in a suitable laboratory host.

Preliminary Safety Tests

Tests of 'attenuated virus' in seronegative natural host species (using at least 5 animals/group) for signs of illness and transmissibility; if transmissible, then a number of passage for 'reversion to virulence' should exceed 5. Stop passages if acceptable level of attenuation observed and prepare stock virus (lyophilize or freeze at <-60C).

↓

Continued passage

If preliminary safety test indicate unacceptable attenuation, passage is continued until acceptable level is reached. When virus is considered attenuated, test for: (1) Pathogenicity at the earliest age an animal is expected to receive vaccine; (2) ability to cause transplacental infections in pregnant animals; (3) 'reversion to virulence' by back-passaging in natural host.

↓

Determination of minimal immunizing dose

Measure immune responses (usually SN or HI antibody) at the highest passage level to be used.

↓

Standardization of vaccine

Determine the ID_{50} for animal species to be vaccinated.

↓

Efficacy tests and safety check in field

Field-test vaccine for acceptability at the highest level to be used in vaccine; observe vaccinated animals for signs of illness due to vaccination and test for immunity in a paired challenge test or unpaired serological tests. Test random vaccine lots for efficacy at intervals, at least annually, to assure continued quality.

QUALITY CONTROL[1]

In the United States, the basic principle of regulation and testing of vaccines has been to maintain production organizations with research capabilities. Research emphasis is directed toward the anticipation and solution of problems in the manufacture and testing of experimental and licensed products, an approach in some ways similar to that in developing countries where vaccines are often produced in National Laboratories which also conduct research. Stringent enforcement by government authorities, coupled with close co-operation between industry and government, is essential to sustained vaccine quality, a process not followed in many countries. A further, and essential element in the regulatory process is continued consultation and technology exchange with the research community through consultants, seminars, workshops and international conferences.

At the practical level, there are several requirements to be met in order to satisfy 'Good Manufacturing Practices' (GMP) (10), which describe requirements for personnel, facilities, equipment, production controls, records and other aspects of vaccine production.

The term 'Standards' usually refers not to vaccine *per se*, but to the specifications and protocols used by a facility to manufacture and release products of assured potency, purity, and safety. United States regulations and requirements are available by written request

[1]Material for this section was obtained largely from references 1 and 13.

addressed to: Director of Biologics Services, USDA, APHIS, Biologics Staff, Federal Center Building, Hyattsville, Maryland, 20782 (USA). The many requirements are complex, frequently under revision and are too numerous to mention here, except in outline (for a discussion of requirements for poultry vaccines in the USA see reference 15).

Listed below are examples of standard requirements for "GMP":

1. Facilities: Floor and wall construction such that thorough cleansing is possible; preparation rooms arranged to prevent cross-contamination; means to prevent contamination of employee or product (biological hoods); freedom from outside contamination (eg, dust, smoke); adequate air handling to insure sanitary conditions; efficient drainage, etc.

2. Separation of production from quality control. Separation of facilities; different personnel. The 'Head of Quality Control' should not report to the 'Head of Production'.

3. Purity. Freedom from adventitious bacteria, viruses, fungi, or *Mycoplasma* sp. Includes test of seed and master seed virus; cell cultures or embryonating eggs.

4. Safety. Toxicity tests in mice or guinea pigs; *in vivo* tests of intended host (cattle, pigs, dogs, chickens, etc).

5. Potency

   (a) Adequate viral titer in final product, based upon minimal immunizing dose (MID_{50}) studies. Random batch testing.

   (b) Vaccine must provoke satisfactory serological responses (antibodies) in vaccinated animals, using pre- and postvaccination sera, usually collected - 3 weeks after vaccination. Serological tests should be those that indicate immune status (SN or HI).

6. Other. Moisture content of lyophilized vaccine; determination of shelf life at different temperatures (thermostability); virus identity tests using fluorescent antibody or neutralization tests with each batch.

In countries with limited or inadequate facilities, several of the above criteria have proven difficult to satisfy. Nevertheless, once safety has been established for the seed viral stock through research during product development, meeting standards of potency and purity are the minimal requirements that must be satisfied to generate confidence in vaccines, whether they are live or inactivated.

REFERENCES

1. ANON. (1980) Basic license requirements for applicants (for biological products). U.S. Title 9, Code of Federal Regulations. Parts 101-114. USDA/APHIS, Hyattsville, MD (USA).

2. BABIUK, L.A. (1985) The use of vaccines for controlling viral diseases of animals. In: Immunochemistry of viruses. The basis for serodiagnosis and vaccines. M.H.V. van Regenmortel and A.R. Neurath, eds. Elsevier Science Pub. (Biomedical Div), Amsterdam.

3. BAKER J.A. and ROBSON, D.S. (1958) Serological tests as indicators of immunity. United States Livestock Sanitary Assoc. (Proceedings) **62**:1.

4. BAKER, J.A. and ROBSON, D.S. (1958) Simplified standards for live virus vaccines. United States Livestock Sanitary Assoc. (Proceedings) **62**:43.

5. BIGGS, P.M. (1974) Desirable requirements for live vaccines used against Marek's Disease. In: International Symposium on Requirements for Poultry Virus Vaccines. Develop.biol.Stand. **25**:127. Karger, Basel.

6. BITTLE, J.L. and MUIR, S. (1989) Vaccines produced by conventional means to control major diseases of man and animals. In: Adv. Vet. Sci. Comp. Med. **33**:1.

7. CARMICHAEL, L.E., JOUBERT, J.C. and POLLOCK, R.V.H. (1981) A modified live canine parvovirus strain with novel plaque characteristics. I. Viral attenuation and dog response. Cornell Vet. **71**:408.

8. CARMICHAEL, L.E. (1983) Immunization strategies in puppies - why failures? Compendium on Continuing Education for Pract. Vet. **5**:1043.

9. CHANOCK, R.M. and LERNER, R.A. (1984) Modern Approaches to Vaccines: Molecular and Chemical Basis of Virus Virulence and Immunogenicity.p.389. Cold Spring Harbor Laboratory, NY.

10. CODE OF FEDERAL REGULATIONS, Title 21, parts 600-680, Subchapter F-Biologics. (1985) US Government Printing Office, Washington, DC 20402 (USA).

11. FENNER, F. (1985) Poxviruses. In: Virology.B.Field, D.M. Knipe, R.M. Chanock, J.L. Melnick, B. Roizman and R.E. Shope, eds. Raven Press, N.Y.

12. HILLEMAN, M.R. (1985) Newer directions in vaccine development. J.Inf.Dis. **151**:407.

13. HOPPS, H.E. MEYER, B.C. and PARKMAN, P.D. (1988) Regulation and testing of vaccines. In: Vaccines, S.A. Plotkin and E.A. Mortimer, Jr.editors.p.576, W.B. Saunders Co, Philadelphia.

14. KIT, S., KIT, M., BARTKOSKI, M.J. and DEES, C. (1987) Genetically engineered pseudorabies virus vaccine with deletions in thymidine kinase and glycoprotein genes. In: Vaccines '87,p.345. Cold Spring Harbor Laboratory, NY.

15. LASALLE, B. (1974) Requirements for Marek's disease vaccine in USA. In: Develop.biol. Standard. **25**, 26l. Ch. Merieux, E.C. Hulse, D. Gaudry, W.H. Allen and Regamey, editors. Karger, Basel.

16. MARINER, J.C. et al. (1990) Comparison of the effect of various chemical stabilizers and lyophilization cycles on the thermostability of a Vero-cell adapted rinderpest vaccine. Vet. microbiol. **21**:195.

17. MURPHY, B. and CHANOCK, R.M. (1990) Immunization against Viruses. In: Virology, 2nd Edition. B.N. Fields, D.M. Knipe et al., eds. Raven Press, Ltd. NY.

18. NORRBY, E. (1983) Viral Vaccines: The use of currently available products and future developments (A brief review). Arch. Virology **76**:163.

20. NORRBY, E. (1989) Modern Approaches to Live Virus Vaccines. In: Advances In Vet.Sci. and Comparative Med. **33**:249.

21. PANVAC Vaccine Bulletin (1991). D. Sylla and M. Rweyemamu, eds. Pan African Vet. Vaccine Centre, Debre-Zeit, Addis Ababa, Ethiopia; Hann, Dakar, Senegal **1**:1.

22. PHILIPS, T., JENSEN, H., RUBINO, M.J. et al. (1989) Effects of vaccines on the canine immune system. Can.J.Vet.Res. **53**:154.

23. PLOTKIN, S.L. (1988) A short history of vaccination. In: Vaccine. S.A. Plotkin and E.A. Mortimer, eds.p.1. W.B. Saunders, Philadelphia.

24. RUPRECHT, C.E., DIETZSCHOLD, B. and KOPROWSKI, H. (1987) Development of an oral wildlife rabies vaccine: Immunization of raccoons by a vaccinia-rabies glycoprotein recombinant virus and preliminary field baiting trials. In: Vaccines '87. (1987) Modern Approaches to New Vaccines: Prevention of AIDS and other Viral, Bacterial and Parasitic Diseases. Cold Spring Harbour Laboratory, NY.

25. TIMONEY, J.F., GILLESPIE, J.H., SCOTT, F.W. and BARLOUGH, J.E. (1988) In: Hagan and Bruner's Microbiology and Infectious Diseases of Domestic Animals. Comstock Pub., Cornell Univ. Press. Ithaca, N.Y.

26. TIZARD, I. (1990) Risks associated with use of live vaccines. Jour. Am. Vet. Med. Assoc. **196**:185l.

27. WILLIAMS, G. (1959) Virus Hunters. A.A. Knopf, NY.

14. KIT, S., KIT, M., KATTROSKI, M.L. and DUBBS, G. (1987) Genetically engineered pseudorabies virus vaccine with deletions in thymidine kinase and glycoprotein genes. In: Vaccines '87 p 345. Cold Spring Harbor Laboratory, NY.

15. LASALLE, B. (1974) Requirements for Marek's disease vaccine. In: I.S.B. In: Develop. biol. Standard. 25, 261. Ch. Merieux, E.C. Hulse, B. Cauldry, W.H. Allen and Regamey, editors. Karger, Basel.

16. MARINER, J.C. et al. (1990) Comparison of the effect of various chemical stabilizers and lyophilization cycles on the thermostability of a Vero-cell adapted rinderpest vaccine. Vet. Microbiol. 21:195.

17. MURPHY, B. and CHANOCK, R.M. (1990) Immunization against Viruses. In: Virology, 2nd Edition. B.N. Fields, D.M. Knipe et al., eds. Raven Press Ltd., NY.

19. NORRBY, E. (1983) Viral Vaccines: The use of currently available products and future developments (A brief review). Archs Virology 76:163.

20. NORRBY, E. (1989) Modern Approaches to Live Virus Vaccines. In: Advances in Vet. Sci. and Comparative Med. 33:249.

21. PANVAC Vaccine Bulletin (1991). D. Sylla and M. Jeggo, eds. Pan African Vet. Vaccine Centre, Debre Zeit, Addis Ababa, Ethiopia, Hann Dakar Senegal 1:1.

22. PHILLIPS, T., JENSEN, H., RUBINO, M.J. et al. (1989) Effects of vaccines on the canine immune system. Can. J. Vet. Res. 53:154.

23. PLOTKIN, S.L. (1988) A short history of vaccinations. In: Vaccines. S.A. Plotkin and E.A. Mortimer, eds. p. 1. W.B. Saunders, Philadelphia.

24. RUPPRECHT, C.E., DIETZSCHOLD, B. and KOPROWSKI, H. (1987) Development of an oral wildlife rabies vaccine: Immunization of raccoons by vaccinia rabies glycoprotein recombinant virus and preliminary field baiting trials. In: Vaccines '87 (1987) Modern Approaches to New Vaccines: Prevention of AIDS and other Viral, Bacterial and Parasitic Diseases. Cold Spring Harbour Laboratory, NY.

25. TIMONEY, J.F., GILLESPIE, J.H., SCOTT, F.W. and BARLOUGH, J.E. (1988) In: Hagan and Bruner's Microbiology and Infectious Diseases of Domestic Animals. Comstock Pub., Cornell Univ. Press. Ithaca, N.Y.

26. TIZARD, I. (1990) Risks associated with use of live vaccines. Jour. Am. Vet. Med. Assoc. 196:1851.

27. WILLIAMS, G. (1959) Virus Hunters. A.A. Knopf, NY.

INACTIVATED VIRAL VACCINES

by

L E Carmichael

INTRODUCTION

In the early 1950's, advancements in methods for large-scale propagation of viruses in embryonating eggs and tissue cultures promoted the development of inactivated vaccines; until that time, most human and animal vaccines were living products.

Once virus could be grown in large quantities, methods which were developed earlier for the inactivation of bacteria and toxins were then applied to viruses - formaldehyde was the common inactivant. This reagent was exploited initially for the production of polio vaccine and, subsequently, for several other human and domestic animal vaccines. It should be noted that the use of formaldehyde, and the production conditions for early whole-virion polio vaccines, was entirely empirical, but success with this vaccine gave rise to the unfounded conviction that formalin was the optimal, universal inactivating agent for the production of killed vaccines - a belief that continues to persist (6). Fortunately, concern was raised over the unpredictability of formalin, and alternate procedures such as use of β-propiolactone (12) and aziridines (ethyleneimines) were explored (7,9). These have greater inactivation efficiencies and are far less destructive of immunogenic proteins.

Several conditions must be satisfied for safe and effective inactivated vaccines: (1) 'Complete' (statistically probable) inactivation of infectivity, determined by inactivation kinetics under different conditions of time, temperature and pH,(6); also preservation of antigenicity. Three main requirements should be satisfied for efficacy: (1) Protective efficiency - determination of the minimal immunizing dose required to protect against challenge with a standard viral dose; (2) Immunogenic efficiency - the extent of immunity (*in vivo* serological responses) engendered by the viral antigen(s) in the inactivated product; (3) Virion immunogenicity - ie the preservation of virion 'potency'; loss of the physical stability of a virion may greatly reduce the capacity of a vaccine to induce an immune response - which also may occur after prolonged storage. Inactivation, by formalin or irradiation, may lead not only to the destruction of native antigens (epitopes), but also to formation of new ('artificial') antigens as a consequence of denaturation (3, 9, 13). Detailed elaboration of these principals has recently been published (6), and should be studied by all involved in the production of inactivated vaccines. Perhaps Lewis Carrol anticipated the process:

"You boil it with sawdust, salt it with glue ...
Condense it with locusts and tape ...
Keeping one principle in view ...
To preserve its symmetrical shape." (viz, structure)

The Hunting of the Snark (1876)

This abstract focuses on general aspects of 'classical' inactivated vaccines, rather than on new technological developments - mainly because virtually all inactivated veterinary vaccines are produced by similar ('old') methods. The newer ones are not adequately developed to the stage where they could be exploited commercially; in developing countries, the technology for their production does not presently exist. Even more critical to subvirion vaccine development is the general lack of knowledge on the repertoire of epitopes required of each virus to achieve effective immunization (6, 14). Also, effective adjuvants, carriers and antigen delivery systems for subvirion vaccines, whether produced from purified virus or through hybrid-DNA technology, are neither perfected nor presently cost-effective (4, 10, 14, 15). In developing countries, cost is a major consideration.

CHOICE OF VACCINE

Attitudes with respect to choice of vaccine have changed on several occasions, partly as a consequence of problems with several viral vaccines - both live and inactivated - and partially because of the accumulation of new knowledge. During the last decade there has developed an increased preference for inactivated vaccines by many vaccinologists, some with vested interests. In developed countries, especially, society-at-large is ever more concerned with safety. The aesthetically satisfying notion that all killed vaccines are innocuous, as well as effective in preventing disease, is also an influence. Inactivated vaccines, however, may not be totally safe, and many fail to generate immune responses (eg mucosal immunity) that completely block infection and subsequent transmission of virulent virus. This is an important factor that should be considered in any effort to control highly transmissible diseases caused by stable viruses (such as parvoviruses) in assembled animals, such as those maintained in herds, zoos or kennels.

The propensity to use inactivated products was encouraged by the success with vaccines such as rabies, polio (in Scandinavia), and, later, human hepatitis B (18) - prior to development of a recombinant vaccine produced in yeast cells. Inactivated products against those diseases have proved highly effective (10). They also have proven safe and effective against several diseases of veterinary importance such as parvoviruses of cats, dogs, pigs and mink, Newcastle disease virus, and several togaviruses such as Eastern, Western and Venezuelan encephalitis and, especially, rabies. The evolution of new technologies for: antigen production and purification, subunit immunogens, the production of viral proteins through recombinant DNA methods in bacteria or eucaryotic cells such as yeast, insect and mammalian cells and, more recently, synthetic vaccines; or possible use of anti-idiotype antibodies as immunogens; delivery of immunogens; and, the discovery of potentially useful novel adjuvants (15) - has also influenced the contemporary interest in non-living vaccines.

ADVANTAGES AND DISADVANTAGES OF INACTIVATED VIRUS VACCINES

Advantages and disadvantages of live versus inactivated vaccines were briefly noted in the previous paper 'Live Virus Vaccines'. The principal advantages of properly inactivated products are their greater safety; no choice is possible with diseases where an attenuated viral vaccine has not yet been developed. With rabies, the risks of postvaccinal illness have been documented (21, 23) and inactivated products are generally recommended. Properly inactivated vaccines with sufficient potency (immunogen content) usually produce efficient immunity in those disease where viraemia is an essential part of the pathogenesis

(16), such as in parvovirus infections, Newcastle disease and viral encephalitides. As noted in an accompanying paper 'Vaccines for Wildlife and Companion Animals', effective inactivated vaccines for canine distemper are possible, but the problem of maintaining potency, which is related to the ability to grow commercial-scale quantities of distemper virus to consistently high titers, has not been solved. This problem also appears to be one that has impeded progress on inactivated vaccines against other morbilliviruses such as human measles, where only small amounts of the principal immunogens (glycoprotein-H and F-protein) are produced in infected cells (17). Wild animals in the United States should not be vaccinated for rabies, even with inactivated products, until vaccines approved for use in wildlife species are available (21).

Several 'inactivated' vaccines have caused outbreaks of disease due to incomplete inactivation. Such events occurred with early poliovirus vaccine lots as well as with several veterinary vaccines. There is a common belief amongst many veterinarians that "a little bit of live virus is necessary for a good vaccine!" (21) - this may have been true for some vaccines, but it hardly constitutes "good vaccinology" - or adherence to "Good Manufacturing Practices" (1). Perhaps the most celebrated recent episodes are those that involved formalin-inactivated foot-and-mouth disease virus (5, 13, 19), where the presence of residual live virus accounted for costly outbreaks. Difficulties in assuring complete inactivation, as well as adequate potency, have lead to the discontinuation of FMD vaccination in several countries (13, 22). Also, inactivated FMD vaccines have a stringent refrigeration requirement; there are additional difficulties in cell culture propagation of some strains as well. Such reasons have inspired the desire to produce recombinant or synthetic vaccines, despite the problems of multiple serotypes. Living virus also has been detected in certain canine and feline parvovirus vaccines[1], but there was no associated illness.

Several inactivated virus vaccines for humans have actually potentiated disease. It is to be noted that the majority of the offending vaccines were inactivated with formalin, a notoriously unpredictable inactivating agent (2). Such vaccines include measles, respiratory syncytial virus, influenza-A and, perhaps, poliovirus (14, 18). Although the mechanisms differ, they involved the destruction, or alteration of some essential immunogens by formalin. Also, poor primary Tc-responses have been noted with inactivated vaccines in animal studies, and unbalanced Td cell responses have led to delayed hypersensitivity reactions upon exposure to virulent virus (14). In the case of polio, virus grown in cell cultures contains an uncleaved outer capsid protein (VP1) that has only limited ability to induce neutralizing antibodies (14). There is, thus, little or no immunity to polio type-3 in the intestine, where the VP-1 has been cleaved by intestinal proteases.

Other 'disadvantages' of inactivated vaccines include a generally shorter duration of immunity; lack of, or diminished, mucosal immunity, which is important with infections caused by viruses such as influenza, coronaviruses or rotaviruses; failures to immunize against infection and interrupt transmission of disease in populations, unless vaccination was frequent, eg parvovirus, polio, coronavirus; the usual requirement for multiple doses ("boosters"); the need for adjuvants for optimal protection; and, the cost of vaccine production, which is higher than that for live vaccines. Fortunately, rabies is an exception to many of the above comments.

[1] L E Carmichael (1979-80). Unpublished data.

GENERAL COMMENTS ON INACTIVATED VACCINES

It is recognised that most inactivated veterinary vaccines produced today have been developed by empirical methods, ones that, nevertheless, have had the benefit of time to prove their worth - or ineffectiveness. Unhappily, lack of effectiveness has often been realized only after a vaccine has been licensed by a government authority. The biological considerations and procedures required for producing optimal inactivated vaccines are complex, perhaps even more so than with living viral vaccines. Amongst the most important development and production factors, and conditions, to be satisfied are:

Choice of inactivant - its selectivity for nucleic acid destruction without destroying essential virion components necessary for immunogenicity. Formalin should be discouraged; use of β-propiolactone (BPL) or aziridines, eg acetylethyleneimine (AEI); binary ethyleneimine (BEI) have proved much more satisfacatory.

Since inactivated vaccines do not replicate in the body, the amount of immunogen received in a vaccine is that which is contained in the inoculum. Many failures have occurred as a result of inadequate immunizing virus.

The kinetic approach should be used to determine the appropriate conditions for each virus, under the conditions of production. Both chemical (inactivation) and biological (destruction of immunogenicity) factors must be considered.

The minimum immunizing dose for vaccines produced under standard conditions must be determined in animals. Most countries require challenge of vaccinated animals, but serological responses are satisfactory where antibody responses have been correlated with immunity.

The sero-conversion rate must be determined in the field for inactivated products. Like their living counterparts, they may be labile to temperature and storage conditions.

Safety must be determined in the laboratory as well as in the field. It is recognized that, in principal, it is not possible to achieve complete assurance of freedom from residual live virus - especially with products inactivated with formaldehyde.

Determination of number of doses required for satisfactory immunity, and duration of immunity.

Determination of allergic or other undesirable reactions.

REQUIREMENTS FOR KILLED VIRUS VACCINES IN THE US

The General Requirements of the USDA/APHIS are noted below. [Satisfying the requirements does not necessarily ensure the safety/efficacy of a product]. The published requirements[1] should be consulted for details. A list of general requirements is given below:

General Requirements - for all vaccines:

1. Killing agent - appropriate test for inactivation.

2. Cell culture requirements - use of approved primary cells or cell lines.

3. Purity tests - freedom from bacteria, mycoplasma and fungi.

4. Safety tests - use of guinea pigs and mice (exempt for poultry vaccines).

5. Viricidal activity tests - if inactivated virus is to be used as diluent for live virus vaccine, it must not have viricidal activity.

6. Formaldehyde content - concentration must be $<0.2\%$. This requirement has been modified to include other approved inactivating agents.

Specific Requirements - differ somewhat for each licensed vaccine type. They generally include:

1. Potency test in animals. USDA requires challenge of vaccinated animals, generally 2-3 weeks after the last dose for many vaccines. The number of animals required for each vaccine varies, and appears to be arbitrary.

2. Serology may be used with certain vaccines where serological test values have been correlated with immunity. In such cases, virus-neutralizing antibody sero-conversions are generally acceptable in lieu of challenge.

In many countries, especially in underdeveloped regions, it is not possible to monitor the quality of many vaccines. A prime factor is costs, especially if production is on a limited scale and does not take into consideration regional needs. Additional problems, encountered also with living vaccines, are storage, distribution and administration of vaccines in the field - factors that negate all efforts to produce effective vaccines.

[1] See: Basic License Requirements for Applicants for Biological Products. U.S. Title 9, Code of Federal Regulations. Parts 101-114, especially §.113,20. Government Printing Office. Veterinary Biologics Staff, Veterinary Services, Federal Building, Hyattsville, MD 5050 (USA).

Table 1. Inactivated Vaccines 'Used For Animals[1]

Animal	Vaccine
Dogs	Canine Adenovirus-2 (for infectious hepatitis)
	Canine coronavirus
	Canine parvovirus
	Rabies
Cats	Feline panleukopenia (parvovirus)
	Feline calicivirus
	Feline leukemia
	Rabies
Swine	Pseudorabies (Aujesky's disease)
	Swine parvovirus infection
	African swine fever*
	Hog cholera*
Cattle	Bovine parainfluenza-3
	Bovine rhinotracheitis (IBR, bovine herpes-1)
	Bovine virus diarrhea (mucosal disease)
	Foot-and-mouth disease*
	Bovine papillomas (warts)
Sheep & Goats	Louping ill*
	Nairobi sheep disease*
Horses	Equine rhinopneumonitis (equid herpes-1)
	Equine influenza
	Eastern, Western, Venezuelan encephalomyelitis
	African horse sickness (9 serotypes)*
Poultry	Newcastle disease
	Avian encephalomyelitis
	Avian parainfluenza-3 (turkeys)
	Avian arthritis (tenosynovitis)
	Infectious bronchitis
	Infectious bursal disease (Gumboro)

[1] Modified from data references 2, (pp. 198-204) and 21 (p.456).

* Vaccines for diseases outside North America.

Table 2. A Model Production And Quality Control Protocol Developed For Newcastle Disease Vaccine[1]

Control		Production step
		Stock Vaccine (seed) Virus
		↓
Control (Sterility)	←	Preliminary passage in SPF eggs (Master Seed Virus)
		↓
		Lyophilize Master Seed
		↓
Control	←	Second passage in SPF eggs (Working Seed Virus)
		↓
		Virus Production in SPF eggs (or eggs from disease-free flocks)
		↓
Control (Sterility & Virus Titration)	←	Harvest of virus-laden fluids (AAF)
		↓
Control (Sterility & Virus(Titration)	←	Inactivation (β-propiolactone, formalin[2]) ~0.3% ~0.1%
		↓
		Emulsion in oil adjuvant
		↓
Control of final product		Sterility; Safety; Extraneous Agents; Viral inactivation; Potency; Stability

Similar protocols are used for other inactivated products, however specific information should be sought when contemplating production of any vaccine.

---

[1]From Palya, V. (1991). Manual for the production of Marek's disease, Gumboro disease and inactivated Newcastle disease vaccines. FAO Animal Production and Health Paper **89**, FAO, Rome.

[2]See above for comments on formalin

REFERENCES

1. ANON. (1985) Code of Federal Regulations, Title 21, parts 600, 601, 630, 211. Subchapter F-Biologics (Human vaccines). Government Printing Office, Washington D.C.

2. BABIUK, L.A. (1985) The use of vaccines for controlling viral diseases of animals. In: van Regenmortel and A.R. Neurath, eds. Immunochemistry of Viruses. The basis for serodiagnosis and vaccines. Elsevier Science Pub., B.B., Amsterdam.

3. BACHRACH, H.L., et al (1957) Inactivation of foot-and-mouth disease virus by pH and temperature changes and by formaldehyde. Proc. Soc. Exp. Biol. Med. **95**:147.

4. BEALE, J. (1982) Synthetic peptides as the basis for future vaccines. Nature (London) **298**:14.

5. BECK, E. and STROHMAIER, K. (1987) Subtyping of European foot-and-mouth disease virus strains by nucleotide sequence determination. J. Virol. **61**;1621.

6. BUDOWSKY, E.I. (1991) Problems and prospects for preparation of killed antiviral vaccines. Adv. Virus Res. **39**:255.

7. DERMER, O.E. and HAM, G.E. (1969) Ethyleneimine and other aziridines. Academic Press, N.Y.

8. ESPESETH, D. (1986) Licensing consideration for New Adjuvants and Carriers. In: Advances in Carriers and Adjuvants for Veterinary Biologics, R.M. Nervig et al., editors: p.159. Iowa State Univ. Press, Ames, Iowa.

9. BAHNEMANN, H.G. (1975) Binary ethylenimine as an inactivant for foot-and-mouth disease virus and its application for vaccine production. Arch. Virology **47**:47.

10. HILLEMAN, M.R. (1985) Newer directions in vaccine development. J. Infect. Dis **151**:407.

11. KING, A.M., UNDERWOOD, B.O., McCAHON, D., et al (1981) Biochemical identification of viruses causing outbreaks of foot-and-mouth disease in the UK. Nature (London) **293**;479.

12. KRUGMAN, S. (1982) The newly licensed hepatitis B vaccine. Characteristics and indications for use. J.A.M.A. **247**:2012.

13. LO GRIPPO, G.A. (1960) Investigation of the use of beta-propiolactone in virus inactivation. Ann. N.Y. Acad. Sci. **83**:578.

14. MANN, J.A. and SELLERS, R.F. (1990) Foot-and-Mouth Disease. In: Virus Infections of Ruminants. Z. Dinter and B. Morein, eds., pp. 503-512. Elsevier Science Pub., Amsterdam.

15. MURPHY, B.R. and CHANOCK, R.M. (1990) Immunization against Viruses. In: Virology, 2nd edition. B.N. Fields, D.M. Knipe et al. eds. p.475. Raven Press, Ltd., New York.

16. NERVIG, R.M. et al (eds) (1986) Advances in Carriers and Adjuvants for Veterinary Biologics. Iowa State University Press, Ames, Iowa.

17. NORRBY, E. (1987) Toward new viral vaccines for man. Adv. Virus. Res. **32**:1.

18. NORRBY, E., ENDERS-RUCKLE, G. and TER MEULEN, V. (1975) Differences in the appearance of antibodies to structural components of measles virus after immunization with formalin-treated and live virus vaccines. J. Infect. Dis. **132**:262.

19. PRINCE, G., et al (1986) Mechanism by which intramuscular inoculation of formalin-inactivated respiratory syncytial (RS) virus enhances pulmonary pathology in cotton rats subsequently infected with RS virus. In: Vaccines 86: New Approaches to Immunization. F. Brown, R.M. Chanock and R. Lerner, editors, p.261. Cold Spring Harbor Laboratory, NY.

20. RWEYEMAMU, M.M., PAY, T.W.F. and SIMMS, M.J. (1982) The control of foot-and-mouth disease by vaccination. In: The Veterinary Annual 1982, C.S. Grunsell and F.W.G. Hill, eds. vol. **22**:63. John Wright, Pub. Bristol.

21. SELLERS, R.R. (1968) The inactivation of foot-and-mouth disease by chemicals and disinfectants. Vet. Rec. **83**:504.

22. TIMONEY, J.F. et al. Hagan and Bruner's Microbiology and Infectious Diseases of Domestic Animals. 8th edition. Comstock Press, Pub., Cornell Univ. Press, Ithaca, N.Y.

23. STROHMAIER, K. (1978) Die Maul-und Klauenseuche. III. Erfahrungen und Folgerungen aus 20 Jahren Bekampfung der Maul-und Klauenseuche. Tierartzl. Umsch. **42**:417.

24. TIZARD, I. (1990) Risks associated with use of live vaccines. J.A.V.M.A. **196**:1851.

VIRAL VACCINES PRODUCED IN EMBRYONATING EGGS

by

L E Carmichael

INTRODUCTION

Before 1931, virologists had variable success in transmitting viruses to experimental hosts, which made the study of viruses onerous and the efficient production of vaccines laborious, expensive and difficult to standardize. Pasteur and Roux developed the first rabies vaccine in 1885, using desiccated rabbit spinal cord material as the source of virus and it took nearly 50 years before animals were discarded as the primary source of virus for such vaccines as smallpox, rabies and yellow fever.

It was not until the early 1930's that rapid progress in the field of viral vaccines was made possible. Rapid advancement in the study of viruses, and in "vaccinology", was greatly facilitated by the demonstration by Ernest Goodpasture and his colleagues, Eugene and Alice Woodruff, that viruses, such as fowl pox virus and, later others, could be grown in chick embryos or in cultured tissue fragments derived from them. Goodpasture's seminal discoveries were not only important to experimental pathology and basic virology, but they proved critical to the development of modern methods of vaccine production, especially vaccines against several viruses that cause serious disease in avian species, as well as influenza, parainfluenza, pox, and some herpesviruses of other species. Those studies also led to an understanding of the nature of "viral inclusion bodies". Almost simultaneously, research by Alexis Carrel, Frederick Parker and Robert Nye on tissue explant culture methods led to the development of modern cell culture methods.

As in the whole animal, viruses have a marked predilection for groups of highly specialized cells in the embryonating egg. While some viruses show little or no host specificity, or tissue tropism, the great majority of them do. Most have been adapted by various procedures to laboratory hosts, chick embryos or host cell cultures. Since the cells and extra-embryonic membranes of the developing chick embryo lack a high degree of differentiation and specialization, they provide a suitable substrate for the growth of viruses from several distinct viral groups. Also, the natural variability of viruses, especially in regard to host-range, has allowed many viruses, some causing important diseases, to be adapted through selection to grow in chicken embryo tissues where they often attain a much higher concentration than in tissues of the natural host species.

A general knowledge of the development, structure, and the physiology of the chicken embryo is important to fully understand the reasons underlying the need for several techniques in order to achieve optimal growth of individual viruses. This is beyond the scope of this discussion, however a brief summary follows.

The extra-embryonic membranes of the chicken embryo arise from three germinal layers; the endoderm mesoderm and ectoderm. The dorsal somatopleure, which consists of a sheet of tissue cells, is composed of ectoderm on one side and the mesoderm on the other, while the ventral splanchnopleure consists of both mesoderm and ectoderm. By a process of folding, the somatopleure gives rise to both the chorion and the amnion, while the allantois and yolk sac membranes develop from the splanchnopleure. The amnion arises from the head and caudal regions of the embryo, the membrane being reflected back to form the serosa or chorion. The amniotic membranes continue to grow rapidly and then fuse dorsal to the embryo by the 5th day to form the amniotic sac. Meanwhile, the chorion continues to grow and, by the 10th day, it has almost completely enveloped the whole of the egg contents and is in contact with the inner shell membrane. The allantois makes its appearance on the 3rd day as a diverticulum from the ventral wall of the hind gut. By the 10th day it has fused with the chorion to form the allantoic cavity which separates the chorion from the amnion. The fused chorionic and allantoic membranes also are referred to as the chorio-allantoic membrane, or simply as the chorio-allantois. The yolk sac arises from the splanchnopleure and envelopes the yolk material. The gross and microscopic structure of the yolk sac membrane closely resembles that of the intestinal mucosa, of which it is essentially an extension.

Because the allantoic sac represents a diverticulum of the gut, it serves as the excretory receptacle for the embryo. The sac contains a variety of solids in solution, the solution becoming very turbid after the 12th day of incubation due to the presence of urates. The chorio-allantois is the primary respiratory organ of the embryo and, hence, is richly supplied with blood vessels. The amniotic fluid, which contains much of the albumen in the egg, appears to serve as a source of protein which is ingested during the swallowing movements made by the embryo from the 9th day onward. The function of the yolk sac membranes is to transport nutrients from the yolk sac to the embryo.

The process of adapting viruses to embryonating eggs has been largely empirical, but selection of the appropriate site of inoculation has been found to be critical in order to ensure optimal viral growth, which is important for the production of several living and inactivated viral vaccines of veterinary and human medical importance.

GENERAL PROCEDURES

Common procedures for the production and quality control of vaccines produced in embryonating hens' eggs are given below. Production of different vaccines requires modification of the general scheme provided here, but abundant references are available for each and only general principals will be given here (1, 4, 5, 6, 9, 10).

1. Procedure for handling eggs upon receipt[1] from an institutional flock or commercial source

a. Upon receipt, eggs should be held at room temperature, away from extreme temperatures. Eggs that have been pre-incubated should be delivered rapidly and moved as little as possible until inoculated.

b. Storage of non-incubated eggs can be done for up to 7 days from the shipping date, but only if held under ideal conditions of 18°C (66°F) and 72% relative humidity.

[1]Excerpted from reference 2.

Further holding of eggs reduces viability sharply. Pre-incubated eggs must be placed in an incubator (Maximum 37.5°C (100°F).

c. Incubation is done at 37.5°C Dry Bulb and 31°C Wet Bulb. It is preferable to use an incubator with a forced-draft circulation and automatic turning apparatus to rotate the eggs. Eggs must be turned at least 1/3 turn at least three, preferably four times each day. Temperature and humidity of the incubator must be checked each day. Lack of sufficient humidity is the biggest problem in small incubators. In such cases, supplemental humidity (eg a large, flat pan of water) is required. Between settings, or at least monthly, the incubator must be cleaned thoroughly with a strong disinfectant such as 0.5 -1% sodium hypochlorite or a quaternary ammonium compound and, if possible, fumigate according to incubator manufacturer's instructions.

Ideally, parental flocks should be 'specific pathogen-free' (SPF) ie negative to avian viruses, screened and found negative to avian endogenous Avian Leukosis/Sarcoma Chicken Helper Factor and to Reticuloendotheliosis Virus as well as Salmonella pullorum (Table 1). For the purpose of cultivating Mycoplasma sp., Chlamydia or Rickettsia, it is essential to use eggs that come from flocks where no antibiotics have been used in the feed. At the very minimum, eggs from SPF flocks should be used for production of seed virus, even though economic conditions in many developing countries limit the purchase or production of SPF eggs for routine vaccine production. This condition, however, might be ameliorated by the creation of regional SPF flocks.

In the United States, fertile, non pre-incubated chicken eggs range in price from \$0.60 each for SPF "Utility" eggs to ~\$1.00 -\$1.20 each for SPF eggs from flocks tested and found negative for all of the agents listed below. Pre-incubated eggs costs about £.30 more.

2. Production of vaccine seed lots

a. With each virus to be used as vaccine, the appropriate strain is selected and cloned by limiting dilution or, where appropriate, plaque selection. A master seed is then established by producing a large volume of infective fluid or homogenized embryo tissue in stabilizing media. Master seed is best stored as lyophilized aliquots (~1 ml), or frozen at -60°C in a freezer dedicated to storage of seed only.

b. For production of vaccine, a working seed is established by expansion of an aliquot of master seed virus to a sufficient amount to allow vaccine production for at least 6 months. Working seed should not be lyophilized, since a loss in titer may occur which results in low titers upon the subsequent first passage. For several viruses, eg influenza, it is important to select an appropriate dilution of virus (generally a 1:100 to 1:1000 dilution of seed) to avoid production of 'incomplete virus' (defective interfering particles).

c. Control of seed-lots requires testing for absence of extraneous agents, especially viruses, bacteria and Mycoplasma spp. (see Table 1). Details of standard requirements for licensing of vaccines and for production of biological products in the

USA are available from the United States Department of Agriculture, APHIS/NVSL, Federal Building, Hyattsville, Maryland 20782.

Table 1. Agents That May Contaminate Eggs Used For Vaccine Production

Viruses

Avian Adenoviruses (Serotypes 1-11	Avian Adeno (CELO)
Avian Adeno Group 2 (EDS-76)	Avian Encephalomyelitis
Avian Influenza	Avian Reovirus (Arthritis)
Fowl Pox	Infectious Bronchitis (various)
Infectious bursal disease (Gumboro)	Infectious laryngotracheitis
Lymphoid leukosis (COFAL (A,B,C,D,E)	Lymphoid Leukosis RSV-A
Lymphoid leukosis RSV-B	Marek's Disease
Parainfluenza	Reticuloendotheliosis Virus
Newcastle Disease Virus	Hemorrhagic enteritis virus

Other Agents

Mycoplasma gallisepticum	Mycoplasma synoviae
Hemophilus gallinarum (Coryza)	Salmonella pullorum-typhoid

3. Growth for bulk production

The growth of each virus, or Rickettsia, in embryonating eggs is influenced by factors such as age of the embryo, route of inoculation, dilution and volume of inoculum, temperature of incubation and time of incubation following inoculation. The common routes of inoculation, and some examples of viruses that grow best by each route are noted below (Table 2). It is important that the fertile eggs are the correct age (time of incubation prior to inoculation) for the different routes of inoculation required by each virus.

Table 2. Optimum Routes for the Growth of Various Viruses in Embryonating Eggs

INOCULATION SITE	VIRUS EXAMPLES
Allantoic cavity Disease Virus	Influenza virus, Newcastle
Yolk sac	Avian infectious bronchitis, avian encephalomyelitis (Chlamydia, Rickettsia)
Chorio-allantoic membrane	Orthopoxviruses, Morbilliviruses
Amniotic cavity	Myxoviruses (eg influenza)
Intravenous	Bluetongue virus

The methods described below for the inoculation of embryonating eggs are those that appear to be most commonly practised. Similarly there are a number of techniques or, variations on the ones given, for each of the inoculation routes listed. After inoculation, the eggs should not be turned.

A. Chorio-allantoic membrane (CAM) inoculation

This method is frequently used for the isolation, growth and titration of several viruses, including several orthopoxviruses of different species and some herpesviruses. Egg-adapted strains of several viruses, including measles, rinderpest, and distemper also may be propagated in the CAM. Introduction of virus inocula onto the surface of the CAM causes lesions to develop as a result of infection with several viruses, some noted above (Table 2). Although the technique described below is a commonly used one, a far simpler and equally effective method "The Gorham Technique" (3) has been used with great satisfaction in the author's laboratory for preparing egg-adapted canine distemper vaccine.

1. Nine to 11 day old eggs are candled and an area about 1 cm^2 is outlined with a lead pencil on the side of the shell that is free of large blood vessels. Many workers prefer to make a 'slit' ~3 mm wide and 8 mm long, which reduces the exposed area and, thus, chance for contamination. The area may be sterilized by applying 5% phenol or a weak solution of tincture of iodine, which is allowed to dry. Care must be taken to use disinfectant sparingly, since alcoholic solutions of iodine are absorbed through the shell and may cause lesions on the CAM which could be mistakenly attributed to virus.

2. Using a carborundum-disk drill, cut through the shell at the area outlined, taking care not to pierce the shell membrane. Also, drill a small hole through the shell over the air cell into the natural air space and disinfect with 70% alcohol.

3. Place the egg on its side in a holder with the drilled side uppermost and place a drop of sterile physiological saline on the side hole and carefully remove the cut portion of the shell, using a dissecting needle or small forceps. Do not damage the underlying shell membrane. When the shell membrane has been penetrated, the drop of saline will be drawn into the egg.

4. Apply negative pressure with a rubber bulb (a teat cup from milking machine apparatus, plugged at the end distal to the teat cup opening has proved useful in the author's laboratory), or by mouth suction with a rubber tube. As the air is removed, the CAM will drop from the shell around the side hole, creating an artificial air space. (A drop of sterile saline will aid in separating the chorioallantois from the inner shell membrane).

5. Deposit up to 0.2 ml of inoculum by carefully passing the needle through the inner shell membrane and dropping the inoculum onto the CAM. A 1 ml 'tuberculin' syringe fitted with a 23- to 27- gauge needle is commonly used.

6. After inoculation, the egg is gently rocked to spread the inoculum uniformly over the surface of the CAM. The window is then closed with cellophane (Scotch ™)

tape. Under strict conditions of sterility, it is not essential to seal the opening if a 'slit' is made.

7. Incubation is carried out at 37°C without turning.

8. Candle eggs daily. Embryo mortality during the first 24 hours is considered due to nonspecific causes. Most viruses produce visible "pocks" on the CAM after 48 - 90 hours after inoculation. The time depends on the virus and the dose inoculated. For vaccine preparation, growth curve studies are essential so that the maximum yields are obtained.

9. Harvesting of tissues is accomplished by candling all eggs prior to harvest and placing the egg in the horizontal position with the window ('slit') uppermost. Eggs are then chilled overnight at 4°C and tincture of iodine or 70% ethyl alcohol is applied to the area with a cotton swab and the tape is peeled off. The surrounding shell is broken away with sterile forceps, detached with scissors and quickly transferred to a sterile vessel.

For production of vaccine, where large numbers of eggs are used, harvest is made into sterile 1- or 2- liter flasks. As the harvest progresses, the containers are removed, closed, numbered and stored at 4°C. After harvest is completed, the contents of each flask are mechanically homogenized and frozen below -30°C, preferably lower, until sterility and potency tests are completed. If test results are satisfactory, vaccine is lyophilized.

B. The allantoic route of inoculation is used for propagation of several important viruses, especially myxoviruses (eg influenza), Group A arboviruses, some coronaviruses (eg infectious bronchitis virus) and parainfluenza viruses (eg Newcastle disease virus, NDV). An excellent technical paper on the production of inactivated NDV vaccine has been published recently (FAO Animal Production and Health Paper #89, ref.9) that provides important details not presented below. As noted above, general manufacturing standards require the use of SPF eggs or, with NDV, embryonated eggs from healthy non-SPF flocks free from NDV antibodies.

1. For allantoic inoculation, 8 - 10 day old embryonating eggs are used. Using a candle, the boundary between the air sac is delineated with a pencil and the position of the embryo is marked. The eggs are held in the upright position with the airsac uppermost. A point is then selected several millimetres above the floor of the air space on the side where the chorio-allantois is well developed, but free from large vessels. The upper surface is cleansed with tincture of iodine, used sparingly, and a hole is drilled, or punched (specialized devices are available), above the air sac.

2. Inoculations are done with a 20 - 24 gauge, 1 inch needle fitted to a 1 - 2 ml syringe. From 0.05 to 0.1 ml amounts of inocula are injected into the allantoic cavity at an angle directed towards the apical extremity of the egg. Holes are then sealed with warm 'vaspar', a mixture of "Vaseline" (petroleum jelly) and paraffin. Some laboratories employ fast-drying glue. Inoculated eggs are placed in egg trays in the upright position in a humidified incubator. Eggs are candled daily, as noted above, and all embryos found dead after 24 hours are discarded.

3. Allantoic fluid is harvested after chilling at 4°C for at least 6 hours in order to avoid haemorrhage while harvesting. Eggs are held in the upright position and the shell over the air sac is removed with sterile forceps. The floor of the air sac (innershell membrane plus chorio-allantois) is exposed. The membranes are then torn away with sterile forceps. In order to facilitate harvesting of allantoic fluid, the embryo is displaced to one side by placing forceps against the embryo with the tips toward the shell wall. The fluid is then carefully aspirated with a 5 - 10 ml sterile pipette, or with a pipette attached to a vacuum device, into large (2 - 3 L) bottles. It is important to avoid contamination with albumin or yolk material.

Harvested allantoic fluids are then centrifuged for 20 minutes at low speed (~2000 rpm in a standard laboratory centrifuge) to sediment erythrocytes and debris. The supernatant is used as the source of vaccine. Bottles are removed, sealed, numbered and maintained at 4°C until tests for sterility and potency (virus titer) are completed. Virus is now ready for inactivation or lyophilization as live virus vaccine.

C. The amniotic route of inoculation is used principally for the isolation of influenza virus and, the Group A arboviruses prior to the development of more efficient cell culture methods. Some parainfluenza viruses (Sendai- and mumps virus) also grow well in the amniotic sac. The embryo, during the course of its development, swallows the amniotic fluid, thereby bringing the inoculated virus into contact with the embryo's respiratory and intestinal tracts. For the amniotic route, 10 - 11 day embryonating eggs are used. Methods for inoculation and harvesting are not discussed here, as this route is used primarily for viral isolation, not vaccine production.

D. Yolk sac inoculation is used primarily for cultivating Chlamydia and Rickettsial organisms. Although several viruses may be inoculated via the yolk sac, they invade the embryo proper and multiply in the embryonic tissues rather than in the yolk sac. There is, therefore, little advantage to using this route for vaccine production, except for the agents noted above. Methods are adequately discussed in the various laboratory texts cited in the references.

Fig 1. Production And Control Of Inactivated Newcastle Disease Vaccine[1]

Original vaccine strain

↓

Control ← Preliminary passage in SPF eggs (Master seed virus)

Sterility

↓

Freeze-drying

↓

Control ← Second passage in SPF eggs (working seed virus)

Sterility

↓

[3]From reference 9, with permission.

Freeze-drying

↓

Multiplication in SPF eggs

↓

Controls ← Harvesting of AAF

Sterility

Virus titration

↓

Inactivation

(Formalin or beta-proplolactone)

Controls ← ↓

Sterility

Virus titration

Emulsion in oil adjuvant

↓

Controls of final product

Sterility

Safety

Extraneous agents

Virus inactivation

Potency

Stability

Table 3. Veterinary Vaccines Produced In Chick Embryos[1]

Disease or Virus	Attenuated (live)	Inactivated
Newcastle Disease	+	+
Avian tenosynovitis (arthritis	+	?
Avian encephalomyelitis	+	+
Turkey parainfluenza-3	-	+
Paramyxovirus infection (pigeons)	-	+
Gumboro (Bursal) disease	+	+
Avian Infectious bronchitis	-	+
Duck viral enteritis (plague)	+	-
Duck viral hepatitis	+	-
Fowl laryngotracheitis	+	-
Fowl pox	+	-
Equine influenza	+	-
Sendai virus infection (rodents)	-	+

[1]Information is compiled from materials provided by the Biologics Licensing and Standards Staff, Veterinary Services, APHIS, USDA (11).

REFERENCES

1. ANON. (1967) Laboratory Methods in Medical Virology. U.S. Dept. of Health, Education, and Welfare. Public Health Service, Bureau of Disease Prevention and Environmental Control, National Communicable Disease Center, Atlanta, Georgia (USA).

2. ANON. (1991) S-SPF Fertile Chicken Eggs and Chicks. Brochure prepared by SPAFAS Laboratory, 67 Baxter Rd., Storrs, CT 06268-1198 (USA.

3. GORHAM, J.R. (1957) A simple technique for the inoculation of the chorioallantoic membrane of chicken embryos. Amer. J. Vet. Res. **18**,691-692.

4. GRIST, N.R., BELL, E.J., FOLLETT, E.A.C. and URQUHART, G.E.D. (1979) Diagnostic Methods in Clinical Virology, Blackwell Scientific Pub., U.K.

5. LABZOFFSKY, N.A. (ed) (1974) Virology Manual, Second edition. Ontario Ministry of Health, Toronto, Canada.

6. LENNETTE, E.H. and SCHMIDT, N.J. eds. (1979) Diagnostic Procedures for Viral Rickettsial and Chlamydial Infections. 5th Ed. Amer. Public Health Assoc. Washington D.C. (USA).

7. Ministry of Agriculture, Fisheries and Food. (1988) Specifications for the production and control of avian virus vaccines. US, ADAS.

8. National Academy of Science. (1971) Methods for examining poultry biologics. Washing D.C. (USA).

9. PALYA, V. (1991) Manual for the production of Marek's disease, Gumboro disease, and inactivated Newcastle disease vaccines. FAO, Rome (Italy).

10. ROVOZZO, G.C. and BURKE, C.N. (1973) A Manual of Basic Virological Techniques. Prentice-Hall, Englewood Cliffs, NJ (USA).

11. TIMONEY, J.F., GILLESPIE, J.H., SCOTT, F.W. and BARLOUGH, J.E. (1988) Hagan and Bruner's Microbiology and Infectious Diseases of Domestic Animals. 8th ed. Comstock Publishing Assoc. Ithaca, NY (USA).

12. WILLIAMS, G. (1959) Virus Hunters. Alfred A. Knopf, Inc. NY (USA).

DISCUSSION

Dr Ozawa started the discussion by raising the subject of the use of established cell lines as substrates for vaccine production. He felt that the time was now ripe for full and detailed discussions on their use for routine vaccine production.

He quoted the objections to the substitution of a cell line for the use of primary bovine kidney cell cultures for the production of rinderpest vaccine. However, experience was showing that an established cell line could prove to be safe and satisfactory. He thought that high level discussions with the appropriate scientific experts and authorities was due, and that the cell lines that could be used, the vaccine viruses that could be produced and the conditions under which such work could be permitted, should be thoroughly debated and the outcome of these discussions published. He could see advantages in the use of cell lines in terms of facilitating production, reducing costs and importantly, offering the possibility of screening for adventitious agents.

Dr Rweyemamu thought that the use of some lines such as BHK 21 was satisfactory for inactivated vaccines such as FMD and rabies for animals, however, he thought that the same was not so in relation to their use for the production of live vaccines. There is a view now that Vero cells are acceptable for human and veterinary vaccines and PANVAC has been encouraging rinderpest vaccine producers to evaluate that cell substrate for routine vaccine production. PANVAC has also recommended that only cells which have been extensively tested for freedom from adventitious agents should be used for that purpose. It has therefore set up a cell bank (with cells obtained from IAH, Pirbright, which have been thoroughly tested) and these cells are now being used widely.

Another point which he raised was whether those who used primary or secondary cultures of fresh tissues had considered the possibility of freezing down these tissues until samples had been screened for contaminants. Provided enough time was planned for this extra step, it was workable and could have advantages in preventing loss from contaminants. With regard to the use of SPF eggs, this had been discussed at a workshop on Newcastle Disease held in Debre Zeit. It is clear that the supply of these eggs in Africa is limited and at present could not be considered for routine production of vaccine. However, a significant improvement could be made by producing the seed virus in SPF eggs, and for the bulk production using only eggs from flocks known to be predominantly disease free.

Dr Wojchiechowski explained the problems to be encountered in developing countries when trying to ensure a steady supply of SPF eggs and other high grade materials for vaccine production. In his opinion there is a need for regional centres to act as supply points for reliable materials and he hoped that the Consultation might be able to suggest ways in which that could be organised.

Dr Doel highlighted the problems which can be met when trying to obtain a steady supply of good quality animal serum, free from adventitious agents, to be used in vaccine production work.

Dr Rweyemamu suggested that the serum used for the preparation of important materials such as small batches of seed viruses could be made with medium containing gamma irradiated serum.

Professor Yilma stated that in the United States it was possible to obtain animal sera which were certified to be free of certain specified agents, he also mentioned that gamma irradiated sera have been found to be affected by the treatment and may not be completely satisfactory for tissue culture purposes.

Dr Pejsak stated that previous experience in Poland with slaughter house derived serum had shown that antibodies to BVD virus occurred frequently in that material and could prove very troublesome in the production of Swine Fever vaccine.

Dr Lombard suggested that another method of treating serum for tissue culture work was by means of beta-propriolactone (BPL). This agent has the advantage that it hydrolyses during the treatment of the serum and virtually disappears.

Dr Doel was somewhat sceptical of this since he thought that some viruses to be found in such sera would prove resistant to the action of that agent. He thought that ethyleneimine (EI) would be a better choice.

Dr Casas-Olascoaga confirmed that EI had been used successfully for that purpose at the PAFMDC in Rio.

Dr Lombard was doubtful about the use of EI since it was not active against orbiviruses.

Dr Carmichael asked how BPL was tested for activity? While there was no clear answer to the question, Dr Lombard stated that it was used by many people for the preparation of rabies vaccine.

Professor Guiyun raised the topic of cell lines again and stated that in China their use for the production of live vaccines would not be permitted but they could be used for inactivated products.

Dr Ozawa took advantage of the subject being raised, to reiterate his belief that there should be a serious examination of the subject and the question of what are the disadvantages in using cell lines should be addressed. Is it the possibility of carcinogenesis or adventitious agents? The safety issue must be comprehensively covered and he would be grateful for advice on how to approach this and who should be asked to participate in such technical discussions.

Dr Rweyemamu stated that there had been discussions on this topic held by WHO about 3 years ago in Geneva. A second meeting had also been held in Washington.

Dr Ozawa agreed that meetings had taken place, but pointed out that only the use of cell lines for human vaccines had been considered.

Dr Carmichael stated that in the US the majority of the vaccines for use in companion animals was produced in cell line derived substrates - but registration of these vaccines was required by the USDA.

Dr Stouraitis agreed with Dr Ozawa that the subject should be thoroughly investigated. In his opinion there had been much mishandling of cell lines in various virus laboratories and in future before extensive use of these materials for bulk vaccine production was introduced there would need to be careful and extensive screening and characterisation of cells. Only then could catastrophes be avoided.

Professor Yilma was also in agreement with Dr Ozawa about exploiting cell lines for production purposes. From experience with early Polio vaccines, which at the time of the Cutter Incident, probably also contained SV40 virus, and the fact that there had been few if any problems attributable to the effects of adventitious agents, he thought that well characterised cell lines had much to offer over the use of primary tissues.

Before moving onto the next section of the programme it was pointed out to the Chairman that although there had been no formal papers on virus inactivation and adjuvants presented to the meeting, it might be useful to have some discussion on these topics. The ensuing discussion centred around the benefits of using an inactivant for Foot-and-Mouth Disease virus which followed first order kinetics.

Dr Doel described the use of the aziridine compound - ethylethyleneimine for this purpose. He also questioned the effectiveness of BPL in the presence of high concentrations of protein.

Dr Rweyemamu agreed with Dr Doel on the usefulness of EEI in the industrial production of FMD vaccine.

Dr Casas-Olascoaga stated that for the last 10 years only the aziridine derivatives had been promoted by the PAFMDC and his colleague Dr Hans Bahnemann had developed the use of a simplified method involving binary ethyleneimine (BEI).

Dr Ozawa was also in favour of first order kinetics inactivants but cautioned that before using on other and previously untried viruses, it was essential to make thorough investigations of the action of the compound on that particular virus.

Professor Yilma suggested that as with polio virus, the combined use of UV irradiation and chemical inactivant could be recommended.

Dr Stouraitis stated that the recommendation from the Research Group of the European Commission for the Control of FMD was for the use of primary inactivants ie aziridine compounds and not formalin, as widely used previously by vaccine manufacturers.

With regard to adjuvants, the first comment was made by Dr Lombard who pointed out that as far as the EEC countries were concerned, the most likely problem would be in relation to adjuvant residues in carcase meat. Already there were inspections of certain tissues such as liver, kidney and muscle for evidence of oily deposits which might occur after the use of oil adjuvant preparations. Developing countries who were dependant upon the export of meat and meat products would do well to keep this point in mind when organising vaccination campaigns.

Dr Nagy thought that the subject of adjuvants was too large for a few minutes of discussion. He made the point that it would be difficult to generalise since there was little in common between many of the adjuvant preparations in common use. As an example he mentioned the use of an oil-in-water adjuvant with rotavirus being innocuous and acceptable, whereas the same adjuvant used with bacterial capsular proteins caused very severe reactions. In consequence he thought that each adjuvant system would have to be discussed individually and that would need more time than was available.

Dr Wojciechowski considered adjuvants and inactivants something of a burning issue. FAO were frequently approached to organise training in these aspects of vaccine production for workers from the developing countries. FAO had in consequence asked him to raise this subject with those attending the Consultation. He needed clear guidance on whether this type of technology could be made available to vaccine producers in developing countries under non-commercial terms, whether it was protected by patents and if so to what extent; also could information be made available, even on limited disclosure? He also wanted to know if training of staff would be possible with established vaccine producers.

Dr Lombard made the point in response, that there was much information concerning the composition and use of inactivants readily available in textbooks and other scientific publications. Apart from minor points of detail there were no restrictions by manufacturers on the use of this type of technology. The same situation applied to adjuvants - particularly the common ones such as saponin and aluminium hydroxide gel. The exact conditions for the preparation of oily adjuvants might be regarded as 'in house' and confidential, but that information could be obtained.

Finally, Dr Rweyemamu made the point that since most adjuvants are not chemically pure there could be considerable variation from batch to batch. He wondered if enough attention was paid to quality control of these materials in the production laboratories or indeed by national control authorities. Good Manufacturing Practise should ensure that was done.

CONTAGIOUS BOVINE PLEUROPNEUMONIA VACCINE PRODUCTION AND QUALITY CONTROL

by

P C Lefèvre

INTRODUCTION

After natural infections, animals that have recovered present a strong immunity to contagious bovine pleuropneumonia (CBPP). Its duration, still unknown, is probably rather long as indicated by field observations. Few data are available concerning the nature of this immunity which involves an humoral component (passive protection can be obtained in mice), as well as a cellular one as shown by Masiga et al. (1973).

To be of practical value, a vaccine has to be inoculated subcutaneously and that means, in the case of CBPP, that vaccine strains have to be sufficiently attenuated to avoid the Willem's reaction.

A. VACCINE PRODUCTION

Since the beginning of the 20th century, many vaccines have been described but the only ones to give satisfactory results are those produced with attenuated strains of *Mycoplasma mycoides subsp. mycoides* (SC). A complete and recent review of CBPP including the vaccines is available (Provost et al. 1987).

The Strains

At present, two vaccine strains are commonly used, the T1 and the KH3J strains. These are characterized by differences in their residual pathogenicity - the T1 strain being the most virulent, particularly for bovine cattle (Bos taurus) and more rarely for zebu cattle (Bos indicus).

T1 strain. Isolated in 1951 by Sheriff and Pierce from a CBPP clinical case, this strain underwent 44 egg-passages and, once attenuated, has remained moderately virulent. Its immunogenicity is very good and the immunity developed lasts for more than 1 year (8 to 10 months in case of primo-vaccination). Unfortunately, not all the vaccinated animals will acquire this resistance.

KH3J strain. The history of this strain is not well-known. Isolated in the Sudan, the strain has undergone many sub-cultures in the Khartoum laboratory and also in the Vom laboratory (Nigeria). The vaccine is produced with the 88th egg passage. Streptomycin-resistant variants of these two strains have been developed and are of major interest for production laboratories since streptomycin-resistance is directly related to attenuation and acts as a marker.

Comment. The attenuation of these two strains is not fixed and further subcultures will decrease the residual pathogenicity and the immunogenicity; it is, therefore, recommended, when producing vaccines, to undertake a minimum of subcultures from the master seed banks which are, for the African laboratories, kept at the FAO Reference Center for Mycoplasmosis of Ruminants (I.E.M.V.T., France).

Production Techniques

Vaccines are produced either in a liquid form or a freeze-dried one.

The liquid vaccine. The main characteristic of the production of this vaccine is that the growth of the vaccine takes place in the bottles used for distribution. The lyophilized master bank is grown twice in serum broth to obtain a seed bank (kept frozen at -20°C or lower); the material for sowing is obtained by two more subcultures, the first one made at terminal dilutions and the second one in flasks. Ten ml of culture is sown into 20 litres of broth and, after thorough mixing, is distributed into 20 ml vials which are plugged with cotton and incubated for 3 days at 37°C. When the growth phase is complete, the vials are sealed with rubber stoppers, labelled and stored at 4°C, before distribution to the vaccine centres.

The expiry date is 38 days after stoppering.

The freeze-dried vaccine (Figure 1). The working seed is obtained by two successive cultures of seed bank material in appropriate medium. Five litres of medium are placed in 10 litre flasks (with a magnetic stirrer) sown with 20 ml of the culture in logarithmic phase and incubated at 37°C. The broth is not stirred during the first 24 hours.

The harvest is usually made after 72 hours (end of the logarithmic phase). Skimmed milk is added to the broth (45g/1) before distribution takes place (5 ml in 20 ml vials). The lyophilization should always be carried out in plate type freeze-dryers to obtain a low residual moisture between 1.5% and 3%. The advantages from this are many - easier storage in deep freeze and longer half life (several years at -20°C and 8 to 10 months at 4°C).

When streptomycin-resistant strains are used streptomycin is added to the medium - 200 μg/ml.

Comment. When starting vaccine production, a laboratory should establish a growth curve of the strain in the medium and under the conditions that will be used for all the production batches, to determine the best time for harvest, since that may vary from one laboratory to another.

B. CONTROLS

As with other vaccines, production laboratories should comply with the international recommendations published by W.H.O.

Requirements for biological substances:

No. 1. General requirements for manufacturing establishments and control laboratories (revised 1965, technical report No 323) and

Figure 1

PROCEDURE FOR PRODUCING CBPP VACCINE FROM STRAINS T_1 and T_1-SR

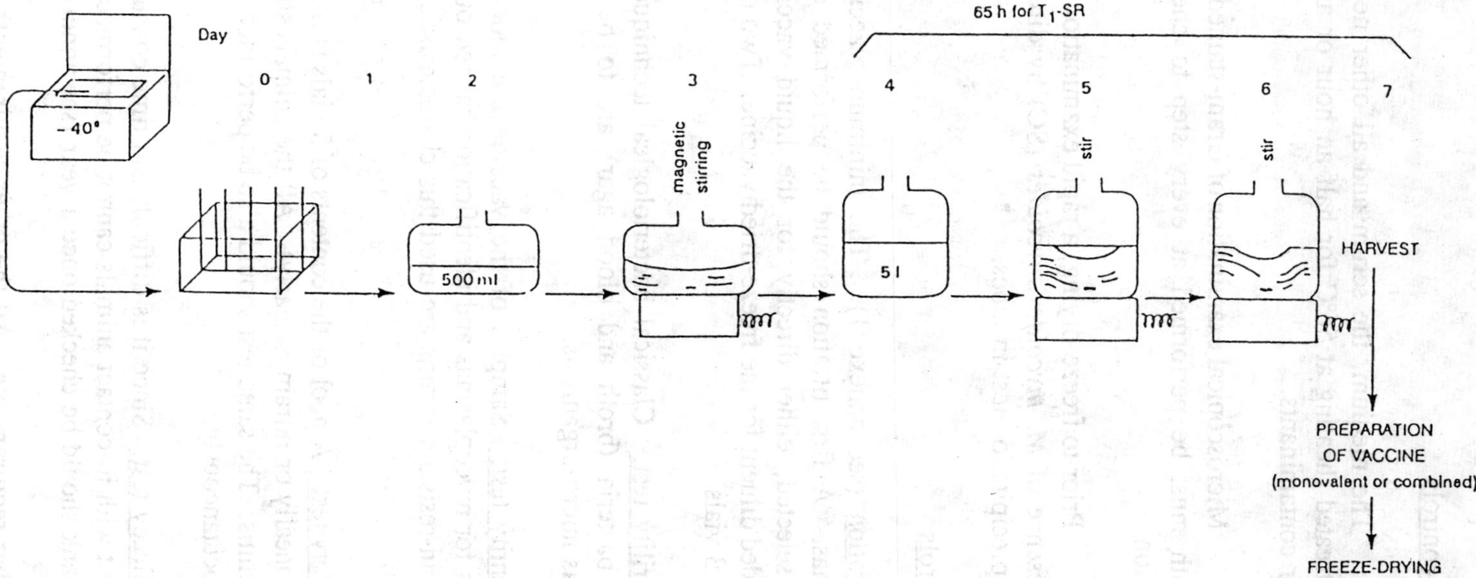

No. 6. General requirements for the sterility of biological substances (revised 1973, technical report No 530).

In-process controls

- The medium, the serum and all other necessary products of animal origin should be treated (heating at 56°C for half an hour or any other treatment), sterilized and checked for contaminants.

- Microscopical examination of Gram-stained preparations or blood agar cultures of the broth must be performed at every step to check for the presence of bacterial contamination.

- Prior to freeze-drying, a rapid examination should also be carried out to check for the presence of *M. mycoides mycoides* (SC) by direct immunofluorescence test or an interfacial precipitation test in tubes.

Batch controls

Titration (see annexe 1). The minimum vaccinal dose for cattle is 10^7 viable mycoplasmas. A first titration should be performed on the mixed contents of 5 vials randomly selected, either directly for the liquid vaccine or after reconstitution in the recommended diluent for the freeze-dried vaccine. Two more titrations should be performed on at least 3 vials.

Sterility test. Classical bacteriological techniques for isolation of aerobic and/or anaerobic bacteria (broth and blood agar) are to be used to indicate the absence of adventitious micro-organisms.

Identity test. Samples of the vaccine are inoculated according to the diagnostic procedures for mycoplasmas and identification carried out by growth inhibition test. When streptomycin-resistant strains are used this characteristic has to be checked as a marker of attenuation.

Safety test. A pool of the contents of 5 vials is inoculated into mice and guineas pigs (intraperitoneally or intramuscularly). All the animals should survive 1 month and show no sign of orchitis. The same test should also be performed on cattle using at least 10 doses per animal subcutaneously.

Efficacy test. Since it is difficult and time consuming to reproduce the disease, the efficacy test with in-contact animals cannot be performed on each batch of vaccine and only the seed bank should be checked once a year (see annexe 2).

Other requirements. All the other requirements described in the W.H.O Standards for Biological Substances are to be applied ie files and dossiers are to be completed, samples of each batch have to be kept for further control work, labelling and information concerning the use of the vaccine are to be clearly indicated.

Conclusion

Apart from the W.H.O General Recommendations, official papers specifically concerning CBPP vaccine production are rather scarce.

Recently, O.I.E has published basic requirements for biological products relating to CBPP (OIE, 1991), and is about to issue in the near future, norms for the production of live vaccine (probably in 1992).

The time is now appropriate for these recommendations and norms to be published so that the production laboratories (as well as the laboratories in charge of vaccine control) can work according to internationally accepted guidelines.

REFERENCES

MASIGA, W.N. and MUGERA, G.M. (1973) Fate of the T1 strain of *Mycoplasma mycoides* in cattle following vaccination. J. Comp. Path., **83** (4): 473-479.

OFFICE INTERNATIONAL DES EPIZOOTIES (1991) Contagious bovine pleuropneumonia. In : Manual of Recommended Diagnostic Techniques and Requirements for Biological Products. Vol. III.

PROVOST, A., PERREAU, P., Bréard, A., LE GOFF, C., MARTEL, J.L. and COTTEW, G.S. (1987) Contagious bovine pleuropneumonia. Rev. Sci. Tech, Off. Int. Epiz., **6** (3): 625-679.

ANNEX 1 Titration

Dilutions (1 in 10) are made in Gourlay's medium. The use of an agitator (vortex type) is useful to homogenize the suspension in each tube. Five ml from the tubes 10^{-6} to 10^{-12} are inoculated in 5 further tubes of medium (1 ml per tube - 5 tubes per dilution). All the tubes are inoculated for 4 days at 37°C and growth is detected by colour change of the indicator.

The 50% end point is estimated by a standard statistical procedure (MacCrady's "Most Probable Number" table or the Reed and Muench method).

ANNEX 2 Efficacy test

Ten cattle are vaccinated subcutaneously according to the recommendations of the manufacturer. The same number of unvaccinated cattle are kept as controls. After 2 months, the 20 animals are challenged by contact with 7 experimentally infected cattle (endobronchial route). The test lasts for 3 months. The seed bank passes the test if the vaccinated animals do not develop clinical signs and if they are free from lesions of pleuropneumonia at slaughter. 80% of the control animals should present lesions at post-mortem examination.

THE QUALITY CONTROL OF VACCINES AGAINST BRUCELLOSIS

by

J De Ryke

Brucella Vaccines Available

Both living vaccines of low virulence, such as B. abortus strain 19 (cattle), B. melitensis Rev. 1 (sheep and goats) and B. suis strain 2 (sheep and other animal species), and killed vaccines in oily adjuvant, such as B. abortus 45/20 and B. melitensis H 38 vaccines, are available. The superiority of live attenuated vaccines in the control of animal brucellosis has been repeatedly demonstrated, both experimentally and in the field, and they should be preferred to killed vaccines. Their main disadvantage is that they provoke a long-lasting serological reaction when regular doses are administered in adult animals, thus preventing the distinction between vaccinated and infected animals. To avoid such interferences, these vaccines should be administered only to immature females, or to adults by the conjunctival route or at reduced dosage (Table 1). The B. suis strain 2 vaccine has also been used successfully in mass vaccination of sheep by the oral route, in China and Libya. Its effectiveness in the control of B. melitensis infection in sheep could not however be confirmed in a recent experimental trial conducted at INRA, Nouzilly, France (WHO Working Group on Brucella S2 vaccine, Rome, September 1991).

Among killed vaccines, 45/20 vaccine has the potential advantage of not producing significant levels of antibodies reacting in classical serological tests, due to the rough phase of the strain. However there are still many uncertainties associated with manufacture, standardization, and conservation of the immunogenic activity of 45/20 vaccines. They cannot therefore be recommended unless effective quality control can be applied. The H38 vaccine provides effective immunity to animals of all ages and at any stage of pregnancy but it produces severe local lesions and induces serological reactions of long duration. It is therefore incompatible with test-and-slaughter control programmes, which make it unacceptable for most countries.

General Manufacturing Requirements For B19 And Rev.1 Live Vaccines

The general manufacturing requirements for B19 and Rev 1 vaccines are very similar and follow the seed lot system of management (see Table 2). They are described in detail in the referenced papers. Only some essential points will be stressed here:

- original seeds should be obtained from Reference Laboratories, ie USDA or Weybridge for B19 strain, and INRA Nouzilly for Rev 1 strain.

- all seed lots should be submitted to the following tests prior to further utilization: purity, identity, dissociation (see Table 3), and biological assays in laboratory animals: ie residual virulence, antigenicity and immunogenicity. These controls should also be carried out on the final product.

- dissociation of the original strain towards rough phase should be rigorously checked at every stage of production, the smooth phase being essential for the retention of full immunogenicity. Seed lots with more than 1%, and final products with more than 5% dissociation should be rejected.

- control of biological properties (residual virulence and immunogenicity) can be performed on guinea-pigs or mice according to recommended methods. Mice should be preferred since their response has been shown to be more homogeneous (see Table 4).

- stability should be tested on the final product. One of the most important factors contributing to stability of freeze-dried vaccines is the level of moisture content. The best viability is assured between 2 and 3% humidity. Under these conditions a freeze-dried vaccine will maintain viability for 12-18 months at 4°C (as against 2-4 weeks for liquid vaccines).

Apart from quality control, the managements of Brucella vaccines should take into account the risk of infection to the staff exposed. Although attenuated, B19 and Rev 1 retain a significant level of virulence for man. Brucella are considered as class III pathogens (WHO Laboratory Safety Manual), ie with high individual risk and low risk to the community. Specific measures should therefore be taken to prevent staff contamination (Joint FAO/WHO Expert Committee on Brucellosis, annex 1).

Conclusions

The effectiveness of live attenuated Brucella strains B19 and Rev 1 has long been recognized in the control of brucellosis in cattle (due to B. abortus) and in small ruminants (due to B. melitensis), respectively. Killed vaccines in oil adjuvant are generally not recommended, although 45/20 vaccine may be indicated for the vaccination of adult cattle in some circumstances. The manufacturing of both live attenuated strains uses the seed lot system and includes several standard control tests on both seed lots and final product. For the production of a good B19 or Rev 1 vaccine, three essential rules should be respected: (1) original seed should be supplied by a Reference Laboratory, (2) dissociation of organisms toward the rough phase should be rigorously controlled at each stage, and (3) the biological activity (residual virulence and immonogenicity) should be assayed on every seed lot before its first utilization, preferably in mice.

REFERENCES

ALTON G.G., JONES L.M. and PIETZ D.E. (1975) Laboratory techniques in Brucellosis, 2nd ed., WHO.

BOSSERAY N. and PLOMMET M. (1990) Brucella suis S2, Brucella melitensis Rev 1 and Brucella abortus S19 living vaccines: residual virulence and immunity induced against three Brucella species challenge strains in mice. Vaccine, **8**:462-468.

Joint FAO/WHO Committee on Brucellosis, 6th Report, Technical Report Series No. 740, WHO, Geneva, 1986.

OIE Manual of Recommended Diagnostic Techniques and Requirements for Biological Products, Office International des Epizooties (OIE), 1991. (Bovine Brucellosis Vol II (BO12), and Brucellosis in Sheep, Goats and Swine Vol III (BO23-24-52)).

PLOMMET M. and BOSSERAY N. (1984) Propositions pour une méthode générale de contrôle d'activité des vaccins antibrucelliques. Dev. Biol. Standard **56**:247-255.

WHO Expert Committee on Biological Standardization, 22th Report, Technical Report Series No 444, WHO, Geneva, 1970. (annex 2: "Requirements for Brucella abortus strain 19 vaccine").

WHO Expert Committee on Biological Standardization, 28th Report, Technical Report Series No 610, WHO, Geneva, 1977 (annex 4: "Requirements for Brucella melitensis strain Rev 1 vaccine").

WHO Laboratory Safety Manual, WHO, Geneva, 1983.

Table 1 Available Vaccines Against Animal Brucellosis

Brucella Vaccine Strains	Strain Characteristics	Reference Laboratory	Animal Species	Immunization Route And Doses
Live Vaccines	Attenuated virulence:			
B.abortus strain 19	Spontaneous	USDA, Ames. Weybridge	cattle	heifers (sc): $5X10^{10}$ adults (sc): $3\text{-}10\ 10^{8}$ (cj): $5\text{-}10\ 10^{9}$
B.melitensis strain Rev 1	laboratory	INRA, Nouzilly (F)	sheep	immature (sc): 10^{9} (cj): 10^{9}
B.suis strain 2	spontaneous	-	sheep, goats	all ages (or): 10^{10}
Killed vaccines in oily adjuvants				
B.abortus strain 45/20	rough strain	-	cattle	adults (sc)
B.melitensis strain H38	smooth strain	-	cattle	adults (sc)

Legend: sc: subcutaneous; cj: conjunctival; or: oral

Table 2 Standard requirements applicable to B19 and Rev 1 Brucella vaccine

STAGE	QUALITY CONTROLS
Original seed	
Seed lot	Purity, Identity, **Dissociation** Residual virulence Antigenicity, Immunogenicity
Single harvest	
Final bulk	Purity, Bacterial content (OD)
Filling lot (final product)	Purity, Identity, **Dissociation** **Viability** Residual Virulence Antigenicity, Immunogenicity

Table 3 Testing of purity and identity

Purity: Gram staining culture in specified media

Identity: Confirmation of morphological, cultural and serological characteristics, by comparison with standard strains

For Rev 1: distinction with B.Melitensis 16M

CHARACTERS	16M STRAIN	REV.1 STRAIN
Phase	S	S
Oxydase	+	+
CO^2 requir.	-	-
H_2S prod	-	-
Serum agglutination:		
anti A	-	-
anti M	+	+
anti R	-	-
Colony size (mm)	1-2	0,5-1
Growth with:		
thionin	+	-
fushin	+	-
penicillin	+	-
streptomycin	-	+

Table 4 Biological assays in mice

(a) Residual Virulence

1 group of 32 female mice CD1 (5 to 6 wk)

subcutaneous inoculation of 10^8 vaccine organisms

spleen counts at 3, 6, 9, 12 weeks

Determination of Persistence Time 50% (PT 50)

(PT50 of reference Rev.1 strain is 7.9 + 1,2 wk)

(b) Immunogenicity

6 groups of 6 female mice CDI

4 groups vaccinated with Rev.1 (10^5), 1 with ref vaccine,
1 unvaccinated

30 days later challenge with $2x10^5$ B.abortus B544

45 days later spleen counts

(log spleen infection controls = 4.5)
(log spleen infection ref vaccine = 2.5)

INDUSTRIAL PRODUCTION AND QUALITY CONTROL OF VETERINARY VACCINES

by

L K Nagy

Industrial production, compared to what might be called "improvised small scale" preparation of vaccines, differs in many ways other than the scale of operation, technologies involved or equipments used.

This paper aims to describe the most important requirements and characteristics of industrial production and quality control of veterinary vaccines, in the framework of the Quality Assurance (QA) system.

1. Siting of Production Facility

It is in the basic interest of the facility that products are safeguarded from apparent sources of contamination. Thus it should be segregated from other activities (animal compounds, diagnostic facilities etc.) within its own secure border, where movement of staff, activities and materials are under strict managerial control.

Services and Utilities

The site must be provided with:

- all weather roads
- water of suitable quality and quantity
- electric power (complete with standby generator)
- safe disposal of contaminated liquid and other wastes (decontamination plant/incinerator) into the uncontrolled environment
- telephone.

2. Building Design and Purpose

Good Manufacturing Practice (GMP) requires that buildings should be correctly designed and located for their particular purpose, allowing proper segregation of activities so as to provide appropriate space and security for any particular activity within. These should include:

Storage of:

- raw material (receipt and quarantine)
- raw material (storage and issue)
- intermediate products, including bulk vaccine under test
- finished bulk vaccine
- filled vaccines under test
- released vaccines

Preparations:

- glassware/equipment, washing, sterilization and storage
- media, solutions, adjuvants etc. preparation and storage

Production:

- culture collection and storage
- cultivation
- downstream processing
- blending
- filling/sealing
- labelling, packaging

Quality Control:

- Animal Testing
- Support Services
- Warehousing
- Offices
- Library
- Canteen

3. Production

(i) Standards

The primary objective of Production is to manufacture vaccines which consistently meet specifications and standards, laid down in the Product Licence, in an environment and under conditions which comply with GMP guide lines.

(ii) Technology

Choice of technology for vaccine production depends partly on the particular product manufactured and partly on economical considerations (scale of operation etc).

(a) Primary Manufacture

For viral vaccines it may be egg or cell culture based. The latter may take the form of static monolayer or monolayer in roller tubes or suspended cultures. For the sake of greater productivity the trend in industry has been the use of established cell lines in cytoculture bio-reactors.

For bacterial vaccines, deep culture/fermentation technology is employed whenever possible.

One of the basic considerations in the choice of technology is that it should be well proven, reliable and capable of regular batch reproducibility. Since parameters of primary manufacture may be best controlled by the use of modern fermenters, their use superseded earlier technologies of primary manufacture of both bacterial and viral agents.

An additional advantage of deep culture technology is that it is readily scaled up to the most economical batch size, leading to greater productivity by reducing the unit costs of quality control.

(b) Secondary Manufacture

Downstream processing of production cultures may vary widely according to the product. It may entail inactivation, detoxification, separation, purification etc. Whatever the process may be, the performance of the technology employed (continuous flow centrifugation, solvent extraction, fractional precipitation, filtration, concentration by ultrafiltration etc) should match the output of primary manufacture.

(c) Blending and Storage of Bulk Vaccine

Once the bulk antigen is ready and tested, bulk vaccine is prepared. Apart from the antigen itself it may involve the use of diluent, adjuvant, preservative, or in the case of lyophilised products, stabilising fluid.

Blending is usually carried out in a large (up to several thousand litres) stainless steel, jacketed in situ steam sterilisable vessel, complete with stirrer to facilitate blending. On completion of blending samples are taken and the bulk vaccine is transferred into stainless steel, steam sterilisable storage vessels and stored under quarantine in the cold room pending the results of tests.

(d) Filling, Sealing, Capping and Labelling

Bulk vaccine which has passed the acceptance tests is ready for filling. In industry, filling and sealing is carried out by an automatic filling line. The bulk vaccine from the storage vessel is often delivered to the filling room by appropriate pipes without the container having to be brought into the filling room. Sterile vaccine containers are usually delivered to the filling room via an air lock and are placed onto the turn table of the automatic filling machine. The latter fills and seals them and the sealed vaccine containers pass, via an air lock, into another room where they are capped and labelled, also automatically.

(e) Storage of Filled Vaccines

Capped and labelled vaccines are inspected, sampled and stored in quarantine pending on the results of tests.

A batch of vaccine which has passed all the tests is transferred for storage to a segregated part of the cold room, devoted to products to be released for distribution and use.

(iii) Environment

GMP requires an environment for vaccine production which integrates product protection, operator's safety and environment protection. These sometimes conflicting requirements are reconciled by careful adjustment of - air filtration, air pressure differentials, physical segregation of activities and operator training and discipline.

GMP guide lines state that it is not acceptable to culture or otherwise handle more than one live agent in a manufacturing area at the same time.

Totally separate and dedicated facilities must be provided for the following organisms of veterinary significance: *B.anthracis; Cl. botulinum; Cl. tetani.*

Other spore forming organisms must also be handled in a dedicated facility.

It is permissible to culture more than one organism within a manufacturing area, provided the activities are segregated in time and that a validated decontamination procedure has been followed.

From the environmental point of view the following stages of production require special consideration:

Cultivation and Harvest of:

(a) Potential pathogens by a large scale fermentation process.

Under such conditions the potential for exogenous contamination or release of pathogens is much reduced. However, preparation of the inoculum takes place in a more "open system", where closures are removed to permit additions and removals. Exclusion of exogenous contamination is achieved by performing all aseptic manipulations in a Grade* A environment (see footnote) in a Grade B/C background area. The whole of the area must operate under a negative pressure (relative to surrounding areas) in order to ensure containment of pathogens. Air should pass through HEPA filters upon entry and exit of cultivation/harvest areas. These areas should be served by dedicated air handling systems. Personnel and materials must enter via air locks.

EC GUIDE (1989) REQUIREMENTS - STERILE PRODUCTS.

GRADE*	Particles/m^3 0.5μ	5μ	Organisms/m3
A	3500	0	<1
B	3500	0	<5
C	350K	2000	<100
D	350K	20K	<500

(b) Live Agents, No or Low Infection Risk.

With these microbes product protection outweighs safety and containment considerations. Thus the area is operated under net positive pressure utilising Grade A for aseptic manipulation with a Grade B/C background.

(iv) Downstream Processing

(a) Inactivated Product Sterilized by Filtration before Filling

Under such circumstances processing is considered "clean" rather than "aseptic" and Grade C environment suffices.

(b) Inactivated Product not Sterilized before Filling

Under such circumstances processing must be considered "aseptic" as there is no means of sterilising the product before filling. Grade A environment is used for all operations where the product is exposed in a Grade B background. Thus the requirements are as for aseptic filling.

(c) Live Product not Sterilised before Filling

Under these circumstances processing must be considered "aseptic". Grade A environment is used for all operations where product is exposed in a Grade B background. There is also a need for containment of the live agent. Thus the processing area should operate under a net negative pressure and be served with a totally independent air handling system. Air is exhausted from the room through a HEPA filter.

(v) Filling and Sealing

These operations constitute "aseptic" processing and should be performed in areas entry to which is through air locks for both personnel and materials. The filtered air supply should maintain a positive pressure relative to surrounding areas and achieve Grade A classification at the point of filling and surrounding critical zones where products and components are exposed and Grade B in the general background areas of the room. Changing rooms should be designed as air locks and should be flushed with filtered air. Similarly, material transfer areas should be designed as air locks.

If the vaccine consists of live agents there is a need for gross containment of these organisms. Thus the filling area should be served with a totally independent air handling system and the exhaust air should go through HEPA filters.

(vi) Planning and Organisation

In relation to vaccine production these are very important for efficient utilisation of manpower, plant and equipment in an industrial environment.

On the basis of demand forecast, the duration of the production cycle and batch size employed for any particular product is planned for the year and phased in according to the seasonal demand for the product.

Harmonisation of the activities of the various groups involved in production and distribution (support services, primary and secondary manufacturing, quality control, warehousing, distribution etc) requires a great deal of organisation by management to maintain the required levels of stock.

(vii) Methods

Production methods must be aimed at consistently delivering products which meet their quality specifications. One of the important factors for attainment of this objective is the use of stable micro-organisms for vaccine production.

(a) Seed Lot System

A seed lot may be defined as "a quantity of viruses or microbial cells, used to seed a cell substrate or growth medium, processed at one time and of uniform composition, adequately characterised as to identity and freedom from contaminants and stored and used in aliquots in such a way as to maintain these characteristics".

Initially a definitive Master Seed Lot must be prepared from a homogeneous suspension of the original virus or microbial culture and must be aliquoted into individual containers for storage.

Appropriate storage conditions for bacteria and fungi: lyophilised and stored at 2-8°C, for viruses: lyophilised or stored at -60°C.

Usually it is not possible to prepare sufficient Master Seed to permit its use for routine production. For this reason it is standard practice to prepare, within finite passage of the Master Seed Lot, another homogeneous suspension of virus or microbial cells. This, too, is aliquoted into individual containers for storage and is known as a Working Seed Lot.

Both Master and Working Seeds must be adequately characterised to ensure that they display certain properties. These include: identity, purity, freedom from contaminating micro-organisms, stability at the highest passage level used for production.

In Europe it is common to perform this testing in depth on the Master Seed and then simply confirm identity and microbial purity of the Working Seed. In the USA, however, great emphasis is placed upon characterisation of the Working Seed.

(b) Process Operating Instruction (POI)

Production methods must be in strict compliance with those described in the Product Licence. These methods and the relevant process-monitoring and quality control tests are outlined in the form of "flow charts" in the Product Licence. However, production methods are described in detail in "in-house" POIs. The POI scheme serves to remind trained staff of important manufacturing operations and also provides a framework for recording production variables.

The POI scheme also simplifies the review of records by production management and provides an easy review for the Q C department at the time of batch release.

(c) Batch vs. Continuous Culture

The traditional method of cultivation involves the seeding of a culture vessel then harvesting the whole culture after a given period of time. This is known as batch culture. Batch culture has the advantage that the harvest represents a discrete, homogeneous entity, which can be processed as a whole and the associated documentation refers solely to that batch. However, it has the following disadvantages: production volume is limited by equipment size; harvesting, cleaning etc. result in significant loss of time.

For these reasons some manufacturers are considering the use of perfusion or continuous culture techniques, especially for cell-based products. The main advantages are that it reduces time loss and yields are also greater per unit volume of the culture. However, there are certain attendant risks (potential for genetic mutation, greater risk of contamination, intrinsic contamination reactivated etc). Because of the attendant risks and difficulties (batch identification etc) of continuous cultivation most manufacturers, especially of bácterial vaccines, prefer batch cultivation.

(d) Campaign Production

With certain notable exceptions (*B. anthracis, Cl. botulinum, Cl. tetani.*) GMP guide lines permit cultivation of more than one micro-organism within a manufacturing area, provided that the activities are segregated in time and that a validated decontamination process has been followed.

Thus the Campaign Method of vaccine production, which can lead to the fullest utilisation of premises, equipment, manpower and other resources, is feasible within the GMP code of practice.

In brief, campaign production means that vaccines which are compatible in production technology are produced, one at a time, in succession, in the same production unit and by the same staff. At the end of each production campaign, the production suite and equipment are decontaminated by approved and validated methods before the beginning of a production campaign of a new vaccine. The campaign method of production is gaining popularity in industry.

4. Quality Control of Veterinary Vaccines.

Quality control of vaccines in an industrial environment is realised within the framework of the Quality Assurance (QA) system. Briefly QA is the sum total of organised arrangements made with the object of ensuring that products will be of the quality required for their intended use.

GMP is that part of QA which aims at ensuring that products are consistently manufactured to a quality appropriate for their intended use.

Quality Control (QC) is that part of QA which is concerned with the sampling specification, testing and release procedures, so that materials or products are not released for use or sale unless they are judged to be satisfactory. Thus QC in the QA framework includes responsibility for:

- Control of starting materials (seed lot, cell bank, media, buffers, containers, closures, cartons, labels, packaging materials etc.)
- Control of cultivation parameters
- Control of downstream processing techniques
- Control of environmental conditions
- Testing of monitoring and control instruments
- "in-process" sampling and testing (process-monitoring)
- Sampling and testing of finished products (QC-tests)
- Documentation, assessment and release of materials and products
- Validation of all QC matters.

It is beyond the limits of this paper to go into details of all aspects of QA. However, a few brief comments on process-monitoring and quality control tests can be made:

- Process-monitoring and QC tests are indicated in "flow charts" of production and quality control. Samples are taken in a prescribed manner at the indicated stages of the production process.

- Samples are submitted to the QC department for testing

- Tests are described in the form of Standard Operating Procedures (SOP) which not only enumerate all that is required for the test, but also described, step by step, how to carry out the test and also provides the criterion for the "pass mark" of the test.

- Technical details of tests and results are recorded in laboratory note books and a copy of the report of results is sent to production management.

- These results, together with all other results generated by the QC department become part of the batch documentation and form the basis of batch assessment by the official "Qualified Person" for releasing the product for distribution and sales.

Discussion

Dr Rweyemamu in response to a question concerning master seeds for CBPP vaccine production in Africa told the meeting that PANVAC does indeed act as a repository of cells and various master strains for distribution. However, PANVAC cannot operate in a vacuum and is in turn dependant upon assistance from the major international reference centres for help in maintaining these stocks - from IEMVT, the Pirbright Laboratory and the Plum Island Laboratory. As an example it obtains rinderpest vaccine seed from Pirbright and is in contact with the others concerning the newer variants of rinderpest virus. Similar arrangements are in operation for cell stocks such as the Vero cell line. With regard to CBPP at a workshop last year for African producers which was held with the assistance of IEMVT as advisers and consultants, it was agreed that the T1 streptomycin resistant strain should be the standard strain for vaccine production.

Also it was agreed at the workshop that the process in the production labs should be directed towards developing a freeze-dried product.

He thought that CBPP was now becoming one of the major cattle diseases in Africa and it might have implications for the success of the PARC. International support for PANVAC's work on this subject was very important. Finding financial support for this was high on PANVAC's list or priorities.

Dr Davies made the plea that holding the master stocks of vaccine strains in only one laboratory was less than ideal and suggested that for African needs, it might be that another stock of the vaccine strains from Kabete could also be kept at PANVAC.

Dr Korir said that he would have no objection to that arrangement if PANVAC could provide the necessary storage space. He thought that a reserve kept in Debre Zeit would be a good idea.

Dr Bhat wondered if PANVAC would have the funds to make such a proposal workable?

Dr Wojciechowski stated that FAO and PANVAC were seeking further financial support to expand PANVAC's activities and had applied for assistance to several potential donors. However, they were finding it difficult to obtain additional funds and FAO were looking for better ways of sustaining the activities of PANVAC and similar organisations in other countries.

Dr Rweyemamu was of the opinion that there should be collaboration between Regional and International Reference Centres on specified projects and that funding for those specified projects should be arranged, and not subsumed into the overall funding for the running of the centre or laboratory.

Dr Wojciechowski stated that laboratories in some FAO member countries with repositories of seed strains and sera were not maintaining them properly, and in consequence they were relatively useless. In many cases the origins of master stocks of vaccine strains could not be determined and in the case of stored sera, they were often found to be haemolysed and unusable. This was not a case of inadequate funds, <u>but bad management</u>! He thought that to improve the situation there had to be encouragement from FAO and PANVAC. He felt it would be helpful to have suggestions from the Consultation on what might be done to improve the performance of these labs.

<u>Dr Bhat</u>, on the other hand, did not agree with the view that money was not the cause of the problem. The IVRI repositories of stocks were costing almost US$ 1 Million to maintain and that was money they did not have! Consequently these banks were unsatisfactory. He was of the opinion that unless there is government funding, things will not improve. Money is needed for repairs, replacements, staff salaries etc and clearly the problem is primarily related to money.

<u>Dr Wojciechowski</u> thought that since India had a large organisation and functioned on behalf of South Asian countries the problem was different to those experienced by the smaller regional centres. Perhaps efforts should be made to help with the Indian situation.

The topic of SPF eggs and their use for vaccine production was raised once again.

<u>Dr Ozawa</u> thought that a system which was perhaps not as rigorous as that used in the industrialised countries, but never the less effective, could be brought into operation for the benefit of the developing countries. He described a system based on the use of imported genuine SPF flocks kept in isolation and the eggs obtained from these flocks used for the production of stocks of seed virus. Such a system has been developed in Hungary and has been tried out in Turkey. The problem is maintaining the isolation.

<u>Dr Carmichael</u> thought a possible definition of SPF was freedom from those agents which have not been tested for!

<u>Dr Bhat</u> agreed with Dr Ozawa and recommended producing master seed in <u>imported</u> SPF eggs and later when the economics of the situation improved, moving to the bulk production of the vaccine in true SPF eggs.

<u>Dr Mabratu</u> stated that it was not just a question of funding the importation of SPF eggs, but also the organisation to exploit an SPF unit and the associated logistics of vaccine production under those conditions.

<u>Dr Davies</u> gave an example of the benefits of using imported eggs. He stated that in one case, the cost of vaccine prepared from imported SPF eggs was only 50% of that of the price of imported vaccine. He also was in favour of the scheme mentioned previously in which bulk vaccine is produced in eggs from 'minimal disease free flocks'. Such a scheme has worked well at Kabete.

<u>Dr Carmichael</u> warned about the price of importing SPF eggs. He stated that the cost of importing eggs from Germany into Uganda was about 10 DM per egg.

PROTOZOAL AND RICKETTSIAL VACCINES WITH SPECIAL REFERENCE TO QUALITY CONTROL

by

F L Musisi, J A Lawrence, J C Quiroga, S P Kamwendo and J Malika

INTRODUCTION

There are four major livestock tick-borne diseases; these are anaplasmosis, babesiosis, cowdriosis (heartwater) and theileriosis. Vaccination is conducted because these diseases have an economic impact on the cattle industry. Significant losses occur when unvaccinated cattle are exposed within the enzootic areas. Outbreaks are usually due to failure of cattle to receive an immunizing natural infection with B. bigemina, B. bovis, C. ruminantium and A. marginale when young. In Theileria parva infections, considerable losses are observed in both calves and adults not previously exposed to these parasites. Cattle become immune to a homologous challenge with these parasites upon recovery from a primary infection. This principle is exploited in practical vaccination in which cattle are inoculated with the living parasites as vaccines.

The purpose of this paper is two-fold:

(i) briefly outline the procedures for producing the major livestock tick-borne disease vaccines; and

(ii) outline steps taken to avoid contamination of the end product and to ensure that it is safe and potent for use.

VACCINES

Tick-fever vaccines

Tick-fever is a term used to refer to an infection with one or a combination of A. marginale, B. bovis and B. bigemina in cattle. Consequently, tick-fever vaccine refers to vaccines that are used to immunize cattle against these infections (Callow and Dalgliesh, 1980). The three components of the tick fever vaccine are all blood vaccines.

The field parasites isolates of the Babesia spp. have to be attenuated first and thereafter seed material is produced. The appropriate attenuated parasite then has to be multiplied in a live bovine calf to prepare the vaccine which is cryopreserved.

To attenuate newly isolated B. bovis, parasites are rapidly passaged at least 11 times, but more commonly, 20 serial passages in splenectomised calves are required to eliminate contaminants (Callow et al., 1979). On the other hand, rapid passage of B. bigemina does not necessarily result in dramatic reduction of the virulence of this parasite. To reduce virulence of the parasite, it is passaged slowly every 3 months in intact calves followed by splenectomy of the calves 3 months after the primary infection. The 'relapse' parasites are of reduced virulence and can be stored as a bank from which susceptible splenectomised calves are infected to produce the vaccine.

The Anaplasma component of the vaccine is A. centrale, a naturally occurring species of low pathogenicity which stimulates an effective immunity to A. marginale.

Heartwater vaccine

This is a blood vaccine produced by infecting a sheep and harvesting and cryopreserving the infected blood at the time the sheep is experiencing a fever. The procedure was developed and described by Neitz and Alexander (1945).

An alternative method of preparing heartwater vaccine was described by Bezuidenhout (1981); the method involves preparation of C. ruminantium infective tick filtrates which can be used for vaccination of sheep and cattle against the disease. This type of vaccine was shown to be highly infective but has not been adopted for general use.

Theileria vaccines

Theileriosis normally refers to diseases resulting from infection with pathogenic theilerias. The most outstanding ones are tropical theileriosis and the East Coast fever/Corridor disease/Zimbabwean theileriosis complex. Tropical theileriosis, caused by Theileria annulata extends from the Mediterranean region through to the Indian subcontinent (Brown, 1990). The ECF/Corridor disease/Zimbabwean complex is confined to Subsaharan Africa although it should be noted that it does not exist in West Africa. Vaccines exist for both these two major theilerioses.

The vaccine for tropical theileriosis is produced by growing T. annulata infected lymphoblastoid cells in culture media such as Eagle's Minimum Essential Medium (MEM) or RPMI 1640. The vaccine contains infected lymphoblastoid cells (Pipano, 1979). The parasites in cell culture vaccine are attenuated by prolonged culture in vitro of cells persistently infected with macroschizonts of T. annulata.

On the other hand, the immunogens for the ECF/Corridor disease/Zimbabwean theileriosis complex are Theileria parva sporozoites (Cunningham et al., 1973). The sporozoites are prepared by infecting clean Rhipicephalus appendiculatus nymphal ticks with T. parva; after moulting the adult ticks are fed on rabbits for four days and then ground up in MEM which is supplemented with 3.5% Bovine Plasma Albumin (Fraction V) to produce a suspension of Theileria sporozoites in the supernatant. Cryoprotectants are added to the supernatant and the parasites cryopreserved at -196ºC as a stabilate (Lumsden and Hardy, 1965) which together with tetracyclines is used to immunize cattle (Radley, 1981). This technique is known as the "infection and treatment method" of immunization.

QUALITY CONTROL CONSIDERATIONS

Tick Fever Vaccines

Measures to avoid or detect possible contamination of frozen tick fever vaccine in Malawi.

Herd of origin.

The herd of origin of donors has to be confirmed to be free from brucellosis and enzootic bovine leucosis (EBL). Annual serology for EBL and brucellosis is conducted to ensure that the cattle are free from these diseases. Also a representative sample of adult cows has to be shown to be free from bovine virus diarrhoea (BVD). The farm is situated in an area free from foot and mouth disease (FMD) and rinderpest; neither of these two vaccines is used in the area. The farm is subjected to periodic veterinary inspection.

The calves on this farm are reared indoors with minimal exposure to ticks until weaning at 8 - 12 weeks.

Donor selection.

A clinical examination of the whole herd is conducted at the time of selection of donors to confirm freedom from contagious diseases. Particular attention is paid to the possible presence of ephemeral fever, foot and mouth disease (FMD), lumpy skin disease (LSD) and rinderpest. Ideally, for mucosal diseases, the dams of the donors should have been confirmed as seronegative before conception.

Calves are confirmed serologically to be free from Anaplasma spp., Babesia bigemina, Babesia bovis and Theileria mutans before purchase.

Donor handling before and during vaccine production.

Calves are transferred directly from the farm of origin to isolation facilities at the Central Veterinary Laboratory, Lilongwe.

The donor calves are isolated for 8 weeks in tick and insect proof accommodation and are treated with acaricides on arrival and weekly thereafter. Access is strictly controlled and feedstuffs are concentrate meal and maize silage only. During this period, calves are subjected to daily clinical examination and rectal temperatures are recorded. Blood smears are taken weekly for examination prior to splenectomy; the exercise is specifically designed to detect the presence of any of the following parasites:

trypanosomes	
Babesia spp.	Anaplasma spp.
Theileria spp.	Eperythrozoon
Ehrlichia	Borrelia

Alongside these observations, the presence of any of the following diseases is also monitored clinically:

FMD	Rinderpest
Malignant catarrhal fever (MCF)	Ephemeral fever
Blue tongue (BT)	LSD
Rift valley fever (RVF)	

The donors are splenectomised shortly after arrival at the CVL, Lilongwe. Thereafter, blood smears are taken and examined every second day to check for the haemoparasites indicated above. The calves are treated for 4 days with penicillin and streptomycin to control post-operative infections and to eliminate possible infection with Leptospira spp. and Borrelia theileri.

The donor calf is inoculated with the seed material after not less than 8 weeks in the isolation facility; the parasitaemia and freedom from contaminating haemoparasites are monitored by daily blood smear examination. At peak parasitaemia, blood is collected by a closed technique, diluted with glycerol buffer, dispensed into tubes and frozen at a controlled rate. Daily clinical examination is conducted to monitor possible development of the viral diseases listed above.

Donor handling after vaccine production.

For two weeks after vaccine production, the vaccine donor calf is subjected to a clinical examination for presence of other haemoparasites and the viral diseases listed above, and also anthrax.

Viability and safety testing of the vaccine.

The blood vaccine is subjected to bacteriological and mycological culture to screen for contaminants. Two tubes of vaccine are checked by culture and laboratory animal inoculation for freedom from contaminating bacteria and fungi.

The vaccine is tested in bovine calves over a period of six weeks; two calves are each inoculated with 4.5 ml (10^7 infected erythrocytes per ml) of the vaccine and subjected to daily clinical examination and recording of rectal temperatures. Blood smears are prepared and examined to confirm viability of the vaccine and freedom from contaminating haemoparasites. Freedom from BVD, EBL and brucellosis is confirmed serologically from pre- and post-vaccination samples of these animals.

The following serological tests are normally conducted:

EBL	-	agar gel immunodiffusion test or ELISA test.
Brucellosis	-	Rose Bengal plate test.
Mucosal Disease	-	virus neutralisation test.
Babesiosis	-	indirect immunofluorescent test.
Theileriosis	-	indirect fluorescent test.
Anaplasmosis	-	indirect immunofluorescent test.

Potency testing.

The potency of the vaccine is assessed by inoculation of 2 ml doses of the vaccine in 3-fold dilutions into groups of at least 5 calves, with an equal number of calves in the control group. Infectivity of the vaccine is monitored by taking and examining blood smears every 1 - 2 days and pre- and post-vaccination serology. Safety of the vaccine is again monitored by clinical examination and rectal temperature every 1 - 2 days together with assessment of the PCV at 14 day intervals starting from day 0. These procedures are in general accordance with those recommended in the O.I.E. Manual.

Procedure for monitoring and controlling the immunization responses to the vaccines.

The aims are:

(i) to ensure that infection/immunization has occurred;

(ii) to detect severe reactions so that they are treated in time.

These are monitored in any group of animals as follows:

(i) daily clinical observation from day 7 to day 42;

(ii) blood smears from a representative sample of cattle on days 10 and 35;

(iii) blood smears from all animals with temperature >39.5°C;

(iv) blood for serology from a representative sample on days 0 and 56.

In the case of valuable animals or animals considered to be highly susceptible, daily rectal temperatures should be taken from day 7 to day 42.

Intervention (treatment) may be indicated based on the following criteria:

(i) temperature >40.5°C for a day or temperature >40.0°C on 3 consecutive days; and/or

(ii) clinical illness (anorexia, depression, weakness).

Heartwater Vaccine

Donor sheep.

Merino sheep are obtained from an area which is free from foot and mouth disease and rinderpest, and vaccines for these diseases are not used. Nairobi sheep disease and sheep pox are not known to occur in Malawi. The sheep are held in concrete floored pens, fed on concentrate meal and maize silage only and kept in isolation from other sheep. The sheep are confirmed to be free from bovine virus diarrhoea by annual serological testing.

Sheep handling before and during vaccine production.

Sheep are transferred to the isolation facilities at the CVL eight weeks prior to commencement of vaccine production. The sheep are sprayed weekly with acaricide and the facilities are maintained proof against ticks and flying insects. Access is strictly controlled. Sheep are subjected to daily clinical examination, and rectal temperature is recorded to monitor possible development of infectious diseases. Blood smears are examined every second day to check for haemoparasites.

Donor sheep are inoculated with seed material. At the time of peak parasitaemia, assessed by the height and duration of the febrile reaction, blood is collected by a closed technique, diluted with citrate-lactose-peptone buffer containing dimethyl sulphoxide (DMSO), dispensed into vials and frozen at a controlled rate. The specificity of the febrile reaction is confirmed by demonstration of C. ruminantium in brain biopsy smears.

Viability and safety testing.

Two vials of the vaccine are checked by culture and laboratory animal inoculation for freedom from contaminating bacteria and fungi.

Two merino sheep are inoculated with 5 ml vaccine each from separate vials and subjected to daily clinical examination and recording of rectal temperatures. The specificity of any febrile reaction is confirmed by demonstration of C. ruminantium in brain biopsy smears taken every 1 to 2 days from the third day of fever.

Potency testing.

Potency of the vaccine is assessed by titration using 3-fold dilutions in groups of 10 calves. Calves are examined clinically and temperatures are taken daily starting on day 12 through to day 24. Calves showing a febrile reaction are treated with tetracycline. Infectivity of the vaccine is monitored serologically using the immunofluorescent test on days 0 and 42 after inoculation. The ID_{50} is calculated. One dose of vaccine should contain not less than $10ID_{50}s$.

Theileria annulata Cell Culture Vaccine

This vaccine is produced in many countries and what is described below is given as an example to illustrate one approach to quality control, developed and adopted by Israel for this vaccine (FAO, 1984).

The Veterinary Institute at Beit Dagan, Israel has adopted a programme for testing the vaccine based on the general principles for testing live cell-culture vaccines against viral diseases.

Extensive testing procedures are, however, considered unjustified for liquid vaccine because of its short shelf-life and also for the frozen vaccine since individual batches are usually not large enough to justify the extensive procedure. Consequently, the full testing routine is run only on each batch of seed material stored in liquid nitrogen. It is recommended, however, that the actual working vaccine be tested periodically for purity only, as a check on the overall production process.

The Full Testing Programme.

Purity.

The standard procedures for detecting bacteria, fungi, mycoplasma and viruses in live vaccines produced in cell culture as described in the U.S. Code for Federal Regulations for Animal and Animal Products (ref. paras. 113.25, 113.27, 113.28 and 113.51) were recommended.

Safety.

The procedure is that a sample of the frozen vaccine is thawed and adjusted with diluent to a final concentration of 10^7 cells per ml. Inoculate each of five calves with 5 ml of the vaccine (ie 5 x 10^7 schizont-infected cells). Check the inoculated animals for 1 month. This would involve monitoring the temperatures and blood smears daily of animals for 2 weeks before inoculation. Sera for serology to be collected on the day of receiving the animals and just before vaccination. Thereafter, daily rectal temperatures are taken, and blood smears, lymph node and liver biopsies are collected during the acute phase of the infection. Sera are again collected 28 days later to assess the seroconversion.

Different breeds of cattle respond differently to the vaccine; safety tests should be performed with animals of the same stock. It is therefore advisable, with a new batch, to start field immunization with small groups of animals (10-15) so that unexpected harmful effects may be identified and corrected with a minimum of damage.

Potency.

The procedure is that 5 calves are each inoculated with either 5 x 10^6 infected cells from the liquid vaccine or 10^7 cells from the frozen vaccine. Keep under observation this inoculated group together with another group of 5 uninoculated calves. Examine all the calves for a period of 6 weeks as described above. Challenge the inoculated and control calves with a T. annulata sporozoite stabilate (10 tick equivalents per animal). The animals should withstand the challenge if the vaccine is efficacious.

Theileria parva Sporozoite Vaccine

Although the infection and treatment method of immunization against ECF was developed in the mid 1970s, detailed steps to address quality control aspects were only initiated in the late 1980s. Guidelines for stabilate preparation, safety precautions (field collected ticks, tick handling facilities and stabilate preparation), and purity of the stabilates were given recently in an OIE Manual (1991). However, a detailed approach to quality control for the ECF vaccine specifically addressing production at the Central Veterinary Laboratory, Lilongwe, was given by Terpstra (1990) in a consultancy report.

Standardization of production procedures.

To standardize production, a dossier has been prepared, detailing the sequential steps of stabilate preparation, the in-line quality control tests, and the tests that must be passed by the monovalent stabilate and the trivalent ready-to-use product.

Purity.

Purity of the product is dependent on ensuring that the ingredients and/or additives used in the production are pure and free from contaminating organisms, and freedom from contaminants in the ticks, the bovines, the rabbits, and the media into which sporozoites are harvested.

The ticks used for stabilate production have been reared under laboratory conditions for many generations (>25 years); they have not been shown to harbour any human or cattle pathogens ever since.

The cattle used for parasite pick-up are cross-breds, originating from known farms in the southern highlands of Malawi where ECF has not been reported. Strict tick control is practised on these farms and the animals confirmed to be free of haemoparasites listed in Annex 1. The animals are transported directly to the CVL, quarantined for 6 - 12 weeks prior to vaccine production and are fed silage, maize and mineral blocks. They are sprayed with acaricides twice weekly. Only clinically healthy animals are used for parasite pick-up. FMD, rinderpest and bovine herpes mammilitis are currently not prevalent in Malawi.

Although all the infectious agents listed in Annex 1, with the exception of bovine herpes mammilitis virus, can be present in the blood stream and thus can be picked up by ticks taking a blood meal, only Ehrlichia bovis and T. parva can actively multiply in R. appendiculatus. The animals are pretested for antibodies to T. parva using IFAT. The method is an in-line control test in the vaccine production process. Theileria mutans is not transmitted by R. appendiculatus.

Cattle can be carriers of Borrelia and very seldom also of Leptospira; an injection of penicillin and streptomycin before parasite pick-up clears these infections. A similar treatment is undertaken in rabbits used for prefeeding the infected ticks.

Enzootic bovine leucosis (EBL) virus and bovine diarrhoea virus (BVD) can only passively be transferred to the stabilate. Most probably the viruses will die out in the ticks during the eight weeks elapsing between parasite pick-up and stabilate preparation.

The RVF virus is not very stable and almost certainly dies out before the adults ticks are used in stabilate preparation, assuming the nymphae became infected during T. parva pick-up. A similar situation would apply to Ephemeral Fever, Akabane disease and Bluetongue viruses whose vectors are present throughout the ECF region.

All media, for stabilate preparation, are tested for sterility by preincubation at 37°C and confirmed to be bacteria and fungi free.

Safety of the stabilates.

Freedom from bacterial, fungal and mycoplasma contamination.

Bacteriological and mycological sterility of the stabilate has been a major problem mainly because of the type of substrate (infected ticks) used. Filtration of the stabilate, without losing Theileria infectivity, is not a feasible proposition except for fungi which may be retained by filters with a large pore size.

All media are tested for sterility by preincubation and all inoculations are carried out under sterile laminar air flow conditions to avoid accidental contamination. Prior to testing, samples are cultured in an enrichment medium under both aerobic and anaerobic conditions.

Briefly, the procedure for bacterial and fungal contaminants is as follows:

(i) Each of four tubes with 40 ml thioglycolate medium per tube are inoculated with 1.0 ml samples of a batch of monovalent stabilate or trivalent ready to use product. Two tubes are incubated at 37°C and two at 22°C for seven days.

(ii) Each of four tubes with 40 ml tryptone-soya broth are inoculated with 0.25 ml samples of a batch of monovalent stabilate or trivalent ready to use product. Two tubes are incubated at 37°C and two at 22°C for seven days.

(iii) Shake the tubes after seven days of incubation for turbidity. Should a tube show turbidity, inoculate one or more blood agar plates and incubate these for 48 hours under the conditions, which have caused turbidity.

(iv) Check the blood agar plates for growth. The cultures should remain sterile.

The proposed protocol for checking for mycoplasma is briefly described below. Prior to testing, samples are cultured in an enrichment medium. Thus the procedure would be:

(i) A 4.0 ml sample of either a batch of monovalent stabilate or trivalent ready to use product is inoculated into 100 ml PPLO-broth and incubated at 37°C for seven days.

(ii) A volume of 0.25 ml is then inoculated into each of five PPLO-agar plates and incubated at 37°C for 14 days.

(iii) Examine the plates for growth. There should be no evidence of mycoplasma colonies.

Tests for mycoplasma sterility have not been done so far.

Freedom from EBL, BVD, LSD and RVF viruses.

Although it was suggested previously that these viruses were likely to die out prior to stabilate preparation, it is important to confirm their absence in the final product. For this reason, two EBL and BVD seronegative calves are vaccinated with 20 cattle doses each of the stabilate to be examined. The animals are tested for seroconversion four weeks after inoculation, using either a serum neutralisation test or ELISA for BVD, and an ELISA for EBL. The same animals should be LSD seronegative and are, thus, also used for checking antibodies to the LSD virus. The infection is very common during certain periods and although the level of viraemia is low, the virus is extremely stable.

As Rift Valley fever is a zoonosis, causing mild to severe infections in man, experimental animals are vaccinated with an inactivated vaccine shortly after arriving at the quarantine stables. Such a policy avoids the risk of animal handlers being exposed to viraemic blood and at the same time removes any doubt about absence of RVF virus in the ECF stabilate vaccine.

Potency testing.

For reasons of standardization, economy on the use of stabilate and confidence in the immunizing potency of the product, the actual titration end-point is determined. The stabilate is titrated at least three times. Each titration is an exact replica of the former, using four dilutions: 1:2, 1:4, 1:8 and 1:16 and four animals per dilution. Experience with the semi-quantitative method has shown that all animals inoculated with 0.5 ml undiluted stabilate will react, the undiluted stabilate inoculation is therefore omitted. As the 50% infective dose (ID_{50}) is assumed to be equivalent to one 50% protective dose (PD_{50}), a decision can be made about the minimum number of ID_{50}s of each Theileria stock to be incorporated in the ready to use trivalent product. In the field a near to 100% protection level is aimed at.

Certification of freedom from contaminants.

Vaccines issued should be bacteriologically, mycologically and mycoplasmologically sterile and free from viral pathogens. In-line sterility tests on e.g. media, glycerol and antibiotic additives are done at the CVL, Lilongwe. Those responsible for the results sign for the correct execution of the tests. The same applies to the prescreening tests of sera from experimental cattle for antibodies against T. parva and T. mutans, as these fall into the same category of in-line control measures.

Previously it was reasoned that stabilates need only be checked for the presence of EBL, BVD and LSD viruses. Certification requires the testing of sera taken before and four weeks after the animals have been inoculated with a high dosage of stabilate. The tests can either be done on each separate component or on the trivalent ready to use product. The latter option is probably the best since it reduces the number of cattle to be used and the number of tests required to a third. The advantages, however, have to be weighed against the small risk that the whole batch of final product has to be rejected.

For overall certification of the product, guidance is being sought from the Malawi Bureau of Standards as to which laboratories, within or outside the country, are acceptable before the bureau can issue a certificate for the product.

REFERENCES

BEZUIDENHOUT J.D. (1981) The development of a new heartwater vaccine using Amblyomma hebraeum nymphae infected with Cowdria ruminantium. In: Tick Biology and Control. Published by Tick Research Unit, Rhodes University, Grahamstown, South Africa. pp. 41-45.

BROWN C.G.D. (1990) Control of Tropical theileriosis (Theileria annulata infection) of cattle. Parassitologia, **32**, 23-31.

CALLOW L.L. and DALGLIESH R.J. (1980) The development of effective, safe vaccination against babesiosis and anaplasmosis in Australia. Proceedings of a Symposium held at the 56th Annual Conference of the Australian Veterinary Association, Townsville, 14-18 May 1979. pp. 4-8.

CALLOW L.L., MELLORS L.T. and McGREGOR W. (1979) Reduction in virulence of B. bovis due to rapid passage in splenoctomised cattle. International Journal for Parasitology, **9**, 333-338.

CUNNINGHAM, M.P., BROWN C.G.D., BURRIDGE M.J. and PURNELL R.E. (1973) Cryopreservation of infective particles of Theileria parva. International Journal for Parasitology, **3**, 583-587.

FAO (1984) Tick and tick-borne disease control: A practical manual. FAO, Rome.

OIE (1991) Theileriosis (B/020), OIE Manual of Recommended Diagnostic Techniques and Requirements for Biological Products. Volume III; Section 16, 1-16.

LUMSDEN W.H.R. and HARDY G.J.C. (1965) Nomenclature of living parasite material. Natural, London, **205**, 1032.

NEITZ W.O. and ALEXANDER R.A. (1945) Immunization of cattle against heartwater and the control of tick-borne diseases, redwater, gallsickness and heartwater. Ondestepoort Journal of Veterinary Science and Animal Industries, **20**, 137-158.

PIPANO E. (1979) Virulence and immunogenicity of cultured Theileria annulata schizonts. Journal of South African Veterinary Association, **50**, (4), 332-333.

RADLEY D.E. (1981) Infection, treatment and immunization against theileriosis. In: Advances in the control of theileriosis. A.D. Irvin, M.P. Cunningham & A.S. Young. eds. Martinus Nijhoff Publishers, The Hague. pp. 227-237.

TERPESTRA C. (1990) FAO Consultancy report on East Coast Fever vaccine production and quality control, Project GCP.RAF/247/NET.

ANNEX 1* <u>Risk Assessment and Relevance of Quality Control of Frozen ECF Stabilates</u>

Infectious Agent	Incubation (days)	Viraemia/ bacteraemia/ parasitaemia	Rh. app. trans- mitted	Prevalence (a)	Screening or pretreatment donor calves	Relevance for checking stabilate
Enzootic bovine leucosis virus	carriers	+	-	++		+
Inf.bovine rhinotracheitis virus	2 - 7	low level	-	?		-
Bovine virus diarrhoea virus	carriers	+	-	+		+
Foot-and-mouth disease virus	3 - 14	+	-	-		-
Rinderpest virus	7 - 14	+	-	-		-
Bovine herpes mammilitis virus	?	-	not appl.	-		-
Lumpy skin disease virus	7 - 10	low level	-	++		+
Ephemeral fever virus	?	+	-	+++		-
Akabane virus	?	+	-	+++		-
Bluetongue virus	carriers	+	-	+++		-
Rift Valley fever virus	1 - 3	+	-	+	vaccination	-
Leptospirosis	carriers	+	-	+		-
Borreliosis	carriers	+	-	?	streptomycin	-
Heartwater (Cowdria ruminantium)	10 - 28	+	-	+	penicillin	-
Typanosoma	carriers	+	-	++		-
Anaplasma	carriers	+	-	+		-
Theileria parva	carriers	+	+	++		not appl.
Theileria mutans	carriers	+	-	++		-
Eperythrozoon	?	+	-	?	ind.IFT	-
Erhlichia bovis	?	+	+	?	ind.IFT	-

* EXTRACTED FROM ECF VACCINE PRODUCTION & QUALITY CONTROL REPORT BY TERPSTRA (1990)

(a) - absent or no evidence + present +++ ubiquitous

? - sporadic or erratic occurrence ++ common

Discussion

Dr Mannathoko enquired whether the CVL, Lilongwe now had an established vaccine for Theileriosis or whether the work was still at the experimental stage.

Dr Musisi in reply stated that they have an immunising preparation which has been used widely in Malawi and also in Zambia. It has recently been under appraisal in Tanzania and it was anticipated that a request for a hundred thousand doses would be received soon. Dr Musisi said that further development work is continuing to improve its use in the field.

Dr Korir stated that in Kenya they have a stabilate which is effective and has given good results against East Coast Fever for the last two years or so.

Specific Issues Related to Veterinary Vaccines

MODERN TRENDS IN VETERINARY VACCINOLOGY

by

T R Doel

INTRODUCTION

Despite extensive cloning, expression and sequencing of the structural proteins of a number of important pathogens over the last decade, there has been relatively little impact at the level of novel vaccine development and application. This owes a great deal to an imperfect understanding of the detailed structure of antigens and the ways in which the immune system of the host deals with and develops an immune response to these antigens. As a result, relatively empirical approaches have been used in the application of synthetic or biosynthetic antigens for novel vaccines.

The detailed structure of potential vaccine antigens can only be revealed through costly and complex crystallographic studies, foot-and-mouth disease virus, rhinovirus and poliovirus capsids and influenza virus glycoproteins being the best known. At the moment, it is not possible to compute reliable secondary or tertiary structures from primary sequence data.

The immune response to synthetic or biosynthetic antigens is poorly understood except at relatively simplistic levels such as neutralising antibody. This is often paralleled by our limited knowledge of the immune response of the target species to the whole pathogen. Indeed, the field suffers from a tendency to compartmentalise the immune response into the various effector mechanisms which, while convenient experimentally and for reasons of comprehension, neglects the importance of these mechanisms acting in concert. This does not mean that a purified antigen which induces only a part of the immune response to the whole pathogen will necessarily be inadequate but rather that it might be considerably more effective if it were able to induce a more comprehensive response.

The Immune Response

The acquired immune response may be considered in terms of antibody and cell mediated mechanisms.

In the case of antibodies, there are the further subdivisions of the humoral and mucosal compartments. Humoral and, specifically, neutralising antibodies attract considerable attention in the development of novel vaccines partly because they can be measured very easily and have connotations of relevance. However, it must be remembered that 'neutralisation' is more often than not an in vitro assay which merely tests the ability of a serum to prevent attachment of virus to cells. It need not bear any relationship to the much more complex situation in vivo where other factors come into play including the extent to which immune complexes are recognised by phagocytic cells. Nevertheless, with certain qualifications, the measurement of neutralising antibody is more or less satisfactory with viruses such as foot-and-mouth disease (FMD) where there is a good correlation between titres induced by whole virus vaccines and protection (Pay, T.W.F. and Hingley, P.J. 1987).

It is perhaps worth commenting further on the control of a disease, FMD, of the upper respiratory tract by an inactivated vaccine given by the parenteral route. The simple priority with FMD is to limit replication as much as possible in the animal and thereby minimise further spread of the disease. The fate of the individual is of little consequence. Because a safe attenuated vaccine for FMD does not exist, the parenterally administered preparation has to give antibody titres which will be sufficient to protect systemically, including by transudation, the mucosal surfaces of the upper respiratory tract. Even the best FMD vaccines often fall short of this expectation.

While mucosal immunity is clearly important with diseases which invade via the respiratory and/or digestive tracts, it has been relatively neglected in comparison with humoral immunity. The situation owes something to the problem of maintaining high levels of mucosal IgA following administration of an inactivated antigen. Thus, intranasal administration of inactivated poliovirus gives a nasopharyngeal IgA response which returns to pre-immunisation levels after two months. This may be contrasted with the long-lived (>two years) IgA response with per oral administered attenuated poliovirus. However, the inactivated poliovirus vaccine given by the parenteral route is very satisfactory because low levels of pre-existing antibody or antibody from recently stimulated memory cells are invariably adequate to prevent the virus reaching the central nervous system. In contrast to FMD, shedding of poliovirus by an individual and mild illness such as gastrointestinal upsets are considered to be of lesser consequence. The mode of action of IgA appears to be primarily by coating and preventing the attachment of pathogens to mucosal surfaces. In the event that the IgA barrier is breached, antigens will encounter IgE bound firmly to mast cells leading to the release of mediators which generate a local acute inflammatory reaction and recruit other agents of the immune response including serum IgG by transudation.

In addition to the direct action of specific IgG on cell-free pathogens, serum antibodies may bind to infected cells which display foreign antigen(s) on their surface and facilitate their destruction. Target cell death may arise by phagocytosis (several mechanisms including opsonic adherence), complement mediated lysis or antibody-dependent cell-mediated cytotoxicity (ADCC). In ADCC, the effector cells bearing the specific antibody bound by the Fc region, link to the antigen bearing cell and kill by an extracellular mechanism. A number of cell types are capable of this method of cell killing including the K and NK cell lineages. ADCC has been reported for a variety of viruses including herpes, rabies, vaccinia and mumps infected target cells.

Cytotoxic T cells (Tc) may act directly on an infected cell in which the foreign antigens are presented in the context of the Major Histocompatibility Complex (MHC). In general, target recognition and killing by class I MHC restricted Tc cells requires de novo protein synthesis, ie replication of the pathogen, within the target cell. That Tc cells are important in the acquired immune response is suggested by a number of studies particularly with influenza virus, It is a fact, nevertheless, that the relative importance of different mechanisms of immunity is a contentious issue because of the complexity of the immune response and the limitations of experimental design.

Another class of T cells, the T helper cells (Th), recognise antigen which has been endocytosed, processed and presented in the context of class II MHC and respond by producing a battery of lymphokines. These soluble mediators of the immune response play key roles in the further development of antigen specific B cells and Tc cells.

Synthetic and biosynthetic antigens

Both small fragments representing single epitopes and larger fragments or whole proteins of pathogens have been used as new generation vaccines. Frequently, they are used as the equivalent of killed vaccines, ie there is no opportunity for the antigen concentration to increase as would happen with a natural infection. More recently, however, several virus and bacteria have been used as vectors of important antigens with the aim of achieving at least limited replication.

SYNTHETIC PEPTIDE VACCINES

With the notable exception of FMD, this approach offers little promise at the moment for the development of new veterinary vaccines. A major problem is that of reproducing an important epitope, many of which are conformational in their natural state, using a linear sequence of amino acids. Possibly the greatest success has been achieved with FMD. Synthetic peptides based on the VP1 protein of the virus and having the sequence C-C-(200-213)-P-P-S-(141-158)-P-C-G raise very high neutralising antibodies in cattle and a number of other species. Although the molarities of peptide used are in considerable excess over that of virus, the antibody titres are often an order of magnitude higher than is obtained with conventional FMD vaccines. In the author's laboratory, it has been possible to protect some but not all cattle given one or two doses of peptide. In contrast, the guinea pig, a small-animal model for FMD, is relatively easy to protect. The discrepancy between neutralising antibody titre and protection with synthetic FMD peptide vaccines has not been resolved but most probably relates to the induction of inappropriate isotypes/affinities of antibodies which are less effective in vivo. One interesting feature of FMD peptides was the unexpected finding that they induced more cross-reactive antibody than whole virus vaccines. Thus, a single dose of an O serotype peptide protects completely against homologous challenge and significantly against challenge with an A or C serotype virus (Doel et al, 1990). This situation is unheard of with whole virus vaccines.

Synthetic peptides have also been suggested as candidate vaccines for rabies but their success compared with recent developments with vaccinia expressed G protein is extremely limited. Residues 253-275 of the G protein of the ERA strain of rabies virus, when linked to a T helper cell epitope of the N protein, protected 75% of mice challenged by the intramuscular route.

The generally negative appraisal of the prospects for synthetic peptide vaccines at the beginning of this section needs qualification. Peptide vaccines face many problems but have a number of significant advantages over other types of vaccine. Firstly, they are easily prepared as very pure materials by conventional solid-phase chemistry although it must be said that the cost of synthesis by this route is still too high to consider for veterinary vaccines. Secondly, the antigen is a highly defined product which can be easily manipulated either following or during synthesis. For example, it might be desirable to conjugate the peptide at a particular position to a carrier protein or another molecule such as a long-chain fatty acid. Only the latter could be done by the peptide approach. Thirdly, it may be possible to induce precisely the desired immune response, for example heterologous protection, whereas a larger protein would probably be processed and presented by the immune system in a different way.

BIOSYNTHETIC PROTEIN VACCINES

This approach has been exploited considerably with many proteins. Once again FMD VP1 was one of the first virus proteins to be cloned in E.coli and the expression products used to immunise experimental animals. Two doses, each of 250 μg of a 44 kDa recombinant trp Δ LE1413-VP1 protein protected cattle and pigs (Kleid et al, 1981). However, the requirement for several doses to be effective was prejudicial to the future of this approach because of the requirement for FMD vaccines to protect with one dose only. The Bluetongue virus proteins VP2 and VP5 have been expressed in baculovirus systems and used to protect sheep as VP2 and VP2/VP5 vaccines. VP3 and VP7 have also been expressed and fold to give macromolecular structures which it is suggested could be used as carrier molecules for other antigens. In the case of immunity to this virus it is important to consider both induction of antibody and cytotoxic T cells, both of which have been implicated in protection. The glycoproteins G1 and G2 of Rift Valley fever virus have been expressed in E.coli and a nuclear polyhedrosis virus of caterpillars of Autographica californica. When inoculated into mice, both induced neutralising antibody and probably a cell mediated immune response.

VECTORED ANTIGEN VACCINES

The concept of delivering a 'foreign' antigen in a harmless viral or bacterial vector which will nevertheless replicate in the host is a most attractive one. It offers the possibility of numerous cycles of replication of the foreign antigen without the associated disease. This would appear to be ideal in terms of inducing an optimum immune response. However, a number of other considerations are important. Firstly, an immune response will be induced against the vector and there is the possibility that it will be rapidly checked before significant replication has occurred. Secondly, administration of the vaccine to an animal with pre-existing immunity to the vector may compromise the desired immune response. Thirdly, there is the issue of what constitutes a safe vector. The risks of reversion to virulence and rescue of virulent strains by recombination.reassortment events in the field need careful consideration. Furthermore an otherwise safe vector may cause considerable problems if the health/immune response of the animal is greatly diminished by disease and/or famine. Unfortunately, few studies have considered and answered all of these questions.

Vaccinia virus has been widely used as a carrier. Perhaps the best example of this is the use of vaccinia-rabies glycoprotein G recombinants given in baits for foxes. The vaccine appears to be safe for a wide range of European mammals, is capable of horizontal transmission and produces immunity in excess of one year. Although evaluated considerably less, the glycoprotein G of vesicular stomatitis virus has been expressed in vaccinia and used successfully to protect mice and cattle. A number of laboratories have expressed the H and F proteins of rinderpest virus in the thymidine kinase gene of vaccinia and protected cattle and pigs (eg Yilma et al, 1988).

Although modern hog cholera vaccines are generally regarded to be safe and effective, there have been attempts to develop recombinant vaccines. DNA corresponding to the entire structural protein coding region of hog cholera virus has been cloned into vaccinia virus and used to protect pigs against a lethal challenge. Vaccinia virus has also been used to express the G1 and G2 proteins of Rift Valley fever virus (RVFV) in immunised mice which developed high titres of neutralising antibodies and were protected. An 11 amino acid long neutralizing epitope of RFVF has been inserted near the NH_2 terminus of the E2 protein of Sindbis virus and multiple immunizations of mice produce partial protection.

Several other viruses offer advantages over vaccinia as vectors of the antigens of other pathogens. Capripox viruses affect sheep, goats and cattle and attenuated vaccines are available which provide immunity for at least two years. The considerable size of the genome of the capripox virus, like the related vaccinia virus, would allow many different antigens to be incorporated. Another poxvirus, fowlpox (FPV), has been used to deliver a number of antigens of other viruses of poultry, notably the haemagglutinin genes of avian influenza and Newcastle disease virus as well as those of non-poultry viruses such as the rabies glycoprotein. The latter constructs were used to vaccinate non-permissive hosts (mouse, rabbit etc) which developed antibody 14 days after inoculation. The herpes virus, infectious bovine rhinotracheitis (IBR), also exists as an attenuated vaccine strain and could equally accommodate large sequences of foreign genetic material. Kit and his colleagues have used IBR as a vector for the FMD peptide described earlier in this chapter and succeeded in stimulating neutralising antibodies in calves.

Several bacteria, notably E.coli and S.typhimurium, have been used to present 'foreign' antigens. In addition to the attraction that both organisms allow presentation at mucosal surfaces, there is the added advantage that they may be controlled by antibiotics should there be any problems following vaccination.

ATTENUATED VACCINES

Despite the reservations of some authorities, attenuated vaccines have proven to be of immense value in the control of disease, offering the prospect of life-long immunity from a single vaccination. Such is the case with rinderpest vaccine developed by Plowright and his colleagues (Plowright and Taylor, 1967) and, while this vaccine has been criticised on the grounds of thermostability, it is likely that it will continue to be the vaccine of choice for many years.

The question of thermostability with rinderpest is being addressed by several approaches. Reference has been made to the use of vaccinia virus as a vector to carry rinderpest antigens. Another approach is to develop more thermostable rinderpest viruses and develop delivery systems which minimise cold-chain problems.

Unlike the related poliovirus, it has not been possible to develop a safe attenuated FMD vaccine. Despite considerable efforts at Pirbright and other laboratories, viruses attenuated for one species either proved to be virulent for another or reverted following immunisation. Indeed very occasional reversion to neurovirulence has been observed with poliovirus and is one of the justifications for the use of killed poliovirus vaccines. Given more detailed knowledge of the FMD genome including its replication and, in particular the recent availability of an "infectious" DNA copy of the FMD genome, it may be possible to genetically engineer a safe attenuated vaccine but it has to be remembered that the virus is capable of recombination-like events in the laboratory and that the widespread distribution of an attenuated FMD virus would be just as disadvantageous in terms of export of livestock and livestock products.

The possibility of a reassortment or recombination event between a wild-type virus and a vaccine strain remains one of the major objections to attenuated vaccines. This problem was addressed with an attenuated Rift Valley fever virus vaccine in which reassortants from a mixture of the live vaccine strain MP 12 and wild type virus were easily generated. However, analysis of the reassortants indicated that virulence was under polygenic control and at least one mutation capable of independently attenuating the virus was found on each of the genome segments. Because of the multiple mutations in MP 12, the authors concluded that reversion to virulence and the generation of virulent reassortants were unlikely events in the use of the virus in the field. Attenuated Bluetongue virus vaccines are subject to the same potential problem. Because the virus replicates in an insect host and is known to increase its pathogenicity, it is recommended that vaccination is not used in non-epidemic regions during the vector season.

As noted above, a number of viruses allow the possibility of controlling more than one disease because of their genomic capacity for "foreign" genetic material. Sheep and goatpox and lumpy skin disease are important diseases of sheep, goats and cattle for which good attenuated virus vaccines exist. They represent, therefore, excellent vectors of other antigens. Another potentially useful group is the herpes viruses, embracing a wide range of important hosts. Mention has been made of the use of IBR as a vector of an FMD peptide. Other candidate viruses include Aujeszky's disease virus (or pseudorabies, PR) for pigs, and equine herpes virus. The former example perhaps illustrates the potential of this and similar viruses as both vaccines in their own right as well as carriers of the antigens of other important pathogens. Kit and his colleagues (Kit, 1990) have developed a PR vaccine in which the thymidine kinase gene has been deleted entirely thereby preventing or greatly limiting replication in non-dividing cells (eg neuronal cells) such that the risk of latency is reduced considerably. A further deletion of a gene coding for a major glycoprotein of the virus (gIII) allows the immune response to the vaccine to be distinguished from that against field isolates of PRV.

<u>Enhancement of Antigenicity and Immunogenicity</u>

This remains a highly empirical area where few rules-of-thumb exist. As an example of this, synthetic FMD peptides (141-160) couples to protein carriers such as Keyhole Limpet Haemocyanin induce reasonable antibody titres when delivered as oil or A1(OH) vaccines whereas the free peptide C-C(200-213)-P-P-S-(141-158)-P-C-G is effective only in oil emulsion vaccines.

A number of other adjuvants have attracted considerable attention over the last few years. These include liposome preparations, ISCOMs, muramyl dipeptide and related analogues and pluronic block co-polymers. There is no question that some of the novel adjuvant/antigen preparations have given good responses as vaccines but it would be incorrect to suggest that any one formulation is of general value. There is also the question of cost in the case of veterinary vaccines. With the possible exception of vaccines for valuable bloodstock, particularly race-horses, the cost/difficulty of manufacture of some of the above preparations would rule out their application in control of animal diseases.

REFERENCES

PAY, T.W.F. and HINGLEY, P.J. (1987) Correlation of 140S antigen dose with the serum neutralizing antibody response and the level of protection induced in cattle by foot-and-mouth disease vaccines. Vaccine, **5**, 60-64.

DOEL, T.R., GALE, C., DO AMARAL, C.M.C.F., BROOKE, G., MULCAHY, G. and DIMARCHI, R. (1990) Heterotypic protection induced by synthetic peptides corresponding to three serotypes of foot-and-mouth disease virus. J. Virol. **64**, 2260-2264.

KLEID, D.G., YANSURA, D., SMALL, B., DOWBENKO, D., MOORE, D.M., GRUBMAN, M.J., McKERCHER, P.D., MORGAN, D.O., ROBERTSON, B.H. and BACHRACH, H.L. (1981) Cloned viral protein vaccine for foot-and-mouth disease: responses in cattle and swine. Science, **214**, 1125-1129.

YILMA, T., HSU, D., JONES, L., OWENS, S., GRUBMAN, M., MEBUS, C., YAMANAKA, M.. and DALE, B. (1988) Protection of cattle against rinderpest with vaccinia virus recombinants expressing the HA or F gene. Science, **242**, 1058-1061.

PLOWRIGHT, W. and TAYLOR, W.P. (1967) Long-term studies of the immunity in East African cattle following inoculation of rinderpest culture vaccine. Res. Vet. Scl. **8**, 118-128.

KIT, S. (1990) Genetically engineered vaccines for control of Aujeszky's disease (pseudorabies). Vaccines, **8**, 420-424.

GENETICALLY ENGINEERED VACCINES

by

T Yilma

INTRODUCTION

Vaccination has been practice by the indigenous peoples of Africa and Asia for hundreds, if not thousands, of years. Modern vaccination began in 1796 when Edward Jenner noticed that milkmaids who had been infected with cowpox did not subsequently develop smallpox. He began to vaccinate people against smallpox by scratching them with scabs from cowpox lesions. The exact origin of vaccinia virus is unknown; the virus used for smallpox vaccination does not exist in nature and is distinct from cowpox virus and the variola virus of smallpox. Vaccinia virus may have originated from horsepox. What is clear, however, is that the vaccinia virus vaccination procedure has protected hundreds of millions of people worldwide from smallpox. Further, it has been shown to have minimal side effects and no adverse environmental impacts, despite release of the vaccinia virus on thousands of occasions under poor hygienic conditions.

The invention of vaccines is one of the most significant developments in the effort to control human and animal diseases. Recently, a remarkable new generation of vaccines has been developed, namely, subunit, synthetic peptide, and virus vector vaccines. One of these recombinant vaccines uses vaccinia virus as a vector. When the vaccinia vector is inoculated into an animal, the virus replicates in the host's cells, and both vaccinia virus and the foreign genes are expressed. If the foreign gene is for an immunogenic protein of an infectious agent, the animal becomes immune both to vaccinia virus and to the agent from which the foreign gene was taken.

Because animals vaccinated with living or killed whole organisms can develop a full range of immune responses, serologic tests may not differentiate vaccinates from carrier animals that have recovered from natural infection. This inability to differentiate vaccinates from naturally infected animals causes problems in disease diagnosis and control, as well as causing significant economic losses due to bans on importation of infected livestock and their products. Finally, many live vaccines are unstable and must be refrigerated; this requirement complicates their use in developing countries.

The nature of the host's immune response to an injected antigen is critical in vaccination. Inactivated vaccines commonly employ an adjuvant of some type to boost the immune response. Live vaccines cannot use adjuvants because they inactivate the immunizing agent; on the other hand, live agents generally do not need additional help to induce immunity.

Conventional Live Vaccines

Live (attenuated) vaccines have advantages over inactivated, subunit, and synthetic peptide vaccines since they replicate in the host to "amplify" the antigen, but they also have drawbacks: (1) often one cannot distinguish vaccinates from those recovered from infection; (2) attenuated strains might revert to virulence in the vertebrate host or arthropod vector; (3) new strains of the agent may arise from the vaccine strain; and (4) the vaccine may induce disease in pregnant or debilitated animals. Many of these disadvantages could be overcome by using subunit or synthetic peptide vaccines, which also are advantageous since the animal's immune system is stimulated with only the relevant antigens. The major problem with subunit and synthetic peptide vaccines, including inactivated vaccines, is that the antigenic mass cannot be greater than the amount of protein injected; there is no amplification of the antigen, for example, as in an attenuated live virus vaccine.

Recombinant Vaccines

Recombinant DNA technology has made it possible to insert and express heterologous genes in a variety of different viruses. Thus far, simian virus 40, bovine papillomavirus, adenovirus, herpesviruses, and members of the retrovirus family have been used most extensively as expression vectors. Although the relatively small size of these viruses facilitates genetic engineering, this property also restricts the amount of DNA that can be inserted into the virus particle. In addition, virus vectors usually have a limited host range and are defective, requiring either helper virus or special cell lines for replication. Furthermore, many of these vectors are oncogenic and therefore may be unsuitable for use as vaccines in humans and domestic animals. Disadvantages of these viral vector systems can be overcome by inserting and expressing foreign DNA in vaccinia virus.

The Vaccinia Virus Vector

Vaccinia virus, a member of the poxvirus family, is a large, double-stranded DNA virus that packages a complete transcription system and replicates in the cytoplasm of infected cells (Moss, 1974). The virus has a wide host range including humans, cattle, horses, swine, sheep, goats, mice, and monkeys, and a large genome which can accept heterologous genes. Recombinant DNA technology has developed convenient marker rescue techniques and plasmid sequences homologous to the virus DNA, allowing recombination within infected cells (Mackett et al, 1985; Yilma et al, 1985).

There are a number of advantages to the vaccinia virus vector system. Similar to subunit vaccines, this system permits expression of single genes coding for immunogenic proteins. There is also amplification of the antigen, as for live virus vaccines, through DNA replication and transcription. It is possible to make a polyvalent vaccine expressing several genes representing various serotypes of the same agent or a number of unrelated agents. Rapid diagnostic kits can be developed to distinguish vaccinated animals from those exposed to the whole agent by infection or vaccination as, for example, kits we have developed for vesicular stomatitis and foot-and-mouth disease (Workman et al 1986). Finally, unlike many live vaccines, the lyopholized form of vaccinia virus is heat stable, obviating the need for maintaining the cold chain. This is a major advantage in carrying out a successful vaccination program in developing countries.

Construction of a Vaccinia Vector

The strategy for using vaccinia virus as a vector first involves the creation of a plasmid carrying a chimeric gene that consists of a vaccinia virus promoter fused to a foreign protein-coding sequence, flanked by DNA from a nonessential region of the vaccinia virus genome. The chimeric gene then is incorporated into the vaccinia virus genome by homologous recombination in tissue culture cells that have been transfected with the plasmid and infected with wild-type vaccinia virus.

Although any nonessential region of the vaccinia virus genome can be used as the site of gene insertion, the thymidine kinase (TK) gene locus provides some advantages, because recombinants are then TK^-, which distinguishes them from wild-type TK^+ virus. The TK^- phenotype provides a simple method of selection and also serves to attenuate viral pathogenicity (Buller et al 1985). Alternatively, recombinants may be selected by their expression of the inserted foreign gene.

Another selection marker that we use in our laboratory for rapid screening of recombinants of interest is the co-expression of the Escherichia coli β-galactosidase (Lac Z) gene along with the foreign gene of interest. Expression of the Lac Z gene leads to the development of blue plaques in the presence of XGal (5-bromo-4-chloro-3-indolyl-β-D-galactopyranoside). One is thereby able to distinguish TK^- recombinants from spontaneous TK^- mutants (Chakrabarti et al 1985).

Recombinant Rinderpest Vaccine

To illustrate the potential for infectious vaccinia virus recombinant vaccines, we describe here one that we have just developed for rinderpest. This disease is not only the single most important disease of livestock in developing countries, but it also has played a crucial role in the development of the veterinary profession. Rinderpest is an acute, febrile, highly contagious viral disease of ruminants, particularly cattle and buffalo, manifested by a rapid course and high mortality. The disease is characterized by inflammation, hemorrhaging, necrosis, and erosion of the gastrointestinal tract accompanied by bloody diarrhoea, wasting, and death (Plowright, 1968).

The Plowright tissue culture vaccine (PTCV) is widely used for vaccination against rinderpest, but there have been difficulties in sustaining the manufacture of the vaccine, delivery to the field, the need for skilled personnel, a lack of refrigeration, and vaccine instability. In contrast, the lyophilized form of vaccinia virus is heat stable, easily produced and transported, and administered by scarification.

The rinderpest virus (RPV), is enveloped and has a single-stranded RNA genome with a minus polarity. The virus is in the family Paramyxoviridae and is a member of the morbillivirus group, along with measles virus of humans, distemper virus of dogs, and peste-des-petits-ruminants virus (PPRV) of goats and sheep. In paramyxoviruses, the hemagglutinin (HA) and fusion (F) surface proteins have been shown to provide protective immunity. We propagated the highly virulent Kabete "O" strain of RPV in primary bovine kidney cells and characterized eight viral proteins (Grubman et al 1988). We made cDNA copies of the HA and F mRNAs, and determined the complete nucleotide sequence of both the HA and F genes (Yamanaka et al 1988; Hsu et al 1988). Standard procedures were used to construct vaccinia virus recombinants expressing the HA gene (vRVH) and the F gene (vRVF) of RPV (Yilma et al 1988).

The Immune Response to Recombinant Rinderpest Vaccine

Protective immune response studies in cattle were conducted in the high containment facility at the Plum Island Animal Disease Laboratory according to proper institutional guidelines. Humoral responses of cattle were assessed by serum neutralization (SN) assay. Two separate studies were conducted in animals that were shown to be seronegative to RPV prior to vaccination. In the first study, two animals each were vaccinated with either recombinant (vRVH or vRVF), a cocktail of both recombinants (vRVH+vRVF), or PTCV as a positive control. An additional two were left unvaccinated as negative controls. Vaccinia virus recombinants were administered by intradermal inoculation and scarification with 4 X 10^8 PFU of virus, and one ml of PTCV (10^6 $TCID_{50}$) was administered subcutaneously. Four weeks after the primary vaccination, a second dose of recombinant vaccine was administered. Positive controls were not revaccinated with PTCV.

In the second study, only a single vaccination was administered. Five animals were used per group for either recombinant (vRVH or vRVF) or a cocktail of both recombinants (vRVH+vRVF). Two animals were vaccinated with PTCV as positive controls, and two were left unvaccinated as negative controls. For a vaccinia virus control, two were vaccinated with v50, a vaccinia virus recombinant expressing the G gene of vesicular stomatitis virus.

Pock lesions developed as early as four days in all animals vaccinated with the recombinants, but were limited to the site of inoculation and were healed completely by two weeks. All animals vaccinated with the recombinants or PTCV produced SN antibodies to RPV. As expected, control animals had no detectable antibody titer.

To evaluate protection, all animals were challenged with a heavy dose (10^3 $TCID_{50}$) of RPV subcutaneously in the prescapular lymph node region. As low as one $TCID_{50}$ will induce clinical rinderpest with 100% mortality. In the first study animals were challenged on day 42, and in the second study on day 35, following primary immunization.

The animals vaccinated with the recombinants or PTCV were completely protected from rinderpest, exhibiting no detectable illness and a normal temperature of 101°F. All controls developed high fever (108°F) by day two after challenge and died by day 6. They also developed lesions typical of severe rinderpest, characterized by sloughing and erosion of the epithelial lining of the gastrointestinal tract and bloody diarrhoea. After daily monitoring for two weeks and a lack of clinical disease in vaccinated animals, the experiment was terminated.

Discussion

Rinderpest is a potential candidate for eradication using the vaccinia virus recombinant vaccine. There is only one serotype of RPV, although there are different strains manifesting different degrees of pathogenicity in the field. A vaccine against one strain will immunize against all, including PPRV of sheep and goats. Because of the close antigenic relationships of the morbilliviruses, the recombinant vaccine for rinderpest may well have protective activity against distemper in dogs and measles in humans (Plowright 1968). The use of vaccinia virus as a vector which can express heterologous viral antigens allows its use as a live virus vaccine for rinderpest, combining the safety advantages of a subunit vaccine with the antigen amplification and native presentation given by a live attenuated virus vaccine.

Thus we have clearly demonstrated, at least for rinderpest, the potential of vaccinia virus recombinant vaccines to protect against a massive challenge dose of virus. It is important, however, that safety considerations be addressed before introducing live recombinant viruses into the environment. With this in mind, we constructed the recombinant vaccines with the attenuated strain (Wyeth) used worldwide in successful smallpox eradication. It has been demonstrated that insertional inactivation of the TK gene further attenuates this virus. We are also investigating the use of lymphokine genes such as interferon-gamma or interleukin-2 to enhance the immune response and to further attenuate vaccinia virus recombinant vaccines (Yilma et al 1987; Anderson et al 1988). It was recently demonstrated that expression of interleukin-2 prevented disseminated vaccinia virus infection in immunodeficient mice (Flexner et al 1987).

In the World Health Organization smallpox eradication campaign, vaccine was produced by extensively scarifying the skin of a calf and seeding the wounds with vaccinia virus. The scabs from the calf were collected after 7 days, ground in saline, filtered, and the filtrate used for vaccination of humans after testing for pyrogenicity. One calf would yield over 250,000 doses of vaccine. Once lyophilized, smallpox vaccine is very stable for several years. Smallpox vaccine was administered by scarifying the skin using a bifurcated needle or an airgun injector. Similar production and delivery procedures could be used for a vaccinia virus recombinant vaccine, or it could be propagated in tissue culture where facilities are available. Nothing needs to be invented or re-invented for developing countries to be able to cheaply produce large quantities of vaccine. Once the recombinant is available, nomadic herdsmen and other livestock owners could independently conduct both the production and vaccination phases of the program. Alternatively, the governments of developing countries could centrally produce the vaccine for distribution, as in the campaign to eradicate smallpox. In either case, it is not necessary to import manufactured vaccine or syringes and needles.

We have developed an effective vaccinia virus recombinant vaccine for one of the most devastating livestock diseases in Africa and Asia, which eliminates many of the economic and logistical problems of vaccine production, distribution, and administration in these areas. This gives us encouragement to pursue similar strategies in developing vaccines for other livestock diseases.

Acknowledgements

This work was supported by Co-operative Agreement DAN-4178-A-00-6040-00 from the United States Agency for International Development of the State Department.

REFERENCES

1. ANDERSON, P.K., FENNIE, H. and YILMA, T. (1988) Enhancement of a Secondary Antibody Response by Interferon-gamma Treatment at Primary Immunization. J. Immunol 40, 3599-3604.

2. BULLER, R.M.L., SMITH, G.L., CREMER, K., NOTKINS, A.L. and MOSS, B. (1985) Decreased Virulence of Recombinant Vaccinia Virus Expression Vectors is Associated with a Thymidine Kinase-negative Phenotype. Nature 317: 813.

3. CHAKRABARTI, S., BRECHLING, K. and MOSS, B. (1985) Vaccinia Virus Expression Vector: Coexpression of β-galactosidase Provides Visual Screening of Recombinant Virus Plaques. Molecular and Cellular Biology 5: 3403-3409.

4. FLEXNER, C., HUGIN, A. and MOSS, B. (1987) Prevention of Vaccinia Virus Infection in Immunodeficient Mice by Vector-directed IL-2 Expression. Nature 330: 259-262.

5. GRUBMAN, M., MEBUS, C., DALE, B., YAMANAKA, M. and YILMA, T. (1988) Analysis of the Polypeptides Synthesized in Rinderpest Virus-infected Cells. Virology 163: 261-267.

6. HSU, D., YAMANAKA, M., MILLER, J., DALE, B., GRUBMAN, M. and YILMA, T. (1988) Cloning of the Fusion Gene of Rinderpest Virus: Comparative Sequence Analysis with Other Morbilliviruses. Virology 166: 149-153.

7. MACKETT, M., YILMA, T., ROSE, J.K. and MOSS, B. (1985) Vaccinia Virus Recombinants: Expression of VSV Genes and Protective Immunization of Mice and Cattle. Science 227: 433-435.

8. MOSS, B. (1974) Reproduction of Poxviruses. In Comprehensive Virology, vol. 3 (ed. Frankel-Conrat, E.), New York: Plenum Press, pp. 405-474.

9. PLOWRIGHT, W. (1968) <u>Virology Monographs</u> 3: <u>Rinderpest virus</u>. Springer-Verlag, Wein, New York. pp. 25-110.

10. WORKMAN, T., SHEN, D., WOODARD, L. and YILMA, T. (1986) An Enzyme-linked Immunoassay for the Detection of Bovine Antibodies to Vesicular Stomatitis. Am. J. Vet. Res. 47: 1507-1512.

11. YAMANAKA, M. HSU, D., DALE, B., CRISP, T., GRUBMAN, M. and YILMA, T. (1988) Cloning and Sequence Analysis of the Hemagglutinin Gene of the Virulent Strain of Rinderpest Virus. Virology 166: 251-253.

12. YILMA, T., ANDERSON, K., BRECHLING, K. and MOSS, B. In Chanock, R.M., Giensburg, H., Lerner, R. and Brown, F. eds. <u>Vaccines 87 Modern Approaches to New Vaccines including Prevention of AIDS</u>. Cold Spring Harbor Laboratory. Cold Spring Harbor, N.Y., pp. 393-396, 1987.

13. YILMA, T., HSU, D., JONES, L., OWENS, S., GRUBMAN, M., MEBUS, C., YAMANAKA, M. and DALE, B. (1988) Protection of Cattle Against Rinderpest with Infectious Vaccinia Virus Recombinants Expressing the HA or F Gene. Science **242**: 1058-1961.

14. YILMA, T., MACKETT, M., ROSE, J.K. and MOSS, B. Vaccinia Virus Recombinants Expressing Vesicular Stomatitis Genes Immunize Mice and Cattle. In: Quinnan G.V. ed. Vaccinia Viruses as Vectors for Vaccine Antigens. New York: Elsevier-North Holland, pp. 187-200, 1985.

ATTENUATION OF VIRULENCE AND ENHANCEMENT OF IMMUNOGENICITY

by

T Yilma

INTRODUCTION

Attenuation of Virulence

Vaccinia virus recombinant (rVV) vaccines have been developed for a number of important diseases of humans and animals. Two outstanding vaccines have great promise for the eradication of diseases that have devastated both the human and the animal population for centuries (Ada, 1991). The recombinant vaccines developed for rabies (Kieny et al 1984; Rupprecht et al 1986) and rinderpest (Yilma et al 1988; Yilma, 1990, Giavedoni et al 1991) are currently undergoing field testing. These recombinant vaccines combine the advantages of antigen amplification of live attenuated vaccines and the immunogenic specificity of subunit vaccines. It is possible to make a polyvalent vaccine expressing several genes representing various serotypes of the same or a number of unrelated agents (Perkus et al 1985). Unlike many live vaccines, the lyophilized form of vaccinia virus is heat stable, and there is no need for the maintenance of the cold chain, particularly in hot and arid regions of many developing countries. Currently, rVVs are being evaluated as one of several candidate vaccines against a number of human and animal diseases. However, there is a major concern with regard to the safety issues of rVV following the report of a generalized disseminated vaccinia virus infection in an army recruit with subclinical HIV infection after vaccination against smallpox (Redfield et al 1987). It is, therefore, important that safety considerations be addressed before introducing live recombinant viruses into the environment. The rapidly expanding epidemic of HIV, particularly in Africa and Asia, demands that live vaccines do not pose a great threat to the population. Here, five approaches are presented for attenuating live recombinant vaccines.

1. Use of an Attenuated Strain of the Virus

Many strains of vaccinia virus have been utilized up to the 20th century for vaccination against smallpox. There was great variation in the incidence of complications to smallpox vaccinations, and this was in part dependent on the strain of vaccinia virus used. For example, high incidence of complication (1 per 4000 primary vaccinees) has been reported for the Copenhagen strain. In contrast, low incidence of complication (2 to 6 per 1,000,000 primary vaccinees) was reported for the Wyeth (the New York Board of Health) strain. The World Health Organization has recommended the use of a number of attenuated stains of vaccinia virus to diminish the chances of producing complications (Neff 1985).

2. Insertional Inactivation of Virulence Genes

It has been demonstrated for a number of DNA viruses that insertional inactivation of the thymidine kinase (TK) leads to the attenuation of the virus. For vaccinia virus, the inactivation of the TK gene was manifested by reduced replication and virulence to mice and reduction in the size of pock lesions at sites of vaccination (Buller et al 1985).

In the course of development of a double recombinant vaccine for rinderpest, our group recently demonstrated that the insertional inactivation of both the TK and the hemagglutinin (HA) genes lead to further attenuation of vaccinia virus (Giavedoni, et al 1991). This was manifested by lack of pock lesions in vaccinated cattle without any detectable reduction in immunogenicity and protective immunity against rinderpest.

3. Co-Expression of Lymphokine and Immunogenic Genes

In 1986, we described a novel approach of expressing immunoregulatory genes in vaccinia virus for modifying the immune response to both homologous and heterologous antigens expressed by the vector (Yilma, et al 1987). Subsequently, our group and others have demonstrated that the expression of lymphokine genes such as interferon-gamma and interleukin-2 by vaccinia virus attenuates the vector and prevents disseminated, progressive infections in immunodeficient, athymic (nu/nu) mice (Yilma, et al 1987; Ramshaw, et al 1987; Flexner, et al 1987). Thus, this approach may greatly reduce the associated risks and permit widespread and safe use of live virus recombinants as human and veterinary vaccines.

4. Expression of Chimeric Proteins of Immunogens and Lymphokines

We have just reported the development of a novel, approach for the attenuation of live recombinant vaccines. This consists of the construction of chimeric genes of immunogens and lymphokines. We illustrated this concept by demonstrating reduced pathogenicity for nude mice of several vaccinia virus recombinants expressing chimeric proteins of human and murine IFN- and various immunogens derived from the human immunodeficiency virus (HIV-I). Furthermore, we provided evidence that the antiviral and attenuating activities of IFN- have different mechanisms of action. Unlike the antiviral activity, we demonstrated that the attenuating activity of IFN- is not species specific. Moreover, we showed the presence of the attenuating activity of IFN- in the absence of any detectable antiviral activity (Giavedoni, et al 1992).

Enhancement of Immunogenicity

The nature of the host's immune response to an injected antigen is critical in vaccination, and it is frequently desirable to employ some form of adjuvant to boost the immune response. However, live vaccines are inactivated by chemical adjuvants, and their use with inactivated vaccines is limited in practice to the few less effective chemical adjuvants, such as alum conjugates. The most effective adjuvant to date, complete Freund's adjuvant (CFA), dramatically increases the response to antigen in most test systems but is not acceptable for clinical use, even in livestock, because of the intense inflammatory response of vaccinates and their conversion to tuberculin positivity.

In our studies in vaccinology and the effective use of adjuvants, we have developed a number of different types of vaccines for vesicular stomatitis (VS) and compared them for antibody response and protective capacity in cattle and mice. VSV is an enveloped, negative-strand RNA virus which causes a severe debilitating vesicular disease in cattle, horses and swine that is characterized by lesions on the oral mucosa, particularly the tongue. Vesicles often develop on the snout in pigs and on the teats in cows. In cattle and pigs, there may also be lesions on the foot along the coronary band and in the interdigital space.

Because of its excellent immunogenic properties and ease of purification (Volk et al 1982; Yilma et al 1985) we have isolated the envelope G glycoprotein subunit of VSV and used it as a successful vaccine. Antibodies raised to G glycoprotein neutralize infectivity of VSV both in vitro (Kelley et al 1972) and in vivo (Dietschold et al 1974). Therefore, an in vitro virus neutralization test can be used to monitor levels of protective antibodies, and the in vivo protective effects of immunization can be evaluated. When administered with complete Freund's adjuvant (CFA), this subunit vaccine provided complete protection against 400X the infectious dose necessary to reproduce the disease.

The best possibilities for effective adjuvants which can be used with recombinant vaccines now appear to be immunoregulatory proteins such as interferons and interleukins. Interleukin-2, one of the most promising, is a lymphokine released from lymphocytes triggered by antigen, mitogen, or allo-antigen, that functions to switch T cells from G1 into the proliferative phases. IL-2 activity is characterized in vitro by its ability to maintain cytotoxic cells and functional T-helper cells in culture (Morgan et al 1976), and acts indirectly to aid in B-cell maturation. Studies in model systems utilizing purified and recombinant DNA-derived IL-2 and IFN-gamma show that IL-2 regulates the production of IFN-gamma by the thymocyte population. While the role of IFN-gamma may be to drive B cells into functional secreting plasma cells, IL-2 is one of the growth factors important earlier in the pathway (Reem and Yeh 1985). Others have also demonstrated the adjuvant effects of interleukin-2 (Nunberg et al 1989).

Interferon-gamma is a secreted polypeptide product of stimulated T-lymphocytes which has potent immunomodulatory properties as well as antiviral activity (Sonnenfeld et al 1978; Gresser et al 1979). Treatment of macrophages and other specific cell types with recombinant DNA-derived IFN-gamma can induce or enhance expression of class II major histocompatibility (MHC) products (King and Jones 1983; Wong et al 1983; Skoskiewicz et al 1985; Chang and Lee 1986), and treatment of purified resting B-lymphocytes can stimulate proliferation and differentiation into immunoglobulin secreting cells (Leibson et al 1984; Sidman et al 1984; Nakagawa et al 1985; Romagnani et al 1986). In addition, in vivo administration of recombinant DNA-derived murine IFN-gamma in conjunction with immunization has been reported to enhance immune responses to specific antigens (Nakamura et al 1984; Playfair and de Souza 1987).

We have investigated the effects of in vivo IFN-γ treatment on the antibody response of mice and cattle to the purified envelope "G" glycoprotein of the VSV virion. Administration of recombinant DNA derived IFN-γ at the time of initial immunization with purified "G" glycoprotein enhances the magnitude of a secondary virus neutralizing antibody response following a booster administration of the same antigen without IFN-γ treatment. This enhancement occurred even in animals in which no significant enhancement of the primary neutralizing antibody response was observed. Furthermore, cattle treated with IFN-γ at the time of a single primary immunization were more resistant to a subsequent viral challenge than those immunized without IFN-γ treatment (Anderson et al 1988).

No signs of inflammation were observed in either mice or cattle treated with IFN-γ, and relatively low doses of IFN-γ were required to elicit enhanced antibody titers. Optimum enhancement of the secondary antibody response in mice occurred at a dose of approximately 15 (OAmg/square meter). This dose is far below that where minimal side effects such as chills and fatigue have been observed in human volunteers following intramuscular injection (50-100 μg/square meter), and is less than the maximum tolerated dose in humans by a factor of 30 (Foon et al 1985; Kurzrock et al 1986). IFN-γ treatment in conjunction with primary immunization therefore has the potential for use as an effective, non-inflammatory, immune adjuvant. Whether IFN-γ can enhance the activity of currently available adjuvants or work synergistically with other cytokines and differentiation factors has yet to be explored.

These studies demonstrate that interferon gamma (IFN-gamma) duplicates the adjuvant effect of CFA when administered with the VSV G-glycoprotein subunit vaccine, and further increases the anamnestic response to G on booster administration (Yilma et al 1989). IFN-gamma treatment in conjunction with primary immunization may therefore provide a practical means of enhancing

protection from viral challenge without inflammatory adjuvants or boosters. It has been demonstrated previously that IFNs have little or no antiviral activity against a number of DNA viruses (Stewart, 1979), a distinct advantage for the use of IFNs with infectious vaccinia virus recombinant vaccines.

Acknowledgements

This work was supported by a Co-operative Agreement DAN-4178-A-00-6040-00 from the United States Agency for International Development of the State Department.

REFERENCES

1. ADA, G. (1991) Nature **349**, 369.

2. KIENY, M.F., LATHE, R., DRILLEN, R., SPEHNER, D., SKORY, S., SCHMITT, D., WIKTOR, T., KOPROWSKI, H. and LECOCQ, J.P. (1984) Nature (London) **312**, 163-166.

3. RUPPRECHT, C.E., WIKTOR, T.J., JOHNSTON, D.H., HAMIR, A.N., DIETZSCHOLD, B., WUNNER, W.H., GLICKMAN, L.T. and KOPROWSKI, H. (1986) Proc. Natl. Aca. Sci USA **83**, 7947-7950.

4. YILMA, T., HSU, D., JONES, L., OWENS, S., GRUBMAN, M., MEBUS, C., YAMANAKA, M. and DALE, B. (1988) Science **242**, 1058-1061.

5. YILMA, T. (1989) Vaccine **7**, 484-485.

6. YILMA, T. (1990) Biotechnology **8**, 1007-1009.

7. PERKUS, E.m PICCINI, A., LIPINSKAS, B.R. and PAOLETTI, E. (1985) Science **229**, 981-984.

8. REDFIELD, R.R., WRIGHT, D.C., JAMES, W.D., JONES, T.S., BROWN, C., BURKE, D.S. (1987) N. Engl. J. Med. **316**, 673-676.

9. NEFF, J. (1985) in Vaccinia Viruses as Vectors for Vaccine Antigens, ed. Quinnan, G.V. (Elsevier-North Holland, NY), pp 187-200.

10. BULLER, R.M.L., SMITH, G.L., CREMER, K., NOTKINS, A.L. and MOSS, B. (1985) Nature **317**, 813-815.

11. GIAVEDONI, L.D., JONES, L., MEBUS, C. and YILMA, T. (1991) Proc. Natl. Acad. Sci, USDA, **88**, 8011-8015.

12. YILMA, T., ANDERSON, K., BRECHLING, K. and MOSS, B. (1987) In: Chanock RM, Giensburg H, Lerne R, Brown F eds. Vaccines 87 Modern Approaches to New Vaccines including Prevention of Aids. Cold Spring Harbor Laboratory, Cold Spring Harbor, NY, pp. 393-396, 1987.

13. RAMSHAW, I.A., ANDREW, M.E., PHILLIPS, S.M., BOYLE, D.B. and COUPAR, B.E.H. (1987) Nature **329**, 545-546.

14. FLEXNER, C., HUGIN, A., MOSS, B. (1987) Nature **330**, 259-262.

15. GIAVEDONI, L.D., JONES, L., GIBSON, H., LEE NG+, C.T., BARR, P.J. and YILMA, T. (1992). Proc Natl. Acad. Sci, USA, **89**, 3409-3413.

16. VOLK, W.A., SNYDER, R.M., BENJAMIN, D.C. and WAGNER, R.R. (1982) J. Virol. **42**;220.

17. YILMA, T., BREEZE, R.G., RISTOW, S., GORHAM, J. and LEIB, S.R. (1985) Adv. Exp. Med. Biol. **150**, 101-115.

18. KELLEY, J.M. EMERSON, S.U. and WAGNER, R.R. (1972) J. Virol. **10**;1231.

19. DIETZCHOLD, B., SCHNEIDER. L.G. and COX, J.H. (1974). J. Virol. **14**;1.

20. MORGAN, D.A., RUSCIETTI, F.W., GALLO, R. (1976) Science **240**;1007.

21. SONNENFELD, G., MANDEL, A.D. and MERIGAN, T.C. (1978) Cell. Immun. **140**, 285-293.

22. GRESSER, I.J., DeMAEYER-GUIGNARD, M.G., TOVEY, S. and DeMAEYER E. (1979) Proc. Natl. Acad. Sci. USA **76**, 5308-5310.

23. KING, D.P. and JONES, P.P. (1983) J. Immun. **131**;315.

24. WONG, G.H.W. CLARK-LEWIS, I., McKINN-BRESCHKIN, J.L., HARRIS, A.W. and SCHRADER, J. (1983) J. Immun. **131**;788.

25. SKOSKIEWICZ, M.J., COLVIN, R.B., SCHNEEBERGER, E.E. and RUSSELL, P.S. (1985) J. Exp. Med. **162**;1645.

26. CHANG, R. and LEE, S. H., J. Immun (1986) J. Immunol. **137**;;2853.

27. LEIBSON, H.J., GEFTER, H.J. ZLOTNIK, A., MARRAK, P. and KAPPLER, J.W. (1984) Nature **309**, 799-801.

28. SIDMAN, C.L., MARSHALL, J.D., SCHULTZ, L.D., GRAY, P.W. and JOHNSON, H.M. (1984) Nature **309**, 801-804.

29. NAKAGAWA, T., HIRANO, T., NAKAGAWA, N., YOSHIZAKI, K. and KISHIMOTO, T. (1985) J. Immunol. **134**, 959-966.

30. ROMANGNANI, S., GIUDIZI, M.G., BIAGIOTTI, R., ALMERIGOGNA, F., MINGARI, C., MAGGI, E., LIANG, C. and MORETTA, L. (1986) J. Immunol. **136**, 513-528.

31. PLAYFAIR, J.H.L. and de SOUZA, J.B. (1987) Clin. Exp. Immunol. **67**, 5-10.

32. ANDERSON, K.P., FENNIE, E.H. and YILMA, T. (1988) J. Imm. **140**, 3599-3604.

33. FOON, K.A., SHERWIN, S.A., ABRAMS, P.G., STEVENSON, H.C., HOLMES, P., MALUISH, A.E., OLDHAM, R.K. and HERBERMAN R.B. (1985) Cancer Immunol. Immunother. **20**, 193-201.

34. KURZROCK, R., QUESADA, J.R. TALPAZ, M., HERSH, E.M., REUBEN, J.M., SHERWIN, S.A. and GUTTERMAN, J.U. (1986) J. Clin. Onc. **4**;1101.

35. YILMA, T., OWENS, S., FENNIE, E.H. and ANDERSON, K.P. (1989) Adv. Exp. Med. Biol. **155**, 145-152.

36. STEWART, W II. (1979) The Interferon System (Springer-Verlag, New York).

Discussion

Dr Rweyemamu asked for guidance on three points:

1. He wondered whether in view of the new types of immuno-propylactics being developed there was not a case for re-categorising vaccines into infectious live agents and non-infectious vaccines. He was concerned about how quality control tests would be implemented for the new recombinant vaccines.

2. He considered the rinderpest and rabies recombinants as candidate vaccines now in the appraisal stage of development which could replace the existing more conventional preparations. He wanted to know under what circumstances they would most likely be used.

3. He also wanted to know if the rabies recombinant vaccine was likely to be of greatest use in controlling rabies in stray dogs and jackals? - What are the target populations for this vaccine?

Prof Yilma in answer pointed out that the rabies recombinant is now being successfully used in Europe and is currently being licenced in some states in the USA for filed application. Africa is an obvious situation where it could be widely used.

In the case of rinderpest there was now the guidelines which had been put together by OIE and WHO for its use in the field.

Dr Mebus added that in the later stages of a rinderpest eradication campaign, the vaccinia rinderpest recombinant could be of value, particularly when there was no obvious circulation of field virus in animal populations. With regard to rabies, the most apparent use for the recombinant was the immunisation of wild species which were not accessible to conventional needle vaccination.

Prof Yilma pointed out that a significant advantage was that the recombinant vaccine stimulated much higher antibody titres than the existing rabies vaccines and in his opinion could and should be used for most species including humans!

Dr Ozawa suggested that since the rabies preparation is an oral one (and generates high antibody titres) and the rinderpest recombinant is applied by needle - if the rinderpest campaigns are not ultimately successful, consideration to a new approach such as an oral vaccine might be of value.

Dr Mowat asked about the possibility of recombinant virus spreading from animal to man, and the associated risk of adverse reactions in a small number of people so infected.

Prof Yilma accepted that there was in theory, a possibility of such an effect, but with the double insertion recombinant virus, that risk was extremely small perhaps in the region of 2 to 3 reactions in 10 million exposed people. The greatest risk would be with immuno-compromised individuals such the T cell depleted HIV positive person.

Dr Stouraitis thought the new vaccines were of great promise, but in exploiting them in disease control campaigns in the developing countries he wondered who would provide the basic technology and the starting materials. He also thought that some countries might want to have this technology before they were able to use it and he cautioned regarding the speed at which it was made available to all.

Dr Doel replied to Dr Stouraitis that the principal advantage at present of synthetic vaccines was their ability to be used as research tools to investigate the key antigenic components of, for example, FMD virus. In his opinion the present work on recombinants will lead to effective vaccines for FMD. Transfer of technology should not present any more problems than those associated with the large scale production of E. coli or other similar industrial products. The speed and availability of this technology will be in the hands of the commercial sector.

Dr Cheneau asked about the duration of immunity to be expected with recombinant vaccines. If repeated vaccinations were required and the vaccine was not inexpensive, then the benefits to be obtained from its use would be uncertain. Dr Cheneau also asked whether the technology would be made available without charge or would the recipients be expected to pay for its use.

Prof Yilma in reply, stated that at the recent meeting at OIE, it was agreed that duration of immunity should be the subject of an investigation that would take up to 5 years to complete. However, it was his opinion that the duration of immunity was likely to be very similar to that found with the tissue culture vaccine, since the specific immunity was a function of the antigen and not that of the vector.

Dr Mebus was of the opinion that since protection against rinderpest was easy to produce there was no reason to think that the immunity generated by the recombinant would be any different to that given by the tissue culture vaccine.

Prof Yilma stated that the only way to be sure, was to do the experiments and perhaps FAO will give support to that! He also told the meeting that the University of California had agreed that the technology should be available free of charge and the reason for patent protection was to ensure that it was not exploited unreasonably by commerce. Transfer of technology in Prof Yilma's terms is concerned with training scientists so that they may apply the new technology for other organisms, in their home situation - and is not concerned with the sale of product.

Dr Bhat stated that the IVRI has been testing the recombinant developed in Japan, and the presence of antibodies after 11 months has been demonstrated. Further work on the same lines will continue for the next 5 years. He wanted to know what happens after the second inoculation of the recombinant.

Prof Yilma replied that there is an anamnestic response to the same foreign antigen, however, if the second application of a recombinant carries a different antigen, then the antibodies to the vaccinia tend to suppress an immune response to the new antigen.

Dr Mannathoko enquired about the cost of the rabies recombinant vaccine in comparison to that of the conventional vaccine. The reply was that it would be approximately the same, but because the new vaccine could generate very much higher titres it could be considered cheaper in terms of results. The original method described by WHO of producing vaccinia by the scarification method with calves is very cheap - about 300,000 doses of material can be produced from one calf by this method.

Dr Wojciechowski told the meeting that as a result of consultations between FAO and OIE, strict guidelines for the conduct of small scale field trials of the new vaccine had been laid down. In addition, countries have their own national committees to advise on bio-hazards, and in consequence there are several stages or barriers which must be passed before there could be widespread application of recombinant vaccines. At present Prof Yilma's vaccine is under assessment in a small trial in Ethiopia, being held under the aegis of FAO and with the technical assistance of PANVAC. Only when this trial has shown satisfactory and safe results, will the next stage - a larger trial be started and only after that will it be released for wider application. There are also other candidate vaccines in the pipeline, some of which make use of other large DNA viruses, such as the attenuated strain of capripox virus. There are, therefore likely to be several possible ways of exploiting the recombinant vector technology in the future.

Dr Ozawa entered a note of caution by stating that the guidelines formulated by OIE and FAO were regarded by some workers as the minimum level of safeguards which should be applied to this work.

Dr Doel made the point that he did not think it was possible to have a small scale field trial with replicating agents. In his opinion there was no such thing!

At that point the Vice-Chairman drew the discussion to a close with the comment that the Consultation had been given a fascinating glimpse into the future of veterinary immunisation and the discussion had been extensive and worthwhile.

Major Vaccination Campaigns in Developing Countries

THE ROLE OF PANVAC IN THE QUALITY CONTROL OF VETERINARY VACCINES FOR MAJOR VACCINATION PROGRAMMES IN AFRICA

by

D Sylla, M Rweyemamu, V Palya and J Prandota

EVOLUTION OF PANVAC

Infectious diseases such as rinderpest, contagious bovine pleuropneumonia, Newcastle disease and foot-and-mouth disease continue to be the most important constraints to the development and productivity of the African livestock industry. The continuing presence of these epizootic diseases in Africa constantly poses a major threat to the world livestock economies. Zoonotic diseases, for example rabies and Rift Valley fever, are also common in Africa. The only realistic approach for controlling epizootic diseases in Africa is by effective and regionally co-ordinated immunization programmes.

It is against this background that the Inter African Bureau for Animal Resources of the OAU (OAU/IBAR) has engaged itself in the co-ordination of two major programmes for the control of rinderpest. The first was the Joint Project 15 (JP 15) which was implemented in phases. In West Africa (1962-69) the campaign progressed in three phases, in East Africa (1969-76) the campaign was implemented in the same way. The JP 15 was very successful since the incidence of rinderpest was substantially reduced. Unfortunately, the follow-up measures were not strictly adhered to and as a consequence, rinderpest reappeared in the early 1980's. A second joint continental campaign, known as the Pan-African Rinderpest Campaign (PARC) was therefore started in 1986. It should be noted that PARC was initiated after two major FAO Expert Consultations. The first, in 1984, was concerned with rinderpest diagnosis, vaccine production and quality control. The second, in 1986, was on Global Eradication of Rinderpest. This latter one was an important technical milestone for such campaigns as PARC, WAREC and SAREC.

Following the 1984 FAO Expert Consultation, a system for international quality control of rinderpest vaccine in Africa was set up. The initial programme consisted of collecting samples from 11 production laboratories and hand-carrying such samples to Pirbright and Paris for testing by the two FAO international reference laboratories. The majority of these samples failed to attain the prescribed level of potency and many also failed in sterility.

Consequently, when the PARC programme was started in 1986, FAO was requested to set up, within Africa, an international system for vaccine quality control. This was established as two independent units based on the national vaccine laboratories at Dakar, Senegal and Debre Zeit, Addis Ababa, Ethiopia. FAO initiated these two units under its own Technical Co-operation Programme (TCP).

The initial emphasis was for the two units to test for vacuum, potency (titration) and sterility of the vaccines held by PARC in the 5 designated rinderpest vaccine banks. Soon it became obvious that this limited programme was likely to be inadequate both in support of PARC and in stimulating vaccine production in Africa utilising the most appropriate and relevant technologies.

Consequently, with the financial assistance of UNDP, in 1988 a new project (UNDP/FAO/RAF/88/050) was set up to take over the work initiated by FAO and OAU under the FAO TCP programme. The title of the new project was: *Production and Quality Control of Veterinary Vaccines in Africa.*

The development objective of RAF/88/050 was clearly broader than that initiated under the previous TCP. The objective was: *"To make Africa self sufficient in priority veterinary vaccines by the year 2000"*. In order to reflect this long-term intention and the Pan-African nature of their activities, the two units originally set up under the FAO project, became jointly named as the PAN AFRICAN VETERINARY VACCINE CENTRE (PANVAC).

The mandate of PANVAC has been defined by all the parties concerned, ie OAU, FAO and UNDP, as comprising the following:

(i) International Quality Control of priority vaccines;

(ii) Promotion of concepts of biological standardization and control in Africa.

(iii) Transfer to Africa of appropriate vaccine production technologies including their adaptation or development to suit African conditions.

(iv) Provide training and such support services as repair and maintenance of vaccine equipment.

There are 23 vaccine producing countries in Africa who participate in the PANVAC project network. Table 1 summarises the list of vaccines produced in Africa from which it will be apparent that there are some 26 different types of vaccines produced under a variety of technologies. A peculiarity of Africa, in this regard, is the almost total absence of private, commercial enterprise in vaccine production. Only one international vaccine manufacturing company has a manufacturing facility in Africa, which is jointly owned by the host government and limits its activity to 2 - albeit major - vaccines. In another country, a fully government owned parastatal company has been set up to be responsible for the production and marketing of all veterinary vaccines. Elsewhere, in Africa, vaccines are produced by the veterinary departments themselves, although it has to be noted that in many countries there are moves to set up vaccine production sections as self accounting units.

ATTITUDES OF THE PANVAC BENEFICIARIES

The goals of PANVAC, as defined above, have been endorsed by all the responsible bodies in Africa, such as the International PARC Technical Committee, the Directors of National Vaccine Laboratories, the Directors of Veterinary Services and, above all, the Ministers responsible for livestock development in Africa. Thus, for example, the directors of national vaccine laboratories identified priority vaccines as:

Table 1: VETERINARY VACCINES PRODUCED IN AFRICA

Country	FMD	RP	LSD	BT	RVF	S/G Pox	ORF	AHS	CSF	ND	F/ Pox	IBD	RAB	RP/ CBPP	CBPP	CCPP	ANTR	BLEG	BPAST	BRUC	ASALM	APAST
Angola																						
Botswana	X	X																				
Cameroon		X								X			X		X		X	X	X			X
Chad		X	X			X				X	X		X	X	X		X	X	X	X		X
Côte D'Ivoire																						
Ethiopia		X				X		X		X				X	X		X	X	X			
Guinea		X								X	X		X		X		X		X		X	X
Kenya	X	X	X	X	X	X	X			X	X		X		X	X					X	
Lesotho										X												
Madagascar									X	X	X		X		X		X	X	X			X
Malawi										X												
Mali		X													X		X	X				
Mozambique										X	X		X				X	X		X		
Niger		X								X					X		X	X	X			
Nigeria		X								X	X	X	X		X		X	X	X	X	X	X
Rwanda																					X	
Senegal		X				X									X	X	X	X	X			
Somalia																						
Sudan		X								X					X		X	X	X			
Tanzania																	X	X	X	X	X	
Uganda										X												
Zambia													X				X	X	X	X		
Zaire										X	X		X				X			X		
TOTAL	2	11	2	1	1	4	1	1	1	14	7	1	9	2	11	2	14	12	11	6	5	5

Abberation
==========

FMD = Foot and Mouth Disease
RP = Rinderpest
LSD = Lumpy Skin Disease
BT = Blue Tongue
RFV = Rift Valley Fever
S/G Pox = Sheep and Goat Pox
ORF = Contagious pustular derumatitis
AHS = African Horse Sickness
CSF = Classical Swine Fever
ND = Newcastle Disease
F/Pox = Fowl pox

IBD = Infectious Bursal Disease
RAB = Rabies
RP/CBPP = Rinderpest/Contagious Bovine Pleuropneumonia combined
CBPP = Contagious Bovine Pleuropneumonia
CCPP = Contagious Caprine Pleuropneumonia
ANTR = Abthrax
BLEG = Blackleg
BPAST = Haemorrhagis Septicaemia
BRUC = Bovine Brucellosis
ASALM = Fowl typhoid
APAST = Fowl Cholera

Rinderpest
Contagious bovine pleuropneumonia (CBPP)
Newcastle Disease
Rabies
Foot and Mouth disease (for Eastern and Southern Africa)
A model bacterial vaccine to be identified on a regional basis.

Also at their meeting held in Nairobi on the 27th and 28th September, 1990, the Directors of vaccine laboratories made recommendations on the following other aspects:

1. *Good Manufacturing Practices (GMP)*

That PANVAC should stimulate the awareness of vaccine producers in Africa to concepts of GMP and Quality Assurance.

2. *Vaccine Manufacturing Laboratories*

That these should be in buildings which are ISOLATED from laboratories for diagnosis and research on infectious diseases.

That within the vaccine manufacturing facilities, there should be separate production and quality control sections.

That countries should take steps to allow vaccines to be produced under commercial (parastatal or private) arrangements while quality control authority should be retained by governments. In any case, vaccine production laboratories should be allowed to sell vaccines and keep funds thus generated and thereby enjoy financial autonomy.

3. *International Quality Control and Certification of Veterinary Vaccines in Africa*

Considering the experience gained by PANVAC in the certification of rinderpest vaccine quality, the Directors recommended that:

PANVAC should be the appropriate agency for international quality control of vaccines in Africa.

PANVAC should extend its work beyond rinderpest vaccine in order to be able to certify all priority vaccines - particularly in relation to export of vaccines from one country to another.

4. *Regionalization of Vaccine Production, Distribution and Marketing*

That countries within the same region should co-operate in vaccine production so as to take advantages of technical expertise available in the region, to maximize on economies of scale and to avoid duplication of small, economically inefficient vaccine production units.

One of the key resolutions of the 3rd Ministerial Conference held in Nairobi October, 1990, urged the Secretary General of the OAU to seek all assistance to convert PANVAC from a project base to a long term activity which strengthens the institutional and technical capability of OAU/IBAR. This has been endorsed by the OAU Council of Ministers and now forms part of OAU policy. FAO has been requested by the OAU/IBAR to assist with the technical aspects.

PANVAC'S PROGRAMME FOR PRIORITY VACCINES

Until now resources have limited the activity of PANVAC to 3 vaccines.

1. Rinderpest

As to be expected, PANVAC has been principally engaged with rinderpest vaccine. This has included testing on behalf of PARC about 320 batches between 1988 and the present, the establishment of reference Master Seed banks for both rinderpest vaccine virus and Vero cells. It should be noted that in Africa only the Kabete 0 strain of Plowright is used for vaccine production. Originally, only the calf kidney cell culture adapted virus was employed. The virus and cell banks were set up with the help and co-operation of the Institute for Animal Health, Pirbright, U.K. Recently, however, through the collaborative effort of PANVAC, the Plum Island Animal Diseases Center and Tufts University, a VERO cell adapted virus has been introduced into some national vaccine production laboratories.

PANVAC has now standardised the quality control testing of rinderpest vaccine to levels comparable with those of the British and European Pharmacopoeia standards for bovine live viral vaccines. A manual for The Standard Operating Procedures (SOP) for rinderpest vaccine quality control testing has been produced and distributed to vaccine producers in Africa. The tests described include:

- test for sterility (bacteria, fungi)
- test for brucella (for Seed virus)
- test for absence of mycoplasmas
- test for potency:
  . estimation of virus content
  . efficacy test in cattle
- test for rinderpest identity and for adventitious agents:
  . staining of cell cultures by H&E
  . test for haemadsorbing agents
  . test for BVD virus by IPX method
- safety tests:
  . in small animals (innocuity test)
  . in cattle

Progressively, countries who participate in the PARC programme have been urged by OAU/IBAR to use for their rinderpest campaign only vaccine certified by PANVAC.

2. Contagious Bovine Pleuropneumonia Vaccine (CBPP)

In spite of the economic importance of CBPP in Africa, there has been no major co-ordinated vaccination campaign for this disease, except for a brief period in West Africa under the aborted JP-28 programme. The control of CBPP, however, has now been identified by IBAR for the next phase of PARC. Therefore, PANVAC has been asked to commence work on this vaccine.

In support of this, PANVAC with consultants from the IEMVT, organised a workshop at the Central Veterinary Laboratory, Bamako, November 1990, to consider the proposed OIE Norms for CBPP vaccine and harmonization of vaccine manufacturing procedures. Thus of the four different strains of Mycoplasma mycoides subsp. mycoides that have been used in Africa (ie the KH_3J, KH_37-SR, $T_1/44$ and T_1-SR), it has been recommended that CBPP vaccine production can be standardised by use of the T_1-SR mutant as the sole standard vaccine strain. This recommendation is supported by the following considerations:

(i) The immunogenic properties of the T_1-SR mutant are indistinguishable from those of its parent, $T_1/44$ strain.

(ii) T_1-SR mutant seems to induce fewer post vaccinal local reactions than $T_1/44$. Even with European cattle breeds only minimum post vaccinal reactions have been reported.

(iii) The yield of the T_1-SR mutant from culture containing streptomycin, tends to be greater (reported as 10 to 100 times) than that of the $T_1/44$ parent strain.

(iv) The best characterized vaccine strain is the T_1-SR. The streptomycin resistance of the mutant can be used as a marker for this vaccine strain.

Another important recommendation was that all producers should endeavour to freeze dry their product (PANVAC Bulletin Vol.1, No.3, p2).

It should be noted that until now no standard operating procedures for the quality control of CBPP vaccine have been developed and so far no international quality control data on CBPP vaccine produced in Africa are available. PANVAC has started routine quality control of this vaccine and hopes to issue SOP's.

3. Newcastle Disease vaccine

As in the case of CBPP, PANVAC's approach has been initially to convene a workshop of African producers of ND vaccine and to invite international experts on the subject to address the workshop. These were from Weybridge (UK), Queensland University in Australia and Reading University, UK. Important outcomes of the PANVAC workshop on Newcastle Disease Vaccines for Rural Africa, have been the desire to harmonize vaccine production methods, to work towards rationalization of vaccination regimes for the different poultry keeping practices in Africa, and to undertake trials to evaluate such systems as have been developed by Australasian groups, for vaccination of free range village chickens. The Australian Centre for International Agricultural Research also generously supported the participation of 3 participants from Africa in a recent workshop in Kuala Lumpur on Newcastle disease vaccines for free range chickens.

It is hoped to initiate some activity on Newcastle disease vaccine during 1992.

GLOBAL STRATEGIES FOR RINDERPEST ERADICATION[3]

by

K J Wojciechowski

INTRODUCTION

The first FAO Expert Consultation on Global Strategy for Control and Eradication of Rinderpest, February 1987 (4) reviewed rinderpest campaigns of the past and the present status of the disease and discussed technical and non-technical requirements, as well as strategies to be accepted. It concluded that ... a final internationally coordinated assault upon rinderpest should be made with global eradication as its target.."

During 1991 rinderpest was officially reported from Africa in: Ethiopia, Kenya, Sudan, and from Asia in Nepal, India (Southern States Andhra Pradesh, Karnataka, Kerala, Tamil Nadu), Sri Lanka, Lebanon, Oman, Yemen and Turkey (1,8). However, there are strong suspicions that the disease can be present in some endemic areas of Africa, Far East/West Asia and South Asia affected by civil strife and political instability - so called: "no-go areas". Also some under-reporting motivated by economic and political reasons may take place. There are numerous countries especially in Asia reporting the absence of rinderpest to OIE/FAO but they continue to vaccinate animals against the disease.

Campaign PARC (since 1987), West Asia Rinderpest Campaign. **WAREC** (since 1989), and advanced preparation for the South Asia Rinderpest Eradication Campaign, **SAREC**. Since the early 1980's, FAO has been actively involved in the preparation of regional rinderpest campaigns and has implemented and coordinated numerous activities on the subject. The FAO Expert Consultation on Rinderpest Diagnosis, Vaccine Production and Quality Control, which was held in Rome, 1984 (3), gave recommendations on specific issues. FAO has arranged for consultancies, meetings, training activities, publications, audio-visual materials, projects in support of regional campaigns, technical aspects involved, and formulation of regional strategies of rinderpest control and eradication. The OIE prepared, with the participation of FAO, the "Requirements for Rinderpest Cell Culture Vaccine (Live)", 1987, "Requirements for Rinderpest Vaccinia Vector Recombinant Vaccines", 1989 and the Report of the OIE "Expert Consultation on Rinderpest Surveillance Systems", 1989 (9,10,11). They are milestones in building up technical capabilities for international rinderpest control. Promotion of several technical issues such as: vaccines, disease surveillance, epidemiology, immunology, resulted in the development of basic and applied research on the subjects. The trained specialists: managers, vaccinators, animal health workers, communicators, diagnosticians, vaccine technologists, as well as institutions, established in Africa the Pan African Veterinary Vaccine Centre (PANVAC) in Debre-Zeit, Ethiopia and Dakar, Senegal, and the Epidemiology Unit for PARC in Nairobi) have strengthened regional veterinary and livestock services and become models for other continents. The Experts Consultation on Global Strategy for Control and Eradication of Rinderpest (Rome 1987) revised requirements and stations by regional rinderpest campaigns.

---

[3] Text revised by author May 1993.

THE PAN-AFRICAN RINDERPEST CAMPAIGN (PARC)

Preparations for PARC. A meeting organized by FAO took place in Nairobi (1981) and proposed that the **Pan African Rinderpest Campaign-PARC** be implemented by OAU/IBAR. FAO played an important role in formulating PARC strategy and arrangements for PARC by preparing project operation and funding documents. Strategy for the Campaign was finally defined in 1984. The Campaign started in mid-1986 and in late 1987 the field activities of PARC were initiated with EEC as the major donor, as well as the FAO, ODA-UK, World Bank, Nigeria, Japan, Italy and France, for campaigns to cover 34 countries of sub-Saharan Africa (6,13).

Apart from the efforts to control and eradicate rinderpest by individual countries,**the first modern attempt to eradicate rinderpest from Africa** began in the 1960's under coordination of the Inter-African Bureau of Animal Resources of the OAU. The campaign known as **Joint Project 15 (JP 15)** with multi-donor technical and financial assistance started in the countries of the Lake Chad basin (22 countries were covered) lasting 14 years (1962-76) at a cost to donors of US$ 50 million. The campaign led to a significant decrease in incidence. However it failed to eradicate rinderpest due to residual foci left in Mali and Ethiopia, as well as the fact that due to a decline in veterinary field activity the annual vaccination of young stock was not strictly implemented and immunity levels against rinderpest also declined.

In 1978 and 1979, **resurgence of rinderpest** started in West Africa (Mali, Mauritania and Senegal). In 1980, the disease spread throughout East Africa and remained enzootic in some parts of Somalia, Sudan and Uganda. Early in 1982 in Tanzania occurred an outbreak in wild buffaloes which then extended to cattle. As a result, the disease spread from 1979 to 1982, and then the virus re-established itself over much of Sub-Saharan Africa. The incidence of rinderpest in Africa reached its peak in 1983, resulting in several thousand of outbreaks affecting millions of cattle in Sudan, the Central African Republic (CAR), Chad, Cameroon, Nigeria, Burkina Faso, Benin and Egypt. The pandemic killed millions of cattle and wildlife throughout equatorial Africa and thousands of farmers and herders lost most of all of their cattle. **Between 1979 and 1988, eighteen countries were again affected by rinderpest** and individual countries mounted emergency campaigns to control the disease.

PARC is now the most advanced regional rinderpest campaign in the World. Its **objectives** are:

- **Epidemiological:** to control and ultimately eradicate rinderpest from Africa through vaccination campaigns, sero-surveillance and animal movement control;

- **Policy reforms**: to improve the national livestock services in order to enhance livestock development programmes in sub-Saharan African countries;

- **Environmental**: to help control the risks of desertification of the African continent.

Responding to an urgent call, FAO'emergency action against rinderpest started, and assistance (over US$11 million) was provided during 1980-88 for 62 national projects in 30 African countries and for 19 regional projects covering the implementation of emergency campaigns and preparations for PARC (Technical Cooperation Programme - TCP). It includes :strengthening of diagnosis, vaccine production/quality control, sero surveillance, communication, equipment maintenance, legislation, coordination and relevant training.

The PARC Project located in Nairobi provides technical assistance to the OAU/IBAR on the implementation of the Campaign, preparation of relevant structures and training. The principal donor to PARC is the EEC. The Joint FAO/IAEA Division of Nuclear Techniques in Food and Agriculture-AGE,. in Vienna has been conducting the **sero-monitoring programme.**

FAO PROJECTS FOR PARC

Epidemiology Project

The FAO Japanese Trust Fund project: "Strengthening of PARC", was implemented from 1986 TO 1991 covering epidemiological data processing, cold chain for vaccines and rinderpest diagnosis. An epidemiology unit for PARC was established. Recently, a follow-up project has been negotiated with a potential donor with the following objectives:

- Re-establishment of an Epidemiology Unit for PARC;
- direction and coordination of the PARC sero-monitoring network and its enlargement to include disease and virus surveillance;
- assistance to PARC and its member states in the implementation and the assessment of the regional strategies.

Vaccine Project-Pan African Veterinary Vaccine Centre, (PANVAC). the PANVAC has been developing since 1984, initially under the name of the **FAO/OAU/UNDP Regional Vaccine Quality Control and Training Centre** (1985-90), under the Technical Cooperation Projects (1984-87) and the FAO/UNDP Regional Project (1988-92). Two PANVAC centres have been established in the hosting national veterinary Institutes of Dakar, Senegal and Debre-Zeit, Ethiopia, to strengthen priority veterinary vaccine production and quality control. It included those against rinderpest and Contagious Bovine Pleuropneumonia-CBPP, Newcastle disease as well as veterinary vaccines in 23 African countries. During 1984-86 FAO arranged for continental examination of the quality of rinderpest tissue culture vaccines produced by 12 African manufacturers. The testing indicated an urgent need for standardization of the test and the necessity to improve the tests by African laboratories as well as the reference testing of vaccines for PARC use. Since 1987, PANVAC has been training senior laboratory staff on advanced techniques of rinderpest vaccine production and quality control (for other details see Sylla et al and Rweyemamu et al of these Proceedings). Activities of the PANVAC have contributed significantly to improving the standard of rinderpest vaccine production and quality control in Africa and to the success of the first phase of PARC. The institution has become a model for other continents with regard to rinderpest vaccine for regional rinderpest eradication campaigns WAREC and SAREC.

It is obvious that a successful and efficient implementation of PARC requires people's participation. Especially designed booklets, flipcharts, posters, leaflets, video, radio-programmes, logos, as well as press campaigns are required. They should help the rural community, herdsmen, general public, field veterinary staff, local authorities and government officials to understand the aims and objectives of PARC. Communication-public information project: A communication campaign to promote PARC objectives was initiated in 1986 under TCP and trust fund regional projects covering preparation of mass media communication training. Communication Projects have been operating through its experts working with the OAU/IBAR/PARC Coordinating Unit in Nairobi and in Bamako and have created a communication policy and strategy, multi-media materials example kit, communication guides, training materials for adaptation at the national level and information materials for international use. The projects also helped national authorities on the issue and conducted numerous forms of training.

The revitalization of livestock/veterinary services: It was considered as a very important and necessary part of rinderpest control and it became a prerequisite for subsequent funding by donors.

Vaccine Banks: At the beginning of PARC five vaccine banks were established in various laboratories in Africa whereby 12 million doses of quality controlled Tissue Culture Rinderpest Vaccine were stored. At present, one vaccine bank remains in the BVI, Botswana.

Research on rinderpest: Preparation and implementation of PARC directly and indirectly promoted applied research on rinderpest. It included:

- For diagnosis: standardization of applied methods of rinderpest diagnosis, preparation of standardized diagnostic reagents, developing of new tests;

- for vaccines: standardization of production and quality control of Tissue Culture Rinderpest Vaccine, testing the rinderpest vaccine stability, testing applicability of VERO cells for vaccine production and quality control, research on how to increase thermostability of vaccines;

- research on immunosuppressive effect of rinderpest virus and the vaccine on bovine immune system;

- research on epidemiology, particularly on the role of wildlife and small ruminants.

The strategy of PARC has been to institute **mass vaccination coverage** in those countries where rinderpest has been confirmed as endemic and switch progressively into eradication through the process of virus elimination campaigns. Areas with persistent outbreaks will be surrounded by sanitary cordons and vaccinations will be continued until an immunity level of 80% is exceeded and sustained for years. Later, the vaccination coverage will be removed to check that eradication has been achieved. If necessary, the enforcement of controlled livestock movement will be introduced together with quarantine and the slaughter of infected flock all of which act as an effective control measure. It has been recommended that an immune barrier should be created around infected and "no go" areas where action is limited due to civil strife.

Results of PARC: As a result of the first phase of PARC (1987-91) and epidemiological factors the rinderpest situation in Africa has dramatically improved resulting in a decrease on a number of rinderpest infected countries from 18 (1983) to 3 in 1990. Since 1988 the disease has not been reported from West Africa (the last outbreak was in April 1988 on the Ghana/Burkina Faso border).

There has been a major change in attitudes by most governments particularly on the liberalization of drug and vaccine importation, production and distribution, privatization of clinical veterinary services, increasing the cost recovery for services rendered, re-organization of public livestock services, liberalization of veterinary practice, establishment of primary animal health care,establishing drug revolving funds. Special attention has been given to a control over the risks of desertification after succesful control of rinderpest and other major epizootics.

Current Constraints in Africa are:

- The great size of cattle populations in the present infected area i.e. Ethiopia with 35 million heads (more than the whole of West Africa), Sudan 21 million, Kenya 14 million and Uganda 4.2 million;
- transhumance movement (difficulties in animal movement control);
- poor vaccine handling and vaccinating techniques;
- political instability in infected areas making difficult or impossible the implementation of rinderpest control programmes;
- lack of confidence of veterinary services in their ability to deal with risks associated with the cessation of vaccination whilst the virus still remains.

The strategy for the Phase II of PARC (since 1991) will have to include:

- the establishment of a strong immune barrier, a "cordon-sanitaire" of immune cattle in Central Africa (Chad and CAR) which will protect West Africa against reinfection from East Africa;
- establishing a second immune barrier in Northern Uganda, Kenya and possibly Somalia;
- continuing effort to improve rinderpest control in East Africa through mass vaccination and increased investigation of the underlining causes of disease persistence in the region;
- improvement of disease surveillance and phased withdrawal of vaccination in West Africa.

THE WEST ASIA RINDERPEST ERADICATION CAMPAIGN (WAREC)

Geographical Coverage

The countries concerned are: Bahrain, Egypt, Iraq, Jordan, Kuwait, Lebanon, Oman, Qatar, Saudi Arabia, Syria, UAE and Yemen. The population of cattle (in million) is estimated at 7.3 and buffaloes at 2.7(2).

Epizootiological Situation in the Region

Prevalence of the disease in the Region, as well as the organization of the campaign, was reviewed by Mathur and Inui in 1991, (7). The Near East Panzootic (1969-73) originated from Asia and affected: Afghanistan, Iran, Bahrain, Turkey, Syria, Lebanon and Jordan. In the seventies the disease was recorded in the West Asian regions, again including: Jordan, Kuwait, Lebanon, Oman, Syria, Saudi Arabia, UAE and Yemen. After national control and eradication efforts and partial elimination of the disease, a large scale recrudescence was reported in the region affecting: Yemen, Kuwait, Oman, Egypt, Lebanon, Syria, Saudi Arabia, UAE, Bahrain, Qatar and Iraq.

At present Yemen continues to be infected, but the position is improving, the number of outbreaks in recent years being: 1989 - 200, 1990 - 208, 1991 - 30. Persistent problems have occurred on the Oman and UAE border (Buraimi/El Alein). Lebanon has reported low levels of disease. There may be continuing foci of rinderpest in no-go areas of the Region.

Regarding the virus isolates from the Region, some strains have been characterised by IAH, Pirbright Laboratory, UK. Yemen isolates were found to be of Asiatic origin. However, there is also direct evidence of importation of a strain from the Horn of Africa.

Constrains on rinderpest control in Middle East-West Asia include the occurrence of a mild form of the disease, the occurrence of sub-clinical infections and difficulties in achieving full sub-regional co-operation of countries; lack of a single political umbrella for all countries of the region. Participating countries financed their own control programmes. Also in the region there are inadequacy of veterinary infrastructure including laboratory and quarantine facilities, vaccination policy, planning and technical support to national campaigns.

The Region lacks of rigorous vaccine quality control system by independent agencies. Many countries have financial difficulties, i.e. funds for campaigns and for compensation to livestock owners; and the whole region is characterized by notorious political instability.

Most rinderpest outbreaks in the past, have been linked to entry of disease in imported animals due to faulty quarantine. Non-vaccinated cattle highly sensitive to rinderpest have been imported from rinderpest free areas such as: Latin America, Eastern Europe, Australia and also from the rinderpest affected parts of Africa and Asia. An ineffective quarantine at many ports of entry, uncontrolled land movement of cattle as well as military movements, are the major factors affecting rinderpest control in the area. Mass vaccination of whole cattle populations, in an attempt to control the disease has been carried out during periods of 2 to 3 consecutive years.

Despite years of effort made by a number of individual countries in the region to control rinderpest through mass vaccination, the disease still remains a major constraint to the livestock industry in West Asia. The economic consequences of rinderpest are not limited to mortality but also include disruption of trade caused by imposition of quarantines, the cost of vaccination, the cost of surveillance and other control measures, and the negative effect of a continued threat of the disease.

Among the Advantageous Features of Rinderpest Control in the WAREC Region are:

- A cattle breeding pattern and the fact that bovine rearing is confined mostly to areas of cultivation;
- relatively difficult inter-country movement of livestock due to natural desert/sea barriers;
- mostly non-nomadic breeding patterns;
- insignificant population of wildlife artiodactyles, and
- lack of limitation to slaughter of cattle.

Initiating the WAREC

The Third Conference of the Arab Ministers of Agriculture of the States of the Gulf and Arabian Peninsula (Qatar, 1978), requested the Near East Regional Animal Production and Health Project (MINEADEP) to prepare a plan for the eradication of the disease. A technical meeting of representatives of member states held in Saudi Arabia (1980) resulted in the formulation of a rinderpest eradication project which was submitted to the Fifth Conference of the Ministers (Oman, 1980). Unfortunately, the necessary funding for implementation of this project was not secured. In response to the deteriorating rinderpest situation, individual members intensified their national rinderpest vaccination programmes. During the 1980's, emergency assistance to the region was provided through the FAO Technical Co-operation Projects and MINEADEP. The MINEADEP Meeting for Heads of Veterinary Departments in Baghdad (1984) proposed that a regional rinderpest and eradication campaign be launched.

The UNDP/FAO Project: Co-ordination of Rinderpest Eradication in West Asia, WAREC (1989-93)

The Project was prepared in 1986 and has been implemented from 1989 to cover 11 countries of the Region. So far only Saudi Arabia has not joined the WAREC. Since the end of 1991 Iran and Turkey have indicated their wish to join the Project. The Project aims at total eradication of rinderpest from the West Asian region through effective co-operation and regional co-ordination among its members.

The objective will be achieved through assessing immunity before and after vaccination. Mass vaccination or other strategies appropriate to the area, surveillance and search for hidden pockets of infection, and strengthening animal health quarantine.

Co-ordination on a regional basis has been implemented by the Co-ordinating Unit of the West Asia Rinderpest Eradication Campaign (WAREC), initially established in Baghdad (late 1989). The Gulf War (1990) disrupted WARECC which was moved to FAO Rome, and from 1991, to Amman, Jordan. The WAREC strategy was to combine mass vaccination with evaluation through a serological survey and the strengthening of movement controls and quarantine. Mass vaccination was prolonged by one year as a result of the Gulf War.

Rinderpest Vaccine for WAREC

Tissue culture rinderpest vaccine of different standard has been produced in Egypt (12 million doses), Iraq (2.6 million doses) and Syria (0.9 million doses). The data on production capacity of the Saudi Laboratory in Riyadh are not available. Laboratories in Baghadad and Cairo were assisted through supply the of CK cells (BVD free), Kabete O seed virus and vero cells. In Amman-Jordan assistance has been planned to start a local preparation of rinderpest vaccine. A close link on the above-mentioned issues has been established with the Pan African Veterinary Vaccine Centre- PANVAC in Debre-Zeit.

The FAO has been assisting laboratories in Egypt and Syria through provision of consultants-experts of rinderpest vaccine production and Q.C. In the Veterinary Sera and Vaccine Laboratory in Abassia the FAO Experts, Y.Ozawa and K.V. Singh, were involved in the modernization of the applied standard of rinderpest vaccine production and Q.C. The laboratory later developed under a supervision of Mr. A. Osman has recently received the new extension, which will definitely facilitate production and Q.C. arrangements. The recent development of veterinary Vaccine Production Laboratory in Damascus, Syria has also been achieved with the participation of the FAO Experts: K.V. Singh, T. Feherevary. In the Veterinary Vaccine Producing Laboratory in Baghdad, the local staff has been independently arranging the improvement of some production procedures. However, the scale of production never high. The laboratories declared to follow the OIE Norms (1987), and their quality control has been done through the manufacturer's units and in some cases independent units. the locally produced vaccines were applied together with the imported ones from Kenya, Turkey, India, Pakistan, Coopers, UK and IFFA Merieux, France. Advise on the use of Veterinary Vaccines to be given during the numerous FAO/MINEADEP training and Seminars/Workshops. In Riyadh, Saudi Arabia, under the Saudi Arabia's FAO Trust Fund Project, the Virologist, S.H. Hafez, has been an Adviser on locally produced rinderpest vaccine.

The constrains of rinderpest vaccine production and Q.C. in the WAREC area are still being assessed. They mostly refer to inadequate laboratory facilities, especially freeze drying equipment, lack of rigorous quality control system by independent agencies. Vaccination campaigns has not always been well planned, and regular sero-monitoring of post vaccinal immunity using ELISA has just been initiated within the region.

Initially, the technical programme of the project envisaged: Preparatory Phase, 1 to 5 years (1989-90), a Vaccination Phase, 2 years (1991-92) and a Surveillance Phase, a year (1993).

Results of WAREC: After a preparatory period, in 1991 a mass vaccination against rinderpest was carried out on cattle and buffaloes (7 million bovines). The vaccination was disrupted later during the Gulf War in all affected countries. The second round was implemented during 1992 (8.2 million). An additional third round of mass vaccination has been planned for 1993 to cover the whole population (8.4 million) in order to compensate for the previous shortcomings in the implementation of vaccination programmes. Sera samples were collected from 1 to 15 % of bovine population and tested by ELISA and Sero-neutralization The Coordination Unit and Regional Rinderpest Laboratory were established in Baghdad and ELISA testing facilities in Amman, Cairo, Baghdad, Damascus and Sanaa. The training on diagnosis, ELISA testing, epidemiology and data processing, animal quarantine and vaccine quality control was implemented.

Epidemiological results: Infection in Yemen has been reduced from 200 outbreaks and 1000 cases per year during: 1987-89 to 33 outbreaks and 92 cases in 1991. In Lebanon, Oman, Iraq and UAE the incidence has declined. It is anticipated that by the year 1993 with a vaccination coverage of 100% herd immunity, the incidence of rinderpest may be further reduced by 80 to 90%

Some countries of the region have embarked upon a plan of privatization of veterinary service with the objective of making it sustainable.

Rinderpest in Turkey

Rinderpest was first reported in October 1991 in local herds of cattle in Hakkari and Van provinces. It is believed that the massive refugee movement between Iraq, Iran and Turkey during the Gulf War and the resulting illegal movement of animals across borders for sale, resulted in entry of rinderpest infection into the country.

It was found that the disease was extending westwards. The Veterinary Department immediately arranged for emergency action. The entire population of about 12 million cattle was vaccinated by 1000 teams during 2 months and surveillance was undertaken using helicopters, for illegal livestock movements on the south eastern borders. Before eradication in Turkey, 6,000 animals died or were slaughtered, US $32 million was spent on control, and total losses were estimated at US $210 million. The Government paid compensation for animals destroyed and imposed restrictions on the movement of cattle and buffaloes. A public information campaign has subsequently been launched including intensive education programmes for farmers on radio and TV. At the start of the emergency in response to a request from the Government of Turkey the FAO provided immediate assistance on the supply of vaccine, strengthening of vaccine production (including freeze drying), quality control, disease diagnosis, monitoring and surveillance, epidemiology and communication.

Considering the initial port of entry of the disease, attempts were made to establish in the South East of the country an immune barrier of multiply vaccinated animals.

Technical Consultation on Emergency Rinderpest Control in the Near East:

A Special Meeting on this topic took place at the FAO Headquarters, Rome in November, 1991 with the participation of Iran, Iraq, Lebanon, Syria, Turkey as well as representatives of EEC, OIE and FAO. The Meeting reviewed on a basis of individual country reports, the epizootiological situation of rinderpest in the Region. The Meeting formulated the Immediate Action Plan for Control and Eradication of Rinderpest in the Region and drafted the **"Regional Agreement on Rinderpest Control and Eradication"** for the Sub-Region (6).

In order to prevent the introduction of rinderpest into Europe, special assistance was provided to Bulgaria in order to create an immune belt for the prevention of rinderpest.

A Strategy for a New Phase of WARECC

The strategy beyond 1994 will aim at achieving a free disease status in the Region and the strengthening of veterinary services in order to sustain rinderpest free status and to promote other than rinderpest disease control and related food losses.

SOUTH ASIA RINDERPEST ERADICATION CAMPAIGNS (SAREC)

Geographical Coverage

The countries concerned are Bangladesh, Bhutan, India, Iran, Myanmar, Nepal, Pakistan, Sri-Lanka (candidates for "SAREC Member Countries") with nearly 265 million cattle and 98 million buffaloes (2).

Regional Organisation (s)

South Asian Association for Regional Co-operation (SAARC),and the Animal Production and Health Commission for Asia and Pacific (APHCA);

Epizootiological Situation in the Region

Endemic occurrence of rinderpest in the Region with different countries affected has been recorded for centuries. The persistence of rinderpest in the Indian subcontinent has not only hampered livestock development in the infected territories, but has also been a constant threat to rinderpest free countries in the Region and to other Regions (West Asia, Middle East) through livestock movement associated with trade.

The rinderpest epidemiological situation in the subregion changes from year to year. In 1986, 1987 and 1988, the disease occurred in nine States in India. In 1984, the disease re-occurred in Nepal where it has since become endemic. Rinderpest had been under control in Pakistan since 1977, but the presence of the disease in a buffalo colony in the Province of Sind has recently been confirmed. Myanmar has been free from rinderpest and is maintaining an immune belt on its border with India. In Sri-Lanka, rinderpest re-occurred in October 1987 after almost 40 years absence of the disease from the country. Since then, the disease has spread into the north and north-east regions of the country, causing the death of over 10,000 cattle and buffalo. Sporadic outbreaks of rinderpest continue to occur in Iran. The latest outbreak took place in September 1989 in the northwest, then spread north and southwards. Rinderpest has not been officially reported from Bangladesh (or Pakistan). However, there is a high possibility of ingress of the disease from neighbouring countries. Disease reporting from the Commonwealth of Independent States - CIS (former USSR), - especially from the Southern Asiatic Republics affected by civil unrest, is not always complete. The same situation relates to Afghanistan. Many South Asian countries not reporting outbreaks still continue mass vaccinations, particularly in border areas. Therefore, the term of "SAREC Associated Countries" has been introduced in preparation for the regional campaign to cover Afghanistan, China, Mongolia, Thailand, Laos, Kampuchea, Vietnam and southern republics of the CIS: Georgia, Azerbaijan, Armenia, Turkenistan, Uzbekistan, Tadshikistan, Kirgizia and Kazakhstan.

Constraints to Control in South Asia

An epidemiological assessment of the situation is incomplete. The status of rinderpest in many countries is not available to any extent and neither are national policies for control clear. Exchange of data between countries of the Region on disease status and control programmes require co-ordination. There are no regional or-subregional reference laboratories for rinderpest diagnosis and quality control of vaccines. There are no suitable repositories for rinderpest strains isolated for further study. Some countries are still using Goat Tissue vaccine. Overall there is no regional co-ordination on the control and eradication of rinderpest and the associated technical requirements.

Initiating the SAREC

The first FAO Expert Consultation on Requirements for SAREC was held in India in 1983. The recommendations were subsequently endorsed by a meeting of APHCA in 1984. The proposed SAREC was planned to be implemented by Bangladesh, Bhutan, India, Nepal, Myanmar, Pakistan, and Sri-Lanka. The Expert Consultation on SAREC 's strategy (organized by the FAO Regional Office for Asia and Pacific in Bangkok,1990,1992, helped to elaborate on many technical issues concerned. The EEC is a major donor prepared to finance country campaigns similar to PARC, and has been negotiating the strengthening of veterinary services with countries involved, as part of the funding conditions. The All India campaign: "Operation Rinderpest Zero", started in early 1992. Due to the epidemiologically important location, Iran will probably participate in both WAREC and SAREC projects.

Prior or Ongoing Assistance

It has already been established, that the EEC as a major donor and assisting agency, for rinderpest eradication and strengthening of veterinary services on a bilateral basis, will provide substantial assistance to India, Bhutan, Nepal and perhaps to other countries in the Region. The EEC is already financing the All India "Operation Rinderpest Zero" Campaign. Under its Technical Co-operation Programme, (TCP), FAO provided emergency assistance to Nepal in 1985 to combat an outbreak of rinderpest, and to Bhutan in 1989 to strengthen the cold chain system for the application of vaccine.

The "All India Rinderpest Operation Zero Programme" aiming at the eradication of the disease by the year 1998 (launched in 1992) places the strategy regarding various States of India into categories:

- States which are declared provisionally free of rinderpest;
- States which are not reporting rinderpest but providing a buffer zone against the spread of infection from the endemic area;
- the five South Indian States that constitute the endemic area are: **Andhra Pradesh, Maharashtra, Karnataka, Tamil Nadu, and Kerala.**

The national strategy proposes mass vaccination of all cattle, buffaloes, sheep and goats in the endemic rinderpest areas of India where the combined animal population includes 70 million of large and 20 million of small ruminants. Infected sheep very often initiate rinderpest outbreaks in cattle and the picture of sheep transmitted rinderpest is complicated by the presence of peste des petis ruminants (PPR) also reported from enzootically infected States. A two-year research programme has recently been launched to study the epidemiology of rinderpest virus in small ruminant population and to decide whether to include small ruminants into a mass vaccination. According to Nair, 1990, during 1980-89 in India there were 13 units producing around 70 million doses of tissue culture rinderpest vaccine, 7 units manufacturing goat tissue vaccine (28 million doses) (8).

Project Proposal for Co-ordination of SAREC

FAO has been formulating since 1990/91 the Project Proposal - "Strengthening of South Asia Rinderpest Eradication Programmes (SAREC)", which after a long dialogue is now being considered as a candidate for EEC funding. The Project will provide assistance for strengthening the co-ordination of national rinderpest eradication campaigns and the delivery of sustainable, targeted veterinary services. The main objectives of this Project include:

- Regional co-ordination for control of infectious diseases, beginning with rinderpest in cattle and buffalo;
- participation of farmers and herders in meeting the cost of most vaccination and professional services;
- support for the creation of private veterinary services;
- human resources development;
- rehabilitation of veterinary infrastructure;
- strengthening disease control programmes;
- support to improve diagnostic capabilities and vaccine production;

- improvement of quarantine regulations and enforcement, support to sero-monitoring;

- provision of technical assistance.

For rinderpest eradication, a common strategy will be adopted for all national campaigns in eight countries. However, implementation may vary considerably as the future workload will differ from country to country, not all being equally affected by rinderpest.

Regional rinderpest vaccine production and quality control will have to be strengthened to comply with international norms and requirements.

GLOBAL RINDERPEST ERADICATION PROGRAMME (GREP)

Factors contributing to the eradication of rinderpest are:

- **Restricted range of the disease**: at present the rinderpest risk area includes Northern Equatorial Africa, the Near East, Indian sub-continent and parts of South-East Asia.

- **Restricted transmission:** rinderpest virus is excreted in aerosols-droplets generated in the breath of infected animals and from splashes of fluid, faeces and urine and is spread by live infectious animals. Therefore a strict control of the movement will stop the spread of disease.

- **Short infectious period:** from 2 - 3 to 10 days. Affected animals shed virus in all their secretions and excretions. The duration of the infectious period is influenced by the strain of virus involved and by the resistance of the host.

- **No latency or persistence:** recovered animals are not carriers. Pregnant cattle who abort after recovery from rinderpest, may spread infectious virus through the fetal tissue and vaginal discharges.

- **Available diagnostic tests**: field diagnosis (if the disease is expected) is relatively easy due to the occurrence of fever, stomatitis and gastroenteritis and availability of quick pen-side tests like AGID. However, mild and clinically aberrant cases may occur in animals with a high innate resistance to disease i.e., such as the water buffaloes in Egypt.

Any condition in cattle buffaloes and other artiodactyls that clinically resembles rinderpest should be regarded as rinderpest and immediate steps should be taken to control and contain the disease.

- **Excellent vaccine:** rinderpest virus is highly immunogenic and the Plowright's vaccine is the best live attenuated vaccine that has ever been developed.

- Economic incentive: rinderpest has always been considered a major cattle killer. The losses of individual stockowners are devastating.

Constraints Affecting Rinderpest Eradication

External factors:

- **The existence of "no-go areas" affected by a civil strife;**

- **Absence of legal and emergency powers:** a legislation to control animal diseases is essential. Veterinary departments and relevant Chief Veterinary Officers are responsible for an emergency disease preparedness and contingency planning for a country.

- **Nomadism and transhumance:** nomads tend to ignore borders and may not respect quarantine. They may be difficult to locate. Cooperation between countries having nomads and a nomadic breeding pattern is essential.

- **Uncontrolled trade animals movement:** examples: (a) movement of African cattle to the Near East, (b) movement of buffaloes and cattle from North to South India from where they may be shipped to the Near East, (c) uncontrolled movement of cattle from Iraq/Iran to Turkey which is believed to be a source of the 1991 epidemic in Turkey.

- **Social and religious attitude**: it concerns difficulties in collecting samples and vaccination as well as the ban on cow slaughter.

Technical Factors

- **Wide host range:** (a) In Africa wild ruminant populations are too small to maintain rinderpest virus and outbreaks usually burn themselves out. In India the role of small domesticated ruminants and pigs in the maintenance of rinderpest should be considered. Infection of these animals may take place and cannot be ignored even if many of the cases in sheep and goats are due to PPR. Sub-clinically infected goats may circulate in a sub-clinical form in goats and may be responsible for infecting of cattle.

- **Vaccine:** a Regional rinderpest control and eradication campaign should be supported by the Rinderpest Vaccine Quality Control Centres similar to PANVAC in Africa providing impartial quality control services. Apart from that, establishment of national vaccine quality control laboratories independent from producers, should be encouraged.

- **Naturally acquired passive immunity:** can be a result of immunisation of dams or in an endemic area where vaccinated cattle are exposed to the virus and react anamnestically including rising of their antibody titres. The progeny of these cattle will acquire a significant amount of antibodies in the colostrum which may protect them for several months against rinderpest. The practical solution is to vaccinate all cattle during campaigns irrespective of age, and revaccinate them the following year.

Sub-clinical (cryptic, sub-clinical, unapparent) infections: Molecular epidemiology methods may be helpful in the identification of the presence of viral genomic sequences in a host.

Rinderpest occurs at present in 3 different geographical areas interconnected through trade routes and animal movement. The disease is being controlled by regional campaigns. Control and eradication of any viral disease is possible where the transmission chain can be broken. In the case of rinderpest this can be achieved by preventing the virus from entering susceptible hosts, through slaughter of infected animals and quarantine, thus preventing susceptible hosts from coming in contact with the virus. Also herd immunity, as a result of mass vaccination campaigns has an important part to play.

Global eradication has been achieved for only one human disease - smallpox. The last case of this disease was recorded in 1977 in Somalia. Its eradication showed that the whole concept of global disease eradication is feasible and broke the major psychological barrier of "impossibility". The FAO started in 1990 preparations for the Global Rinderpest Eradication Programme (GREP). The second Experts Consultation conducted by FAO in 1992 (5), on the Strategy of Global Rinderpest Eradication examined the justification for, and feasibility of, global eradication, review past and present campaigns, chart the progress made, identify success and constraints and draw relevant conclusions from progress in other eradication programmes. It concluded that attempts will be made to coordinate technical and other inputs provided under regional campaigns PARC, WAREC and SAREC with a **target** of global eradication of rinderpest by the year 2010 and launching the Global Rinderpest Eradication Programme-GREP. The matter of outmost importance is the improved capacity of modernized veterinary service during rinderpest campaigns. Only this can guarantee sustainability of the programme.

Every effort should be made towards the final outcome of the eradication: declaration of "disease free" status followed by declaration of "free from infection" status should be achieve as close as possible to the target date or before.

REFERENCES

1. FAO-OIE-WHO Animal Health Yearbook, 1991.

2. FAO Production Yearbook, (1990), Rome 1991.

3. FAO Report: Expert Consultation on Rinderpest Diagnosis, Vaccine Production and Quality Control, Rome, 1985.

4. FAO Report: Expert Consultation on Global Strategy for Control and Eradication of Rinderpest, Rome, 1987.

5. FAO Report (Draft): Expert Consultation on Strategy for Global Rinderpest Eradication, Rome, 1992.

6. FAO Miscellaneous Documentation on Rinderpest Control and Eradication, AGAH, Rome, 1982-91.

7. MATHUR, S.C. and INUI, K. "West Asia Rinderpest Eradication Campaign (WAREC)", in: Proceedings of the Regional Expert Consultation on Rinderpest Eradication in South Asia, Bangkok, Thailand, June 1990, FAO/RAPA Publication: 1991/8, pp. 93-110.

8. NAIR, R.P.N: Status of Rinderpest in India, idem, pp 27-32.

9. OIE: "Requirements for Rinderpest Cell Culture Vaccine (Live)", OIE Monograph, Paris, 1987.

10. OIE: Report of the Expert Consultation on Rinderpest Sero-surveillance Systems, Paris, 16-18 August, 1989.

11. OIE: Report of the Expert Consultation on Requirements for Vaccinia - Rinderpest Recombinant (VRR) Vaccines, Paris, 21-24 August, 1989.

12 Wojciechowski, K.J. "Rinderpest Campaign in Africa", in Proceedings of the Regional Expert Consultation on Rinderpest Eradication in South Asia, Bangkok, Thailand, June 1990, FAO.RAPA Publication: 1991/8 pp. 111-118.

13. Wojciechowski, K.J. "Global Strategies for Rinderpest Eradication", as above, pp. 78-90.

Discussion

<u>Dr Sizaret</u> enquired of PANVAC: (a) were all the vaccines reported upon, produced in Africa? (b) how many producers are involved? (c) what was the mode of sampling - direct from the producer, or samples from a central depository? (d) what are the relationships between producers and the testing organisation - do they share premises and are they linked in any way?

The answers to these questions were (a) Yes, (b) 11 producers at present, There were 13 previously but two have dropped out and others may also do so, (c) vaccine is shipped directly by the producer to Dakar or Debre Zeit and is taken from the producers stock and not a central store, (d) PANVAC is totally independent of all producers and has no links with them or government laboratories.

<u>Dr Mannathoko</u> also asked of FAO (a) if any producing laboratory had been rejected for poor performance by an FAO consultant and (b) why is Turkey not included in WAREC?

<u>Dr Wojciechowski</u> replied that FAO only appointed consultants to deal with specific technical problems such as equipment maintenance or process problems eg freeze drying. In general terms, FAO's attitude is not to condemn but to encourage, however if problems of performance arise then after suitable warnings, FAO would be prepared to advise Donors not to continue support for that particular producer.

FAO is participating in an emergency rinderpest control plan for Turkey and some 6 million doses of vaccine have been used in the last two months. In future, Turkey will probably be included in WAREC. Since the advent of rinderpest there, the epidemiology of the disease in the region will have changed. Iran is also negotiating to participate in both WAREC and SAREC - however, in the opinion of FAO it would be better to combine their efforts in one unified plan such as that suggested for the GREP.

<u>Dr Sylla</u> in continuation of an earlier question asked for clarification of the policy for vaccine banks, - are PARC stocks to be kept separate from producer's stocks and are they to be checked on a regular basis? If they are used and replaced by new vaccine, will it be confirmed as acceptable and treated in the same way as the material it replaced?

<u>Dr Khoury</u> was sad when he compared the performance of WAREC with that of PARC. In his opinion, WAREC was of little value since nothing had been achieved and there was no activity other than minor correspondence regarding the handling of vaccine or recommending a manual etc. He thought that the co-ordinating unit should be moved away from Baghdad.

<u>Dr Wojciechowski</u> stated that the strategy for WAREC was now to be revised. The efficiency of the project had been badly affected by the advent of the Gulf War. During a period of 10 months, experts involved in WAREC could not visit the Head Office in Baghdad and since then the Office has been moved to Amman. FAO is now considering asking Syria to take on the function of Quality Control Laboratory for WAREC - this has to be negotiated with the co-ordinators of WAREC.

Dr Cheneau in response to the points raised by Dr Sylla indicated that in many cases the vaccine for PARC will remain in the producer's cold rooms, and although ear-marked for PARC will remain the property of the producer. In the contract drawn up between the producer and the EEC it is clear that the funding agency is paying 50% of the value of the stock to have immediate access to it when required, (and the value is re-assessed every year). With regard to monitoring the storage conditions, manufacturers undertake to maintain stocks of vaccine at -22 C. In many labs this is satisfactorily achieved but in others the performance is less satisfactory.

Regarding replacement of vaccines, the contract states that since the vaccine is the property of the producer or government, they may use a particular stock, provided it is replaced within one month of the time the previous stock was removed, and provided there is immediate notification to PARC of the replacement having taken place, together with the details of the new vaccine for quality control assessment. Some 5 vaccine banks have been established and in some cases eg in West Africa there has been no great urgency to make use of them. It has been decided that for the future, there will be only one vaccine bank for PARC and that it will be located at the Botswana Vaccine Institute.

OFFICE INTERNATIONAL DES EPIZOOTIES

ACTIVITIES RELATED TO VETERINARY VACCINE QUALITY CONTROL

by

Y Ozawa

1. Volumes I - III of the OIE Manual of Recommended Diagnostic Techniques and Requirements of Biological Products (for List A and B diseases) has already been published.

2. A consolidated manual (of Vols I - III) will be published in 1992. This manual will be revised and updated every 4 years. This new version of the Manual will be considered as the OIE "Bible" for laboratory personnel.

3. The Standards Commission of OIE will meet once a year to review the Manual and assess the necessity for the development of new standards.

4. The OIE is currently in the process of establishing networks of Reference Laboratories for some 36 diseases of major importance to international trade (selected by the OIE Code and Standards Commissions). When required, the OIE will request the Regional Laboratories to develop standards either for diagnostic techniques or for biological products in collaboration with other appropriate international organisations such as FAO and WHO.

5. The OIE also takes advice from its Expert Group on Veterinary Biotechnology. The Group meets once per year for discussions on various issues related to OIE's activities. The main task of the Group is to review progress made in the field of biotechnology throughout the world and to publish its findings in the "OIE Veterinary Biotechnology Newsletter". The first issue has just been published. The Group will also deal with developing standards or guidelines for biotechnology products in close collaboration with OIE's Expert Group on Veterinary Drug Registration which also meets once per year.

CONTINENTAL STRATEGY IN THE FIGHT AGAINST FOOT-AND-MOUTH DISEASE IN LATIN AMERICA

by

R Casas Olascoaga

INTRODUCTION

RIMSA-V, the Fifth Inter-American Animal Health Meeting at the Ministerial Level, held on April 27-30, 1987, in Washington, D.C., resolved to "request that all the countries of the region, in accordance with the objective of HEALTH FOR ALL IN THE YEAR 2000, commit themselves to taking all the action necessary to eradicate foot-and-mouth disease within that time frame".

That same RIMSA-V meeting also asked the PanAmerican Health Organisation (PAHO) Director to set up a "Hemispheric Committee for the Eradication of Foot-and-Mouth Disease." With PAHO acting through the Pan American Foot-and-Mouth Disease Center (PAFMDC) as the Secretariat, the Committee --COHEFA-- seeks to ensure the countries maintain their political agreement to eradicate the disease. COHEFA also conducts the evaluation of the progress of the continental programme and pursues alternatives to ensure adequate financing. The Committee is composed of one representative of the national governments of each of the following subregions: Southern Cone, Andean Subregion, Amazon Subregion, Central America, the Caribbean, and North America. The cattle raisers in each of those regions are also invited to appoint a representative to the Committee.

The division into subregions takes into account not only the presence of large ecological, cultural and social "units", but also the existence, on the continental level, of two major areas: the first, unaffected by foot-and-mouth disease, comprises Central America, North America and the Caribbean. The other, affected by the disease, comprises almost all of South America.

For the first area, RIMSA-V proposed to establish a "Commission of the American and Caribbean Countries Free of Foot-and-Mouth Disease Virus". The purpose is to unite efforts to prevent the introduction of the disease into the zone (Resolution VI). For the second area, Resolution XIII was approved with the title of "Eradication of Foot-and-Mouth Disease in South America". It asked the PAHO and COSALFA (South American Commission for the Control of Foot-and-Mouth Disease) to draw up a Hemispheric Program for Eradication of Foot-and-Mouth Disease and to submit it to the approval of the XV Regular Meeting of COSALFA.

COSALFA XV, held in March 1988, gave full approval to the "Subregional Project for Control and Eradication of Foot-and-Mouth Disease in the River Plate Basin". Also approved was the document entitled "Subregional Foot-and-Mouth Disease Project in the Andean Pact Countries". Both documents were drawn up by a group composed of technical personnel from the PAFMDC and from the countries involved. COSALFA then decided to submit the documents to the consideration of COHEFA for implementation and funding.

The COHEFA met for the first time on July 6-7, 1988, in Washington, D.C. The PAMFDC submitted to the Committee a proposal for a "Hemispheric Plan of Action for Foot-and-Mouth Disease Eradication in South America". The plan analysed the main limitations currently noted in the programmes now underway in this part of the Continent. It also included a description of the purposes, objectives and strategies, as well as their programme components, plus an overall schedule and an initial approach to financing for the Plan. COHEFA, in addition to approving the proposed Plan of Action, made a series of recommendations to the countries, urging them to lend maximum support to their national programmes in order to move ahead toward eradication of the disease within the proposed time frame.

JUSTIFICATION

The economic crisis now confronting the majority of the Latin American countries is such that the trade balance, albeit favourable and on the upswing since 1982, hardly generates surpluses sufficient to service the countries' debts. In this scenario, a large segment of the region's population continues to suffer from chronic undernutrition.

On the other hand, the majority of the Latin American countries do have the vocation, and the conditions, to produce and breed excellent quality livestock at relatively low cost. All told, those countries together can muster approximately 257 million head of cattle. However, the yield of that total cattle herd - when compared to herds in the developed countries - is extremely low. Several factors account for this situation, such as: (a) limitations regarding the accessibility and use of appropriate technology; (b) inadequate handling; (c) inadequate implementation and improvement of pastures; (d) lack of clear, stable and coherent policies with respect to the subsector's role in those countries' economic and social development. Also there is the interference that various diseases exert on the bio-economic productive process.

Because of the significant repercussions it exerts on the international markets for animals, products and byproducts of animal origin, foot-and-mouth disease has been one of the diseases causing constant concern among the governments and sectors involved in livestock production. The occurrence of the disease has in turn generated two trade flows, clearly differentiated according to whether the animals, or animal-origin products and byproducts come from countries free or not free of the disease. Thus countries such as Australia, New Zealand and others, considered disease-free, have not only obtained much more favourable prices for their products, in comparison with the non-disease free countries, but neither do they confront a series of restrictions and sanitary barriers that affect agricultural and livestock products, including animal species not susceptible to the disease and its derivations.

Foot-and-mouth disease in South America causes average annual losses estimated at US$210 million. This amount is in addition to what the public and livestock-raising sectors spend just to keep the disease at its present levels, (approximately some US$70 million and US$230 million, respectively). However, it should be remembered that the annual total of economic losses physically caused by the disease prior to the 1970's was much higher than currently. The reason is that several countries in the region, at that time, decided to commence formal development of national foot-and-mouth disease control programmes. Funding was provided by the Inter-American Development Bank (IDB).

In the majority of cases, those control programmes became the basis for the organization of the national animal-health services. The prevention programmes have been the catalyst for animal-health activities in Panama, Central America and Mexico.

In 1972, at the Fifth Inter-American Meeting at the Ministerial Level on the Control of Foot-and-Mouth Disease and Other Zoonoses (RICAZ-V), the Ministers of Agriculture of the Americas resolved to create the COSALFA. The objectives were co-ordination, promotion and regional evaluation, harmonization of the sanitary standards and bilateral and multilateral agreements for the control of foot-and-mouth disease. The Commission is composed of the Animal Health Directors of Argentina, Bolivia, Brazil, Chile, Colombia, Ecuador, Guyana, Paraguay, Peru, Uruguay and Venezuela. The PAFMDC (PAHO/WHO) acts as the Secretariat of the Commission, which has met annually without interruption since 1973. In 1985 COSALFA became a Permanent Institutionalized Commission at the Regional Level, a status which brings recognition by the Foreign Relation Ministers of all the member countries.

Today, the member countries have duly developed epidemiological surveillance and information systems, and diagnostic laboratories. They form a veritable regional network and a field infrastructure composed of approximately two thousand operational units. In addition, the region has official and private foot-and-mouth disease vaccine-producing laboratories that, taken together, are able to meet the needs for that type of biological product. The substantial improvement in the quality and potency of the vaccine presently produced is worthy of mention.

As a direct consequence of those national animal-health programmes, foot-and-mouth disease has been eradicated in Chile and in the northwestern region of Colombia. Argentina, Patagonia, Guyana, French Guiana and Surinam have been kept free of the disease. The annual incidence of the disease has been significantly reduced in those areas where the control programmes

have been implemented. During the first years of the national programmes, 13 to 20 cattle herds per thousand were affected by the disease. That average has been cut more than 90 per cent, to less than one herd per thousand. Morbidity has similarly decreased, from 200-300 cases per 10,000 head/year to the current level of 7-8 per 10,000 head.

The foot-and-mouth disease virus-free area - Panama, Central America, the Caribbean and North America - has maintained its status, with the incalculable benefits shared by the different countries therein. Prevention programmes are considerably cheaper than control programmes, as experience has shown.

Nevertheless, except for those disease-free areas, accomplishments have remained static during the last few years. In turn, this situation has eroded the functioning of the services entrusted with conducting the programmes. In part this may be a consequence of the domestic economic crises confronting those countries and of a series of factors which, due to their enormous influence on the programmes' development, have seriously constrained their action. Some of those factors are:

(a) the majority of countries have not formally implemented the approach of applying selective, specific regional strategies for each foot-and-mouth disease ecosystem;

(b) after more than ten years of actions that have significantly reduced the disease, but without actually eradicating it, the programmes are suffering from sluggishness and an ensuing general loss of credibility. The technical personnel, the livestock raisers and the authorities have become frustrated at not fully attaining the initial expectations;

(c) the goals require exclusive dedication, but the lack of suitable material incentives has engendered personnel cutbacks, partial utilization of specialized personnel, and control actions have become mere routines;

(d) the administrative structures of the animal-health services have become bureaucratically disjointed, and the decision-making process becomes bogged down in the administrative hierarchy. There is a lack of administrative strength to maintain the continuity in the sanitary management that would enable the programmes to reach their goals;

(e) there is insufficient inter-institutional co-operation and co-ordination between the animal-health services and others in the livestock and agriculture sector. Integration of those services would bring mutual benefits;

(f) community sectors directly related to animal health - such as the livestock raisers, field hands, meat and dairy products processors, biological firms, cattle traders and dealers, and organized consumers - have not joined up and/or not actively and systematically participated in the foot-and-mouth disease programmes;

(g) within major community sectors, the lack of awareness and concern regarding the disease-control programmes' importance in terms of the country's overall interests has fostered the continuation of isolated interests that tend to counteract the programmes' efficacy;

(h) sanitary risk situations have been generated by virus escapes due to deficiencies in the biological security procedures at both public and private laboratories handling foot-and-mouth disease virus.

SUBREGIONS IN SOUTH AMERICA

The knowledge available today about the modalities of foot-and-mouth disease behaviour in South America shows that its behaviour is intimately related to the forms taken by the productive and economic organization of the livestock sector predominant in an area or region. Likewise, there is undeniably a commercial and epidemiological interrelationship normally produced between and among neighbouring countries. This has been a determining factor in the experience that shows that isolated actions, or actions solely within a given country, will rarely be crowned with success. And success in this case means nothing more than the permanent absence of the disease within the territory concerned.

Therefore the national programmes should necessarily be complemented by on-going co-ordination among countries. In this respect, concrete experiences in the region, involving bi- and multi-lateral integration in the animal health field, have been noted in the region. The seventeen border agreements currently in force in South America are proof of this. One of the foremost is the agreement by which Argentina, Brazil and Uruguay joined efforts in a project to eradicate foot-and-mouth disease in the southeastern region of the River Plate basin. The project encompasses Argentina's Mesopotamia, all of Uruguay, and the State of Rio Grande do Sul in Brazil.

With the goal of foot-and-mouth disease eradication, South America was divided into three subregions. In some cases, parts of a country may belong to different subregions. Likewise, it is certain the "borders" of these subregions will certainly be altered as the Hemispheric Plan undergoes implementation:

(a) RIVER PLATE BASIN-SOUTHERN CONE SUBREGION. Includes Argentina, Chile, Paraguay, Uruguay and the Brazilian states of Rio Grande do Sul, Santa Catarina and Parana.

(b) ANDEAN SUBREGION. Comprises Bolivia, Colombia, Ecuador, Peru and Venezuela. Excepting Ecuador, parts of these countries also lie in the Amazon Subregion.

(c) AMAZON BASIN, BRAZIL AND GUIANAS SUBREGION. This subregion covers Guyana, French Guiana, Surinam, Bolivia's Department of Pando, Peru's Departments of Loreto and Madre de Dios; Colombia's Amazonas Federal Territory and the Intendencias of Vaupes and Guainia, Venezuela's states of Amazonas and Bol.Var, and all of Brazil excepting the states of Rio Grande do Sul, Santa Catarina and Parana.

PURPOSES AND OBJECTIVES OF THE HEMISPHERIC PLAN

1. Purposes

(a) Increase the availability of meat and milk for the Region's inhabitants.

(b) Improve the economic and social efficiency of the livestock-raising activity.

2. Specific Objectives

(a) Eradicate foot-and-mouth disease on the Continent of South America.

(b) Prevent the disease from entering the present disease-free areas, and prevent its causal agent, as well as other pathogenic agents, from entering and thriving in new livestock-raising areas. This applies especially to the Amazon subregion, with awareness of the full ecological integrity of these zones.

3. Intermediary Objectives

Achievement of the specific purposes and objectives mentioned above implies that "intermediary objectives" have been accomplished or maintained in the various countries and regions. Due to a series of factors - such as the epidemiological situation of the disease, the degree of development of the livestock industry and of the infrastructure of the existing services, the community's commitment and participation, etc. - those "intermediary objectives" will not be homogeneous throughout the entire region when the Hemispheric Programme is begun.

These intermediary objectives are:

(a) protection of existing disease-free areas;

(b) creation of new disease-free areas;

(c) advanced control to achieve epidemiological conditions for eradication in the final stage;

(d) formation of animal-health infrastructure in regions where programmes are only slightly developed;

(e) elimination of endemic foci.

Three stages are proposed for accomplishing the gradual eradication of foot-and-mouth disease. By the end of the first two stages, each lasting six years, the infrastructure and epidemiological conditions required for the third and final stage will have been attained. During that final stage, due to work in the last eight years, it will be technically and economically feasible to eradicate the disease throughout South America. Undoubtedly, the time frames envisioned for attaining the intermediate objectives, both in the subregion and in the areas within the subregions, will vary.

STRATEGIES

If the objectives mentioned above are to be attained, two requirements are indispensable. The first is to maintain and encourage the governments' decision in favour of the Plan; the second is to achieve and secure the on-going, active participation of the rural producers during the entire process of programming, executing and assessing the Hemispheric Plan.

The strategies anticipated - one a general strategy, the other selective in its concentration on the ecosystem predominant in an area or region - should necessarily focus on three levels. The first is regional, the next subregional, the third at the level of the countries and based on the national animal-health programmes. The general strategy includes the 'regionalization' of the continent and of the sanitary actions based on (1) characterization of the disease, (2) securing new virus-free areas, (3) technical-administrative co-ordination of the programmes, and (4) obtaining community participation.

With regard to the selective strategies, they will be, within certain limits, specific for each ecosystem existing in an area or region. The following strategies are foreseen:

1. For Primary Endemic Ecosystems

   (a) Break the permanent endemic cycle by means of broad, continuous immunization of the cattle population during a three-five year period.

   (b) Break the cycle of disease transmission to the secondary endemic ecosystem.

2. For Secondary Endemic Ecosystems

   (a) Reduce the entry of infection by means of rationalized control of the entry of animals into these regions.

   (b) Reduce the risk of internal transmission by means of vaccinations having adequate and frequent coverage in terms of the periods of animal transit and the early detection of foci.

3. For Para-endemic Ecosystems

   (a) Strict control of the entry of possible sources of infection.

   (b) Early detection of foci, extinction and control of their spreading.

4. For Disease-Free and Virus-Free Ecosystems

   (a) Establish sanitary restrictions to prevent the introduction of the foot-and-mouth disease agent.

   (b) Create buffer areas.

   (c) Strict sanitary control of the regions of potential livestock influence.

   (d) Strengthen the prevention programmes in the virus- and disease-free countries and regions.

COMPONENTS OF THE PROGRAMME

In accordance with the experience acquired and the new technological advances, the Hemispheric Plan will incorporate the following programme components:

Control and Foci and Animal Transit

This control must be developed with obvious epidemiological criteria, and should implement measures that tend to cut the virus-transmission cycle at any point on that cycle. The early detection of foci, their complete and thorough investigation, and timely attention to them, are vital to prevent the appearance of secondary foci. The most appropriate tactical procedures should be defined continually in each case, taking into account the ecosystem with other ecosystems. The breadth of the quarantine zones and the necessity, or not, of ring vaccination, should seek to reduce the risk of virus diffusion. The efficacy of the measures outlined is largely conditional on the degree of co-operation from the community and the agility and speed of the actions taken by the animal-health services.

The control of animal transit has a decisive influence on the spreading of animal diseases. In the case of foot-and-mouth disease, transit control is especially vital, given the dependence existing among regional ecosystems.

The exit of animals from breeding zones should be controlled with epidemiological criteria that assess the ecosystems existing in those zones as well as the characteristics of the receiving zones. In these latter zones, conditions normally emerge that become propitious for the creation of a secondary endemic ecosystem. Therefore, vaccination of the existing animals must not be the only factor considered for the exit authorization. Other vital factors must also be studied, such as the purpose of the mobilization, the production cycle and the over-all epidemiological situation.

Immunization and Vaccine Quality

The immunization of herds, using different tactics appropriate to the prevalent epidemiological situation and in harmony with regional strategies, must utilize officially approved vaccines which have recognized potency and innocuity. This consideration is of utmost importance, since the success of eradication in regions where the strategy includes vaccination -such as in the primary and secondary endemic areas - is closely related to the quality of the vaccine used.

The type and volume of vaccine to be produced, as well as the appropriate times for it to be produced and furnished, should meet the pertinent requirements as set by the official sanitary services and the rural producers. In this regard, full co-operation with and from the vaccine-producing laboratories is vital to success. The quality control of the final product is the State's full and entire responsibility; it should set the technical standards for achieving the proper efficacy, stability, innocuity and safety. Likewise, the State, jointly with the biological products industry, must establish and supervise the adoption of the most suitable biosafety measures in order to ensure minimum risk of virus escapes from the vaccine diagnosis, production and control laboratories.

At present, current vaccine production capacity meets the needs of the national programmes. Almost all the vaccine is produced with inactivated virus and with aluminum hydroxide adjuvant; this provides up to four months immunity in cattle. A small part of the vaccine production uses oil adjuvant, which yields longer immunity: six months in young cattle, a year in adults.

Storing and Distributing Vaccines

It is of fundamental importance to ensure that the vaccine has retained all its qualities when applied. This means that an efficient mechanism for storing and distributing the vaccine is fundamental, duly oriented and supported by both the vaccine industry and the official animal-health services.

Control of Vaccination in the Field

This control aims to ensure that the vaccine is handled and administered in the appropriate established time and manner, guaranteeing useful vaccination coverages that generate good immunization of the population. It is the responsibility of the official services to set the standards and guidelines for control procedures. However, that responsibility may and should be shared with the private sector, especially with respect to the operational aspects.

Epidemiological Surveillance

Here, the objective is to propose alternatives for action as efficacious as possible. Such alternatives are to be, in this case, targeted on disease eradication, for which they require complete, accurate and timely information.

It is also necessary to encourage and strengthen the active exchange of epidemiological information among epidemiologically related areas. This applies to areas within and/or shared by countries and regions, as well as to the use of the information to make decision-making more objective.

Diagnostic Laboratories

Whereas the confirmation and follow-up of disease occurrence in the field is decisive for control, it is necessary to collect a sufficient number of good-quality samples for the subsequent isolation, identification and characterization of the agent. Therefore, although the region has established an extensive network of vesicular-disease diagnostic laboratories, that network's potential must be strengthened and implemented with both human and physical resources.

Attention to Other Species

Due to its preponderant role in the maintenance and spreading of foot-and-mouth disease, the bovine species is the main one on which the disease-control and/or eradication measures are concentrated. Nevertheless, other susceptible populations will be the subject of tactical and strategic control actions if they are involved in risk situations and/or interfere in the control and eradication process.

Research Applied to the Programmes

Research must be oriented to overcoming the problems that come up as the prevention, control and eradication activities are put into effect, whether the problems are operational or of a technical or administrative nature. Research must also be oriented to supporting the advancement and development of scientific knowledge.

Training of Human Resources

The frequent movement of manpower and staff and the rotation of personnel in the animal-health programmes, as well as the inadequate use of trained personnel, generate a series of demands for training and upgrading of laboratory and field personnel at various levels, including managerial, consulting and executive positions.

Sanitary Education and Community Participation

There is absolutely no possibility of accomplishing and consolidating the eradication of foot-and-mouth disease in the region if the various sectors of society are not encouraged to participate concretely in each and all of the stages in the process. This applies especially to the rural organizations and livestock producers.

Integrated Programmes

In order to utilize the human, material and financial resources as rationally and efficiently as possible, the activities related to foot-and-mouth disease should be as closely as possible, co-ordinated and integrated to other programmes of livestock development. This is particularly valid in regions where the subsistence and very extensive pre-entrepenurial types of livestock production are predominant, since the services' infrastructure involved is generally weak.

Prevention in Virus-Free Countries or Regions

Maintaining the foot-and-mouth disease virus-free status requires prevention programmes wherein five factors are especially relevant: (a) laboratory diagnosis, (b) epidemiological surveillance, (c) community participation, (d) personnel qualification, and (e) co-ordination among the countries. In this respect, the following should be borne in mind: (i) the RIMSA-V recommendation about establishing a "Commission of American and Caribbean Foot-and-Mouth Disease Virus-Free Countries"; (ii) the outstanding efforts that the International Regional Organization for Animal Health and Agriculture (OIRSA) has made in prevention; (iii) the existence of several bilateral agreements on prevention that various countries of the region maintain with the U.S. Department of Agriculture; and, finally, (iv) the impetus that Argentina and Chile, with the participation of the PAFMDC/PAHO, have given to foot-and-mouth disease prevention activities.

Border Agreements

The inclusion of this component within the respective national programmes of special interest, not only as an instrument to facilitate subregional integration and technical co-operation among developing countries, but also to ensure the effectiveness of the sanitary actions applied by each country in the border areas.

Evaluation of the Hemispheric Programme

This evaluation will be conducted within the framework of the COSALFA and the COHEFA when it refers to regional and continental scope. Each country should take the appropriate measures so that all the sectors involved are informed and participate in the evaluation of their national programmes.

ORGANIZATION AND ADMINISTRATION

The accomplishment of the Hemispheric Programme's specific objectives - eradication of foot-and-mouth disease on the South American continent and prevention of its entry into virus-free areas - requires that the national programmes be made suitable for co-ordinated action among the region's countries. Therefore, all countries have undertaken foot-and-mouth disease control programmes that are presently in varying stages of development.

According to the division of the region into three subregions, which were explained previously and which, for purposes of simplification, we shall call Southern Cone, Andean and Amazon, the Hemispheric Programme contemplates three subregional projects. Each one will have a general body of guidelines under a Committee for the Control and Eradication of Foot-and-Mouth Disease. The Committee is composed of the directors of the veterinary or animal-health services of the countries in the particular subregional project, and the Director of the PAFMDC/PAHO, who will act as the ex officio secretary.

The countries have been and are currently still developing concrete measures of bilateral and multilateral integration and co-ordination as they seek to unify criteria, strategies, goals and time frames in the fight against foot-and-mouth disease. Examples are the agreement for the control and eradication of foot-and-mouth disease in the River Plate basin, the co-operative ICA-USDA project involving Colombia and the USA, and the numerous animal-health border agreements involving several of the countries. As the first stage of the Hemispheric Programmes is initiated, the trend is to intensify work related to such activities.

But the foregoing in no way implies that the action and measures not involved in activities cited in the preceding paragraph should be "suspended, reduced or discouraged". Quite the contrary. It is expected that countries, to the extent allowed by their respective economic situations, will strengthen their national programmes so that throughout their territories, conditions may be created so that the disease can be finally eradicated in successive stages.

Moreover, efforts should also pursue maximum coherence at the different levels where actions against foot-and-mouth disease are planned and carried out. In countries, therefore, the initiatives and tasks performed within their territories must be consistent with the definitions stated in their national programmes. In turn, these programmes must be coherent with the hemispheric proposal for eradication of the disease from the whole continent. For this purpose the instances of intra- and inter-country co-ordination should be encouraged and strengthened, as for example, with the national committees of support to the foot-and-mouth disease programmes, such as COSALFA and COHEFA. This also occurs with the PAFMDC/PAHO/WHO, to which the tasks of technical co-operation and co-ordination have been assigned, through its status as secretariat of COSALFA and the role it plays as the reference, training and consulting centre for the countries of the region.

It was mentioned earlier that subregional initiatives have been drawn up and approved by both COSALFA and COHEFA. Those initiatives, which signal the commencement of the subregional projects, are briefly described below:

River Plate Basin - Southern Cone Subregion

The Project for the Control and Eradication of Foot-and-Mouth Disease in the River Plate Basin initially encompasses the provinces of Corrientes, Entre Rios and Misiones in Argentina, the state of Rio Grande do Sul in Brazil, and all of the Republic of Uruguay. Later on, as the financial resources and organization and infrastructure requirements become available, other areas will be incorporated into the Project. The anticipated expansion will commence with the provinces of Chaco and Formosa in Argentina, the states of Santa Catarina and Parana in Brazil, and the southeastern region of Paraguay.

Similarly, Argentina and Chile have agreed to co-ordinate and jointly strengthen their prevention and control programmes on the major-risk borders. In other primary endemic areas, Argentina is also implementing control actions and strategies that go beyond those usually employed.

Andean Subregion

Taking into consideration the diversity of characteristics observed in the epidemiological situation within and among the countries composing this region, the varying development and degree of execution of their programmes and their unequal institutional and financial situations, "six zonal projects" were outlined in an attempt to integrate the five countries into a combined effort to reach the hemispheric objective. In a first stage, and excepting the case of Peru, the six projects only partially cover the territory of the remaining countries. In a later stage, the activities will gradually branch out from those initial zones to the entire subregion.

The following names, given to the zonal projects, identify the areas involved:

1. Atlantic Coast of Colombia-Lake Maracaibo Basin
2. Peru
3. The Colombia-Ecuador Border
4. Beni, Bolivia
5. Plains of Apure (Venezuela) and of Colombia
6. Coast of Ecuador

Amazon Basin, Brazil and the Guianas

Although each country in this subregion conducts its own animal-health projects and the Amazon countries have engaged in border agreements, no specific, multi-national foot-and-mouth disease project has yet been drawn up for the region. Proposals are being considered, and a final plan will be made in the first stage of the Hemispheric Programme for Foot-and-Mouth Disease Eradication in South America. The base project will be Brazil's national programme, which covers most of the livestock zones in this subregion.

The specific subregional project will emphasize the protection and expansion of the virus-free areas. It will likewise seek to ensure that the development of new cattle-raising areas does not affect the regional ecology and takes steps to prevent the introduction of animal diseases, obviously including foot-and-mouth disease.

NEWCASTLE DISEASE CONTROL IN RURAL POULTRY - OVERVIEW ON QUALITY CONTROL OF FOOD BASED NEWCASTLE DISEASE VACCINE

by

A L Ibrahim

INTRODUCTION

Newcastle disease has always been a major disease of poultry in South East Asia. Although the disease is under control, outbreaks have been reported from time to time. In parallel with modern poultry farming, there also exists backyard poultry keeping in which 20 to 30 chickens are raised per household. Chickens that are reared under the backyard system are seldom vaccinated as they are let loose during the day making it difficult to vaccinate them. The local veterinary authority also provides a vaccination programme under which farmers can take their chickens to the veterinary center to be vaccinated. The problems encountered in transporting these chickens normally discourages the farmers from making use of this facility.

The village chicken plays an important role in the ecology of virulent Newcastle disease virus which can be responsible for frequent outbreaks of the disease in rural areas. Virulent Newcastle disease virus is also a threat to large commercial poultry farms. A new method of vaccine production and application needs to be developed. Effective control of Newcastle disease can only be achieved if village chickens are vaccinated. The approach described here was to isolate an avirulent strain of Newcastle disease virus which is immunogenic and heat resistant, and to incorporate that virus in the feed offered to village chickens.

VACCINE PRODUCTION

Selection of heat resistant V4-UPM

The vaccine virus was cloned according to the method described by Aini, (1990). Progeny virus from the last cycle of selection was purified by the limiting dilution method in embryonated eggs. The subsequent pool of purified virus was tested for sterility, purity, safety, identity and antigenecity by standard procedures.

Seed lot system

If the purified candidate virus satisfied all of the above criteria, a seed lot system was established. In the case of V4-UPM the seed was established as follows:

(i) Master seed - prepared by inoculating purified virus into embryonated SPF eggs, harvesting after 2 days, testing and dispensing into ampoules which were stored at -70°C.

(ii) Primary seed lot - prepared by passaging master seed virus in SPF eggs, harvesting, testing and storing as before.

(iii) Secondary seed lot - prepared from primary seed lot in SPF eggs and processing as before.

(iv) Working seed - prepared from secondary seed lot in SPF eggs and processed as before.

Quality Control Testing

A. Master Seed Lot - (MSL)

(i) Sterility
The MSL should be free of bacterial, mycoplasma and fungal contamination.

(ii) Purity

The MSL neutralised by a specific immune antiserum does not contain any contaminating virus after innoculation in embryonated eggs.

(iii) Identity

The MSL is tested by neutralization using a specific immune serum. The neutralization index is at least equal to 2 (log 10).

(iv) Virus titration

The MSL should have acceptable infectious and hemagglutination titres to enable satisfactory production of the seed lot.

(v) Safety

3-week-old chickens vaccinated with $10^7 EID_{50}$ of the vaccine should not exhibit local or general reactions.

(vi) Potency

80% of 3 week old chickens vaccinated with 1 dose of the vaccine should resist challenge with virulent NDV, while 80% of challenge controls should display clinical symptoms or die of ND.

B. Primary and Secondary Seed Lot

The seed lot must be free of bacterial, mycoplasma and fungal contamination.

C. Working Seed Lot (WSL)

The WSL is controlled as for the MSL.

Production Food Based ND Vaccine

Preparation of feed vaccine

The vaccine is prepared in batches of 50 kg of wheat in a feed mixer. The wheat is placed in the mixer housing chamber and 1.25 litres of an aqueous solution of 1% polyvinyl pyrohdoinc (MW 44,000) containing 5 x $10^{10}EID_{50}$ of V4-UPM virus is sprayed into the chamber while the chamber is rotating. When spraying is complete, rotation is continued for another 15 minutes to allow the feed to dry. The dried wheat is stored in plastic bags at 4°C.

Quality control

Virus titration

10 gms (1 dose) of the wheat must contain at least $10^{6}EID_{50}$ of the virus.

Stability

The titre should remain unchanged for at least 4 weeks when stored at 25° and 4°C.

Safety

Safety is tested by observing the behaviour of 3 week old chickens after feeding 10 doses (100 gms) of the vaccine. Results are satisfactory if none of the chickens show abnormal local or general reactions for a period of 1 week.

Potency Test

The potency of the vaccine is evaluated by comparison of the immunity of 3 week old chicks vaccinated with one dose of vaccine with that of similar controls. The vaccine is satisfactory if at least 80% of the vaccinated chicks resist challenge with virulent NDV when 80% of the challenge control chicks display clinical symptoms or die of ND.

Packaging and labelling

(a) Name of produce - Newcastle Disease Vaccine, V4-UPM strain.

(b) Presentation - for 20 chickens - to be given early in the morning by placing the vaccine in the feed trough or by scattering on the ground. The vaccine is packed in plastic bags containing 100 gm of food vaccine - 10 gram per chicken.

C0nclusions

A new food based Newcastle disease vaccine for village chickens has been developed. It is effective, safe, cheap and has a moderate shelf life. Extensive trials conducted in Malaysia over a number of years using this vaccine (including laboratory tests, a simulated field trial, field trials and control trials in pilot villages), has established that chickens vaccinated with it were protected against virulent ND. The vaccine is being used by the Department of Veterinary Services, Malaysia, for its national vaccination programme in the rural areas. Laboratory and field trials carried out in Thailand, Indonesia, Philippines and Sri Lanka have also demonstrated the effectiveness of the food based ND vaccine.

REFERENCES

1. AINI IDERIS, A., LATIF IBRAHIM and SPRADBROW, P.B. (1990) Vaccination of Chickens Against Newcastle Disease With A Food Pellet Vaccine. Avian Pathology **19**: 371-384.

RINDERPEST VACCINE QUALITY CONTROL BY THE PAN AFRICAN VETERINARY VACCINE CENTRE (PANVAC)

by

M Rweyemamu, D Sylla, V Palya, J Prandota and K Wojciechowski

INTRODUCTION

One of the key recommendations of the FAO Expert Consultation on Rinderpest in 1984 was to set up a system of quality monitoring of the vaccine made by 13 rinderpest vaccine producers in Africa. As explained in an accompanying paper, this culminated in the setting up of the Pan African Veterinary Vaccine Centre (PANVAC) (see Sylla et al, these Proceedings).

The purpose of this paper is to present the results of this centralized rinderpest vaccine quality control testing system in Africa between 1988 and October 1991. Testing was set up initially for assessing the quality of vaccine kept as emergency vaccine bank stocks which by definition would be used at short notice in any part of Africa. Progressively the programme has reached a stage whereby the Pan African Rinderpest Campaign (PARC) is urging all veterinary services under the programme to purchase only PANVAC quality certified vaccine.

MATERIALS AND METHODS

Vaccines

Initially, there were 13 rinderpest vaccine producers. Currently only 10 are in active production. All producers employ the cell culture technique and the Kabete O (RBOK) strain of Plowright. Primary/Secondary calf kidney cells have been the traditional substrate. Recently several producers are switching to the user of VERO cells.

Sample Collection

At the beginning of the scheme, vaccine samples were hand carried from the production laboratory to the PANVAC laboratories either in Dakar or Debre Zeit, Addis Ababa depending on western or eastern location. Since then, however, through the UN-host country agreements both centres are able to receive vaccines directly from the production laboratory. In both Senegal and Ethiopia, PANVAC has been accorded the privilege of collecting vaccine samples from the airport with the minimum of delay. The package must be clearly addressed to PANVAC, labelled as vaccine and clearly marked "to be refrigerated during transit". In Eastern Africa sometimes vaccine samples have transitted in Nairobi over weekends. Experience has shown that clearly marked vaccine samples are refrigerated at both Nairobi and Addis Ababa airports, should there by any delay of whatever cause. Consequently, we have not had any recent experience of vaccine spoilage in transit.

A PANVAC vaccine submission form has been distributed to all manufacturers and each submitted vaccine batch is intended to be accompanied by a duly completed form.

PANVAC Quality Control Testing Procedure

The testing procedures employed by PANVAC, which are also recommended to all rinderpest vaccine producers in Africa, have been published as a PANVAC manual and distributed to all the 23 PANVAC vaccine network countries in Africa. Copies are available from either FAO AGA Division, Rome or the PANVAC laboratories in Dakar or Debre Zeit Addis Ababa.

Because the two PANVAC units were initially set up as independent units, methodologies tended to differ in detail. With the development of the PANVAC manual both centres now employ the same test protocols.

It should be noted that the PANVAC manual has been drawn up to conform with the OIE Norms for rinderpest vaccine as well as the European Pharmacopoeia and the procedures of the FAO/WHO Biological Standardization laboratory at Weybridge for testing bovine live viral vaccines.

Thus PANVAC examination is carried out for: vacuum, titration (3 replicates), sterility (3 replicates using the full and undiluted contents of one vial on each occasion), identity, contamination with adventitious viruses and Mycoplasma, innocuity in laboratory animals.

Comparison of the Vaccine Virus Titration Methods

At the time of the FAO Expert Consultation in 1984 only one titration method was in use, namely titration of the virus in primary calf kidney (CK) cell cultures, inoculated at the time of seeding and incubated for up to 11 days rolling. With the advent of new techniques such as the microtitre and cell substrates, eg VERO, it became important to evaluate their effect on virus titre assessment. Furthermore, the centre in Dakar had been forced in 1989 to adopt the microtitre technique using VERO cells, simply on account of irregular availability of CK cells. The following experiments were, therefore, set up at Debre Zeit.

In the first experiment a pool of 20 vials of reference vaccine preparation was made, aliquoted in 1 ml amounts and frozen at -80°C. *On 15 occasions an aliquot was serially* diluted. The same dilution set was inoculated into calf kidney and VERO cell cultures in tubes and microplates. All cells were inoculated in suspension. For tube cultures 5 replicates were used per dilution while 10 replicate wells were employed per dilution in microplate titration. Tubes were rolled while microplates were tape-sealed and incubated in a CO^2 incubator. Both sets of cultures were incubated at 36° ±0.5°^C for 11 days.

In the second experiment vaccines received over a 1 year period at the PANVAC laboratory of Debre Zeit were titrated in parallel, in tubes and microplates and in VERO and calf kidney cells. Also one vial of a reference vaccine preparation was titrated similarly in parallel on each occasion.

RESULTS

Analysis of Titration Methods

The variation in the titre of the reference vaccine pool used for the first experiment is shown in Table 1. Fifteen rounds of comparative parallel titrations were successfully carried out. It can be observed from Table 1 that the test variance was similar for all 4 permutations. There was no significant difference between results from tubes or microtitrations. There was, however, a highly significant difference between the cell systems; VERO cells were found to be more sensitive to rinderpest virus than CK cells ($p = 0.0001$).

The same superiority of VERO cells was evidence in the second experiment (Table 2) in which a vial of reference vaccine was titrated in parallel with the test vaccines ($p = 0.007$). It will be noted from Table 2 that the test variance was higher than in the results from the first set of experiments. This is because variance was dependent both on the vial-to-vial variation in virus content and on the intrinsic error of the test.

Potency Trends in Africa

Tables 3 and 4 demonstrate the number of batches tested in Africa on a regional and producer laboratory basis. A total of 171 and 147 batches respectively for Western and Eastern Africa were tested by PANVAC. It can be observed that the mean titre per field dose for the PANVAC 'passed' vaccines in both Eastern and Western Africa was above 3.0 logs except for vaccine from laboratory N-4. It should be noted that the OIE minimum requirement is log 2.5 with a value of log 3.0 given as a recommendation. Furthermore, for the vaccines which failed, the mean titre was only marginally below the OIE minimum requirement of log 2.5 per field dose, with the exception of vaccine from laboratory S-7. It should be noted that this laboratory no longer produces rinderpest vaccine. Producers A-8 in Western Africa and MB-8 in Eastern Africa, so far, have had a 100 per cent pass record. Figure 1 compares the potency of vaccine from these two laboratories. The similarity of consistency in results from these two producers is evident.

Table 1: VARIATION IN THE TITRATION RESULTS OF A POOL OF A REFERENCE VACCINE PREPARATION

Test Cycle	CK Tube	CK Microtitre	Vero Tube	Vero Microtitre
Round 1	4.50	4.90	5.10	4.70
Round 2	4.70	4.90	5.10	4.80
Round 3	4.50	4.70	5.30	5.30
Round 4	4.70	4.40	4.70	5.00
Round 5	4.50	4.90	5.50	5.30
Round 6	4.70	4.60	5.10	4.90
Round 7	4.70	4.70	5.50	5.00
Round 8	4.70	5.00	4.90	5.20
Round 9	4.70	4.20	5.10	5.40
Round 10	4.70	4.80	5.30	5.30
Round 11	5.10	4.30	5.10	5.00
Round 12	4.70	4.70	4.90	4.90
Round 13	4.30	4.40	5.50	5.40
Round 14	4.50	4.50	4.70	5.10
Round 15	4.70	4.40	4.70	4.90
MEAN	4.6467	4.6267	5.1000	5.0800
Std Deviation	0.1767	0.2492	0.2828	0.2242
Std Error	0.0456	0.0643	0.0730	0.0579

Table 2: **VARIATION IN THE TITRATION RESULTS OF AN FAO REFERENCE VACCINE PREPARATION**

Test Cycle	CK Tube	CK Microtitre	Vero Tube	Vero Microtitre
Round 1	4.30	4.80	5.50	4.70
Round 2	4.70	4.90	5.70	5.80
Round 3	4.90	4.50	4.90	5.10
Round 4	5.10	5.10	5.10	5.30
Round 5	4.70	3.90	4.90	4.60
Round 6	4.50	4.50	4.90	5.00
Round 7	3.40	3.70	4.45	5.30
Round 8	3.40	4.10	4.40	4.60
Round 9	4.80	4.80	5.20	5.00
Round 10	4.60	4.30	4.60	4.20
Round 11	4.60	3.80	5.40	4.50
Round 12	4.50	4.30	5.90	5.40
Round 13	5.10	5.40	5.30	4.90
Round 14	4.90	5.00	5.50	5.30
Round 15	4.90	4.70	5.20	4.70
	4.70	4.60	5.70	5.00
	4.70	4.20	5.10	5.40
	5.40	5.60	5.80	5.80
	5.10	5.10	6.50	5.50
MEAN	4.6474	4.5947	5.2658	5.0579
Std Deviation	0.5103	0.5286	0.5292	0.4388
Std Error	0.1171	0.1213	0.1214	0.1007

Figure 2 shows the evolution of vaccine potency in Africa. For Eastern but not Western Africa, data on manufacturing date was available to PANVAC. It can be seen that between 1986 and now there has been a progressive improvement in the potency of the vaccine batches tested by PANVAC. This is not evident for Western African producers.

Figure 3 shows the highly significant producer to producer variation in the potency of rinderpest vaccine made in Africa. It should be noted that one major producer in West Africa has not submitted vaccine for testing by PANVAC since 1988. Consequently no data for this producer is available for analysis. Laboratory S-7 in Eastern Africa no longer produces rinderpest vaccine. Laboratory DAM-5 has recently had a major overhaul of its vaccine production with a dramatic improvement in the potency of the vaccines recently submitted to PANVAC. Laboratory N-5 is currently undergoing structural modifications. It is too early to assess the impact of this on the potency of vaccine from this producer.

Table 3: RINDERPEST VACCINE QUALITY CONTROL IN EASTERN AFRICA, 1988 TO NOVEMBER 1991

Producer Lab	Batches Tested by PANVAC	Overall Mean Titre/ Dose	Batches Passed	% Pass	Mean Dose Titre for Passed Batches	Mean Dose Titre for Failed Batches
N-5	7	2.54	3	43	3.08	2.13
S-7	13	1.93	4	31	3.11	1.34
M-8	12	3.08	8	67	3.44	2.36
DAM-5	72	2.56	28	39	3.06	2.22
MB-8	43	3.57	43	100	3.57	N/A

Table 4: RINDERPEST VACCINE QUALITY CONTROL IN WESTERN AFRICA, 1988 NOVEMBER 1991

Producer Lab	Batches Tested by PANVAC	Overall Mean Titre/ Dose	Batches Passed	% Pass	Mean Dose Titre for Passed Batches	Mean Dose Titre for Failed Batches
A-8	24	3.58	24	100	3.58	N/A
D-7	41	3.16	28	68	3.50	2.40
K-5	14	3.55	10	71	3.40	3.90
N-4	39	2.49	21	54	2.83	2.09
T-4	53	3.01	37	70	3.15	2.69

Causes of Rinderpest Vaccine Quality Failure in Africa

Table 5 shows the causes of vaccine failures encountered in Eastern and Western Africa. It should be noted that potency has been the most frequent cause of failure followed by sterility. Until recently the range of tests employed in West Africa has been smaller than in East Africa. It is therefore not surprising that the Eastern African centre has isolated BVD from a vaccine sample on one occasion. Also in a collaborative study between the Ethiopian National Veterinary Institute and PANVAC, the screening of CK cell cultures has revealed a 20% incidence of CK contamination with BVD virus (Table 6).

Table 5: CAUSES OF RINDERPEST VACCINE FAILURE IN QUALITY CONTROL TESTS IN AFRICA, 1998 TO NOVEMBER 1991

Region	Total Batches Tested	Total Failed	Potency Fail	Sterility Fail	BVD Fail
Eastern	147	61	54	21	1
Western	171	51	30	24	Not Done

So far no batch has been failed on account of either Mycoplasma contamination or loss of Identity or Innocuity.

Effect of Cell Substrate on Vaccine Potency

Following the demonstration of the superior sensitivity for rinderpest virus of VERO over CK cells, PANVAC encouraged all producers in Africa to evaluate this system. This was also helped by the efforts of the IEMVT and Tufts University, who not only had published data on superior virus yields by VERO cells, but also made similar personal recommendations to the Directors of laboratories. In some cases the switch from CK to VERO cells was dictated by the lack of availability of neonatal calves.

So far PANVAC has tested a total of 25 batches (13 from Western and 12 from Eastern Africa) of vaccine produced in VERO cells. Student 't' analysis of titres per field dose show a significant improvement in potency both in Western Africa ($p = 0.007$) and Eastern Africa ($p = 0.001$). This improvement in potency has been most dramatic for producers who were operating at relatively marginal levels of vaccine potency. Fig 4 demonstrates the effect on the mean potency of vaccine from 2 producers. It can be seen that the results from DAM-5 are more dramatic than those of the MB-8 producer.

Table 6: SCREENING FOR BVD VIRUS IN CALF KIDNEY CELLS INTENDED FOR USE IN VACCINE PRODUCTION

YEAR	Number of Calves Tested	Number Positive	Per Cent Positive
1990	16	3	19
1991	13	3	23

(Collaborative Study Between the Ethiopian National Veterinary Institute and PANVAC)

DISCUSSION

Vaccination campaigns are costly undertakings. Yet, often the vaccine represents one of the cheapest components of such a campaign. It is, therefore, imperative to ensure the quality of the vaccine so as not to nullify the huge operational costs. This, of course, is aside from the purely veterinary medical objectives. The experience of PANVAC has shown the importance of independent centralised testing, particularly in identifying trends towards poor results. Subsequently it is possible to encourage producers to take appropriate action.

In Africa when the concept of independent external testing was put forward there was some resistance by some national laboratories and veterinary services because they tended to view this development as an encroachment on national sovereignty. Now PANVAC testing is fully accepted as an essential component of the Pan African Rinderpest Campaign. At a recent conference (11-12 Nov 1991) of Directors of Veterinary Services and National PARC Co-ordinators from Eastern and Central Africa, the participants passed a unanimous resolution that:

> *"All PARC member countries in the region should only purchase vaccines with a PANVAC quality control certificate"*

As PANVAC has consolidated its programme, so the range of quality control testing has expanded. Inevitably this has resulted in rejecting some vaccines that would have been released at the beginning of the programme in 1985/6. On the other hand it can be said that the vaccines currently passing through PANVAC scrutiny are indeed of a high quality. It is evident that most vaccines now attain the OIE recommended level, which is 3 times higher than the OIE minimum requirement. This is in sharp contrast to the beginning of the programme when only a minority of vaccine batches tested, was attaining the OIE minimum requirement (data not shown).

It is important, however, to reflect on some of the causes of failure. Sterility continues to be a problem. Some of this is accounted for by technique and practices, but there are still several vaccine producers in Africa with inadequate provision of properly functioning laminar flow units for sterile environment operation.

The increasing use of VERO cells in rinderpest vaccine production should, as has been demonstrated, result in improvement of vaccine potency. We believe, however, that the greatest benefit will come from an over all improvement in attitudes to quality control work, in that rinderpest vaccine producers will operate both cell and virus seed banks on seed lot systems. This paper has also shown the danger of BVD contamination. PANVAC has detected the virus in one vaccine batch and through our work with the Ethiopian National Veterinary Institute we have shown some 20% of calf kidneys to be unsuitable for vaccine production on account of BVD contamination. In one country in East Africa a BVD outbreak which possibly had some association with rinderpest vaccine or vaccination caused quite a public outcry, primarily because of the fear of rinderpest. This is yet another reason for recommending the use of VERO cells for the production of rinderpest vaccine, since VERO cells are non-permissive to BVD virus

Fig. 1

BATCH TO BATCH POTENCY OF RP VACCINE FROM BEST TWO AFRICAN PRODUCERS

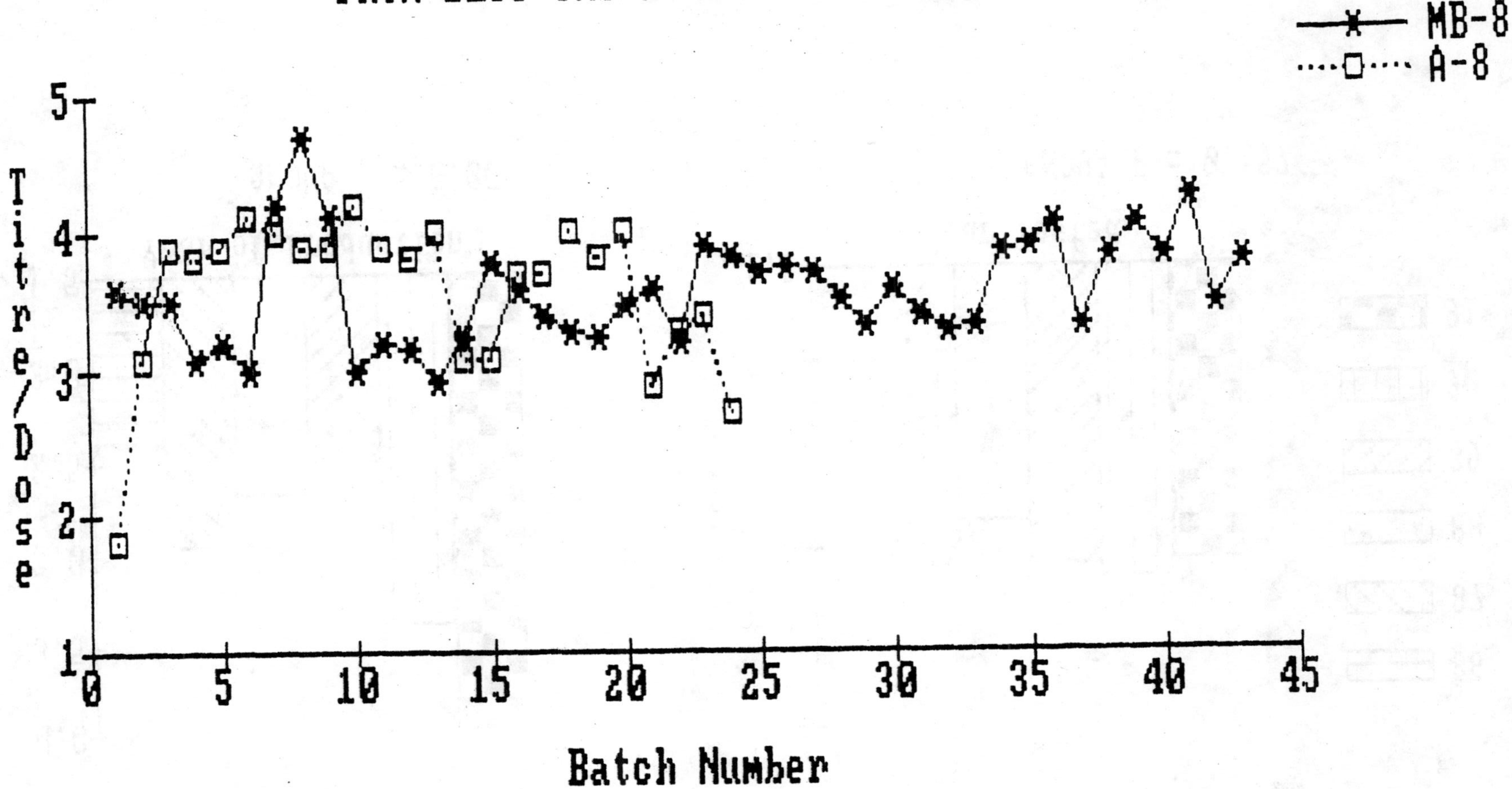

Fig. 2

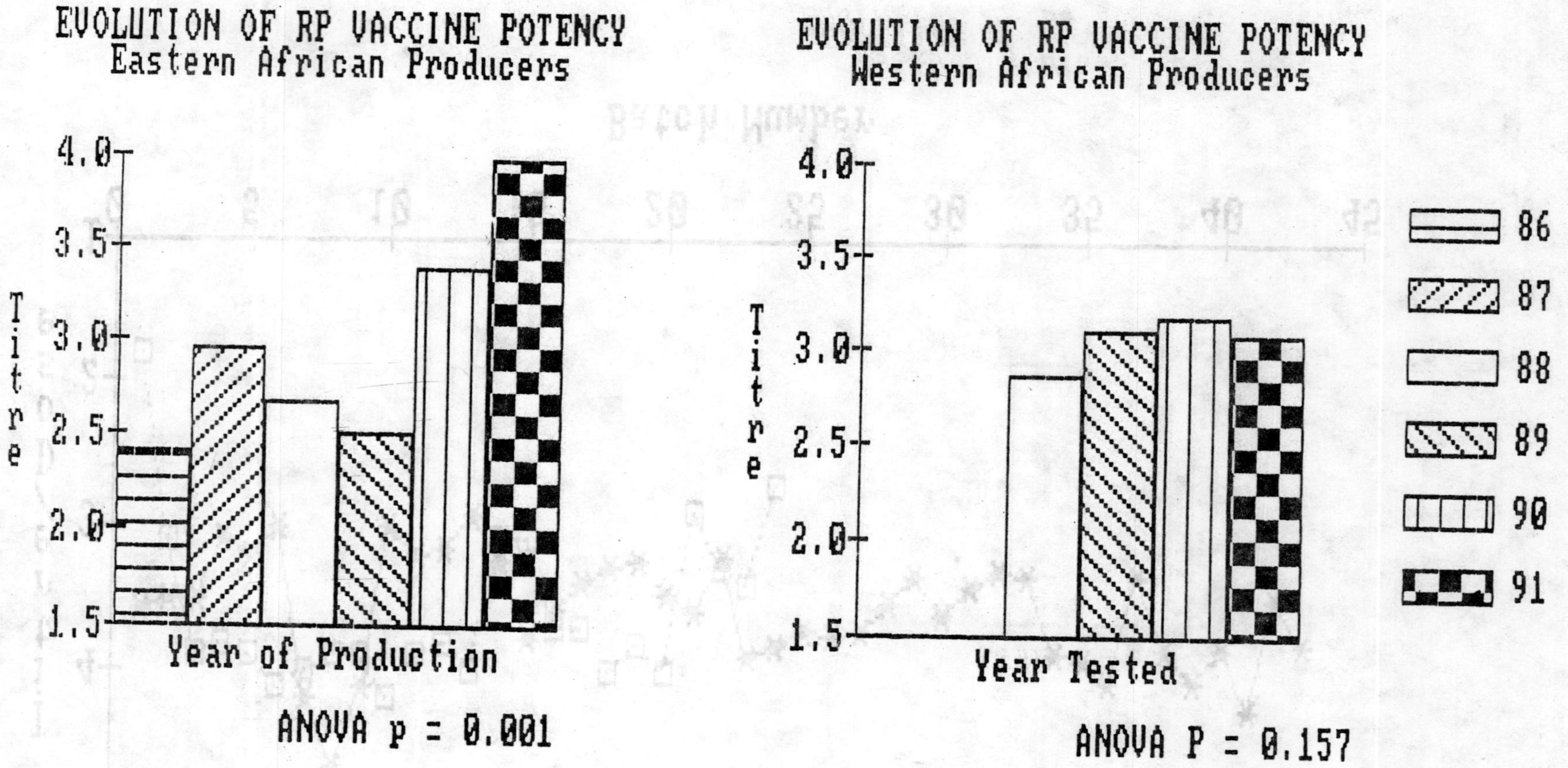
EVOLUTION OF RP VACCINE POTENCY
Eastern African Producers
Titre
4.0
3.5
3.0
2.5
2.0
1.5
Year of Production
ANOVA p = 0.001
EVOLUTION OF RP VACCINE POTENCY
Western African Producers
Titre
4.0
3.5
3.0
2.5
2.0
1.5
Year Tested
ANOVA P = 0.157
86
87
88
89
90
91

Fig. 3

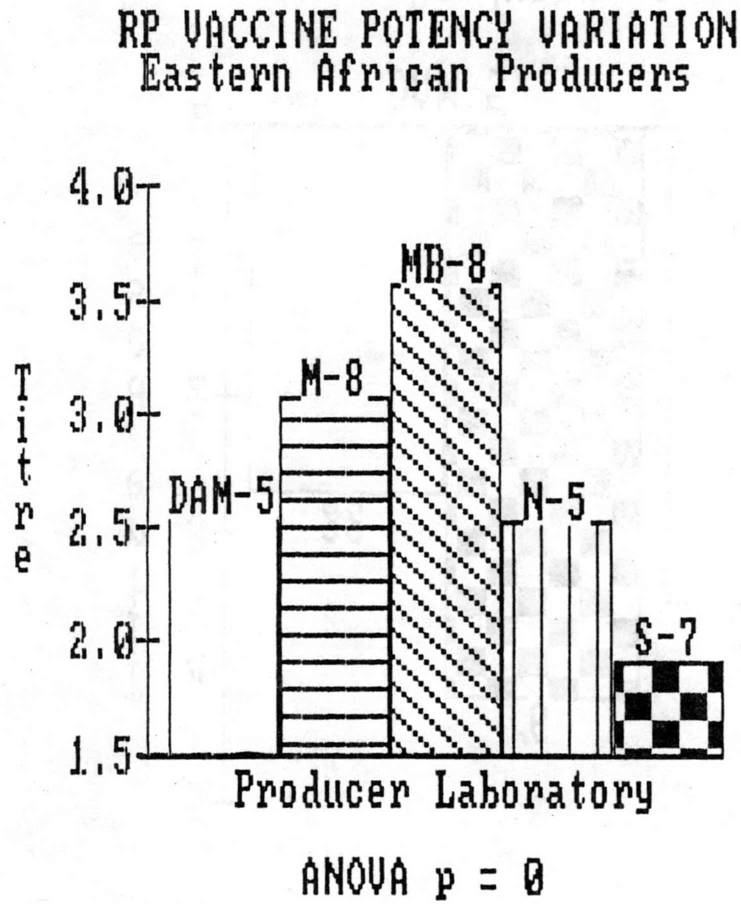
RP VACCINE POTENCY VARIATION
Eastern African Producers
4.0
3.5
3.0
2.5
2.0
1.5
Titre
DAM-5
M-8
MB-8
N-5
S-7
Producer Laboratory
ANOVA p = 0

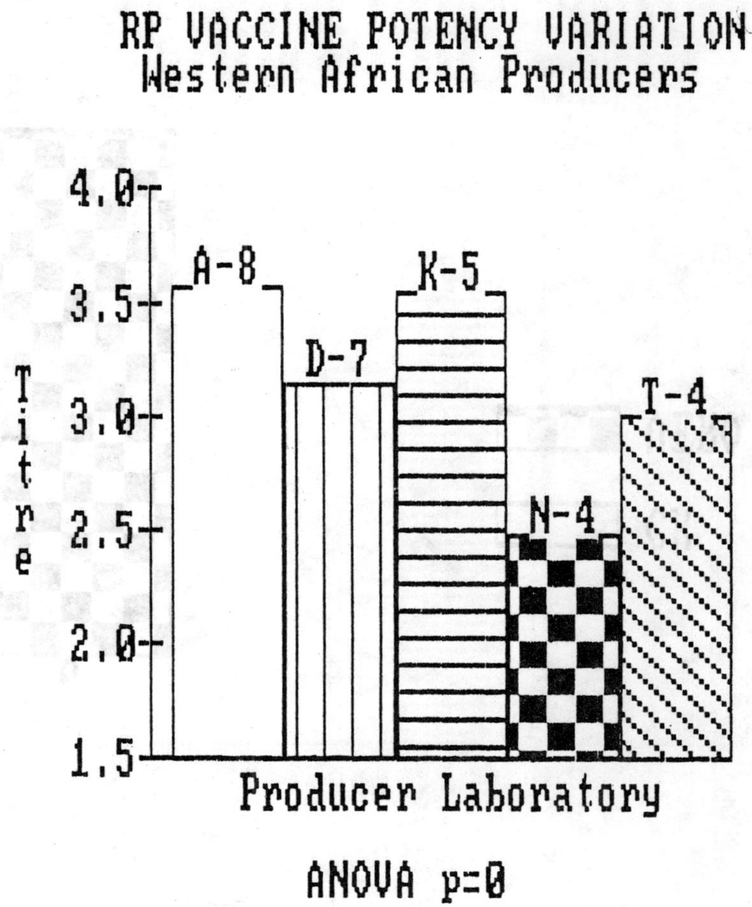
RP VACCINE POTENCY VARIATION
Western African Producers
4.0
3.5
3.0
2.5
2.0
1.5
Titre
A-8
D-7
K-5
N-4
T-4
Producer Laboratory
ANOVA p=0

Fig 4 POTENCY OF CK AND VERO PRODUCED RP VACCINE

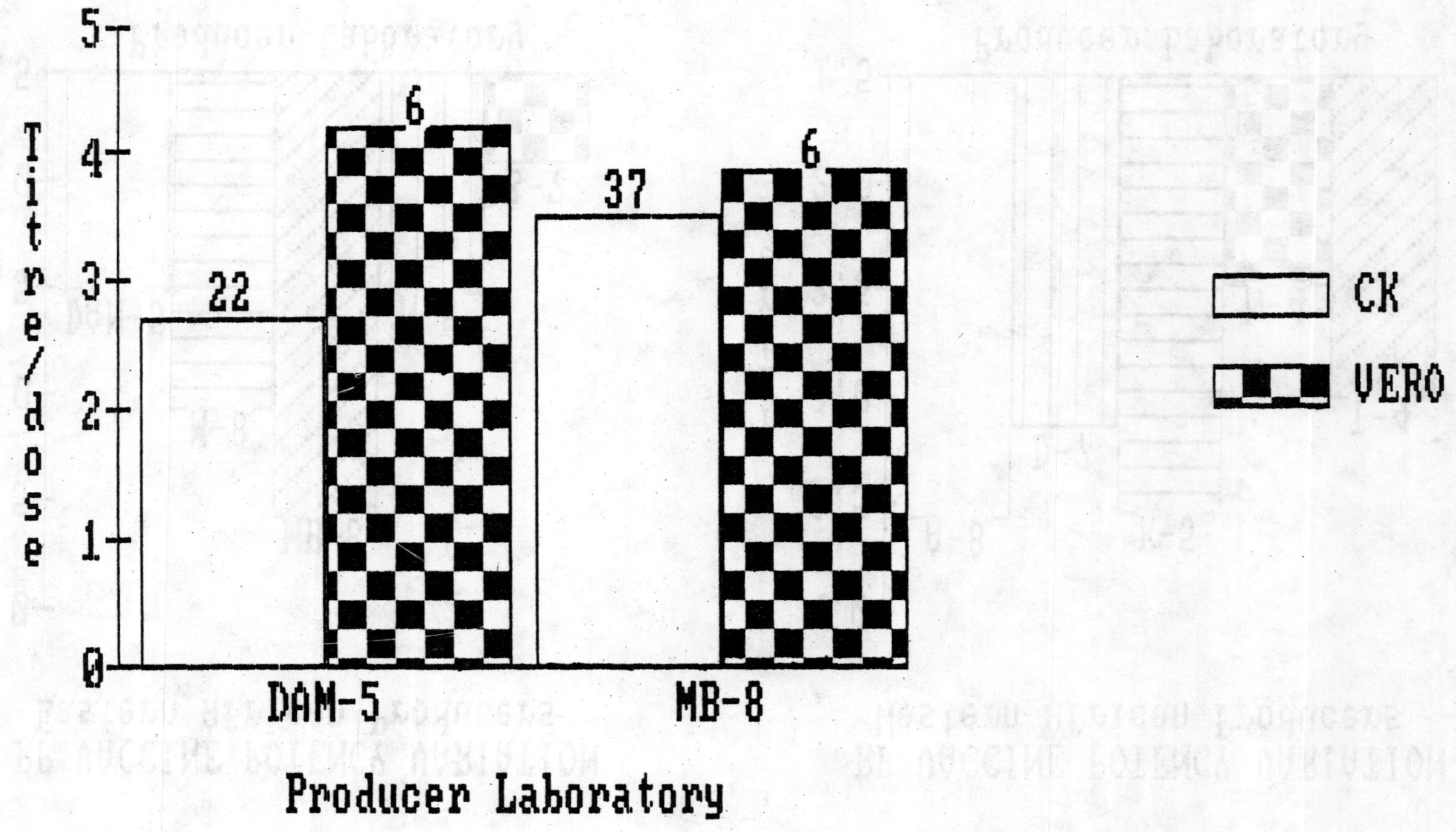

SEROMONITORING OF POSTVACCINAL IMMUNITY

by

M H Jeggo

INTRODUCTION

Seromonitoring of the postvaccinal response is one of the approaches that can be used to measure the success or otherwise of a vaccination programme. If the serological response measured is that which confers protection, or correlates exactly with immunity then seromonitoring can be considered the ultimate quality assurance procedure. Not only does this approach ensure that the vaccine as a product is efficacious but it ensures that the method of administration is adequate and that the population being vaccinated is responding. The major limiting factor of this approach is a frequent inability to sample all the animals in a population. In these cases the value of the results will be dependant on the suitability of the sampling frame adopted.

Serology has been used as the basis for many disease control and eradication campaigns but often vaccination responses have served to confuse rather than assist this process. A notable example would be that of brucellosis where a number of serological tests are frequently employed to separate a vaccine from a field challenge immune response [1]. The situation can become further confused if the serological response being measured identified group-specific antibodies as opposed to a type-specific response.

More recently the use of recombinant technology has enabled vaccine producers to develop products that have been altered in such a way that the response to vaccination can be easily separated from that to a field challenge using serological techniques such as ELISA. One such case is the latest generation of vaccines against Aujeszky's disease [2].

Africa is at presence involved in the largest ever animal disease control and eradication programme, the Pan African Rinderpest Campaign (PARC). Seromonitoring has been an integral part of this campaign from the outset. This paper will detail the introduction and use of an ELISA-based system for seromonitoring during the past six years of this campaign. It is intended that this account will serve to illustrate the advantages and pitfalls of seromonitoring along with the many problems that must be overcome in introducing an international and standardized approach to the process.

The Rinderpest seromonitoring network in Africa

PARC aims to control and eventually eradicate rinderpest from Africa through a process of mass vaccination. A previous campaign, JP15 had set out with a similar aim, but although it was highly successful at control it failed to eradicate the disease. A number of factors were responsible for this failure although of paramount importance was an inability to maintain adequate levels of immunity in the cattle whilst the virus persisted in the region. To avoid this pitfall, PARC included from the start seromonitoring of the vaccination programme to ensure that adequate levels of immunity were reached in each participating country for control and eradication of the disease. It is also intended that this same mechanism of seromonitoring can be used in the later stages of the campaign when vaccination ceases, to carry out serosurveillance to detect seroconversion occurring in a population through the presence of undetected foci of residual virus.

How to achieve this? The PARC approach has always been to operate at the national level and it was not envisaged that one central laboratory would test all the sera in the region but rather that in each participating country one or a number of laboratories would be designated to carry out the testing. However, if the results were to be meaningful on a regional basis it was imperative that similar sampling and testing procedures be adopted in all participating laboratories.

The Joint FAO/IAEA Division in Vienna has operated Co-ordinated Research Programmes (CRP) for several years. Through these programmes research contracts are awarded to scientists in developing countries on an annual basis for up to five years. Each programme has a common research topic and scientists within a programme are brought together several times over the five years to discuss their results and plan future work. This approach appeared ideal for the seromonitoring needs of PARC and in 1987 the FAO/IAEA/SIDA/PARC CRP entitled "The seromonitoring of rinderpest throughout Africa" was established. This CRP was concerned with providing support to individual institutes — in most cases — the central veterinary laboratories of countries participating in PARC.

Programme Support

The programme was initially funded for five years with the majority of the research contracts being supported by funds provided by SIDA. In 1990 SIDA agreed to fund a follow-on programme (Phase II) for a period of at least a further three years.

IAEA also operates a technical co-operation programme aimed at providing support to its Member States for the peaceful use of nuclear and related techniques. In a large number of Member States, technical co-operation projects serve to provide equipment, training and expert services to assist in technology transfer. In animal health, these are mostly concerned with the introduction and use of the ELISA to improve national diagnostic capabilities. This activity is carried out in many of the laboratories responsible for rinderpest seromonitoring and in receipt of FAO/IAEA research contracts under the SIDA-funded programme. In most cases therefore there was an integration of the support provided through research contracts and individual country technical co-operation activities (see Table I).

In these cases, IAEA technical co-operation projects provide the bulk of the equipment, supplementary training fellowships for laboratory staff, and expert services for more extensive technical backstopping, whilst the research contracts provide the ELISA kits and funding for the annual meetings and training courses. It should be noted that wherever possible these two support mechanisms are integrated with support provided through other organizations and in particular FAO, EEC, ODA and GTZ.

Programme Co-ordination

Overall co-ordination of activities conducted under this programme is carried out by the FAO/IAEA regional technical co-operation expert for animal production and health in

Africa. At all times a close dialogue is maintained between the IAEA, FAO and PARC. Numerous visits are undertaken by the programme co-ordinator to PARC headquarters Nairobi and to the participating laboratories. In keeping with the duality of language found in the region, the programme operates both in French and English with the major publications being available in both languages.

Research Contracts

During Phase I of the programme, 21 research contracts were awarded to scientists involved in rinderpest seromonitoring (Table I; Fig. 1). These contracts however, were not all awarded at the commencement of the programme in 1987. Some were incorporated later as the need for a seromonitoring capability arose in individual PARC participating countries.

In a number of cases, individuals initially identified as research contract holders became inappropriate and it was necessary to identify a new person. Research contracts were awarded on an annual basis with the sums provided ranging from $1,000 to $10,000 per year, and in many cases a portion of the grant has been made available locally to provide funds for sample collection.

As part of the FAO/IAEA/SIDA/PARC Co-ordinated Research Programme, research agreements were awarded to scientists from developed countries whose primary task was to oversee and assist the work carried out under the research contracts. Under the Phase I programme, research agreements were awarded to Dr J Anderson of the Pirbright Laboratories, Institute for Animal Health, UK; and to Dr G Libeau of the Institut dElevage et de Médicine Vétérinaire des Pays Tropicaux, Maisons Alfort, France. Both these scientists have been involved for many years in the use of ELISA in developed and developing country situations. Under Phase II research agreements have also been awarded to Dr L Tyler of the Epidemiology Department of Reading University, UK and Dr R Lancelot attached to the French aid programme in Chad. These awards reflect the change of emphasis away from assay introduction and toward improving sampling strategies.

Research Co-ordination Meetings

Research co-ordination meetings are held each year, and in conjunction with training courses. This has proved invaluable in maintaining a close link with all those in the network and developing a standardized and uniform approach.

Contract holders joining the programme after it had commenced were able to learn at these meetings from more experienced members and avoid many of the early pitfalls. These meetings also serve to identify general problems with the kit and accompanying equipment, and enable improvements and the introduction of new components (eg computer software) to be rapidly assimilated into the network. At each research co-ordination meeting, contract holders are required to give a presentation of their work during the last twelve months. A generalized workplan for the following 12 months is agreed upon, taking into account the different situation in each country. Equipment and further training requirements are also dealt with on an individual basis.

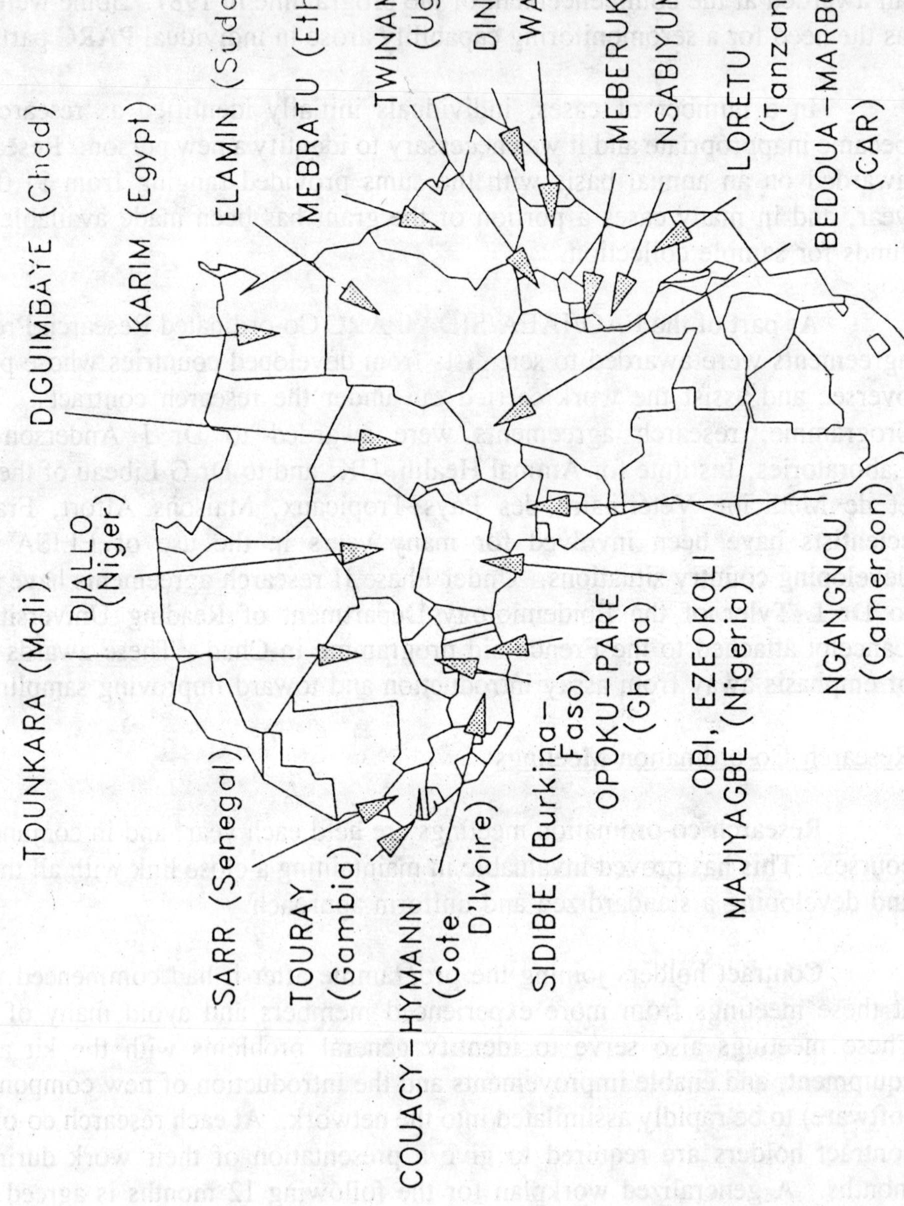

Fig. 1 FAO/IAEA/SIDA/PARC Network for Sero–monitoring of Rinderpest

At the final meeting of the Phase I programme in Cote DIvoire (November 1990) each participant produced an account of all activities conducted under the programme during the first five years [3].

Training

A key component of this programme is the provision of adequate and appropriate training. This is carried out both at the annual co-ordination meetings and through the provision of extensive technical backstopping in individual laboratories. Technical officers and outside FAO/IAEA experts visit each laboratory in the network at least once a year. This has proved invaluable in providing local training to a number of staff of a particular laboratory and augments greatly that provided to contract holders at the research co-ordination meetings.

The subject matter covered during training has been introduced in a stepwise logical manner. Initial emphasis was therefore on the use of the ELISA both as a general diagnostic tool and more specifically as used in the FAO.IAEA rinderpest ELISA kit. Once it was clear that contract holders could reliably test samples using the ELISA-based system the training emphasis moved towards basic and applied epidemiology to ensure that the samples collected would provide the information required. Towards the completion of the first programme, training was provided in the use of computers and specialized computer software to store and manipulate the data.

Crucial to the success of the network is the frequent visits by FAO/IAEA technical officers and experts to participating laboratories. This serves to identify many of the difficulties experienced locally and provides considerable impetus to solve these.

Finally, and perhaps most importantly, it is now possible to utilize the more experienced contract holders from within the programme to act as IAEA and FAO experts to other laboratories. Within the region therefore, the programme has built up a pool of experienced scientists who can technically backstop others in the region.

Two important factors should be taken into account when considering the rinderpest seromonitoring network. Firstly it was never envisaged that the FAO/IAEA/SIDA Co-ordinated Research Programme would provide the primary funding for the serological surveys. Thus under the programme, research contracts were awarded to individuals in each participating country primarily to provide the ELISA kits and some basic laboratory equipment. In many cases though, funds for the laboratory equipment were augmented through IAEA technical co-operation projects, the EEC and national government organizations (ODA, GTZ). The programme also provided for annual research co-ordination meetings which were often held in conjunction with specialized training courses, and for technical backstopping by FAO.IAEA and FAO technical staff and outside experts. In essence therefore, the FAO/IAEA/SIDA programme provided the primary support for the laboratory aspects of seromonitoring.

It was foreseen from the beginning that funds for the actual collection of sera (involving transport, staff per-diems, sampling tubes, refrigeration equipment etc) would be provided by national governments with assistance from PARC. In most cases this assistance would be EEC-funded. In reality, the accompanying activity of sera collection has taken considerably more time to organize and become operational. Hence in many participating countries, the sera collected to-date for rinderpest seromonitoring has often been carried out by laboratory staff including the FAO/IAEA research contract holders in an attempt to get seromonitoring underway before a fully functioning field sample collection system is in place.

The second factor to be noted is that the PARC programme is a gradual event. No two countries are at the same stage of PARC implementation. Thus proposals for inclusion in the rinderpest seromonitoring network can be received throughout the life of the programme and the programme itself thus has to take account of the varying abilities and experience of individual contract holders. Although the network approach tended to bring the expertise in individual laboratories to the same level much more quickly, it did create some organizational problems and frustrations on the part of contract holders. Individuals fully conversant with the techniques and with their laboratory poised to test thousands of sera became understandably disappointed when the sera did not arrive. This varying rate of seromonitoring implementation in each country is clearly visible from the reports contained in the proceedings of the meeting in Cote DIvoire [3].

Clearly, at the end of Phase I the task of seromonitoring was not complete and although nearly all the participating laboratories were capable of using the assay, routine testing of sera had only commenced in 4 or 5 laboratories within the network. Thus SIDA were approached and once again were generous in supplying funds for a Phase II CRP. In the majority of cases the same persons are involved in this new programme (Table 2) and thus a continuity has been maintained. The first meeting under the new CRP took place in Cameroon in October 1991 at which participants were trained in the use of the new FAO/IAEA Competitive ELISA kit [3].

The FAO/IAEA Rinderpest ELISA Kit

Central to success of a seromonitoring programme is the selection and use of the most appropriate serological assay.

In the detection of antibodies against rinderpest virus, neutralization has been the most widely used diagnostic test. This was used in two forms, the tube neutralization test [4] and the virus micro-neutralization test [5, 6]. A large number of sera were tested using the tube neutralization system during the 1960's at the Kenya Agricultural Institute, using many animals of known disease status [7]. This established the tube neutralization as the "bench-mark" test and it still occupies that position today [8]. However, because of the cost and the difficulties of routinely carrying out a tube neutralization system, the microtitre plate assay became more widely used. Although this system is easier to use than tube neutralization it still requires tissue culture facilities, is time consuming, cannot process sera that are contaminated and more importantly shows considerable variability in its sensitivity and specificity between and even within laboratories [8].

The use of an ELISA system for the detection of antibodies to rinderpest virus was first described in 1982 [9]. This system clearly has a number of unique advantages for the wide-scale testing of sera as envisaged under PARC and was the natural choice for use in the FAO/IAEA/SIDA/PARC seromonitoring network. Although details of the validation of this

ELISA against the virus micro-neutralization test and its use to detect antibodies in animals of known disease status have been published [9, 10] a number of the national laboratories within the network (Kenya, Sudan, Senegal, Egypt) also carried out comparative studies of the ELISA with the neutralization test. In all cases a high level of agreement was achieved and in all cases the ELISA was adopted as the test of choice.

In preparing this ELISA kit it is necessary to consider a number of important factors relating to its supply and use:

(a) The reagents should be able to withstand prolonged exposure to high temperature (20°C - 30°C) and high humidity as the kits may well have to spend some time in transit to laboratories in Africa (ie at airport customs holding areas).

(b) The reagents should comply with regulations governing the transport of chemicals by air as laid down by the civil aviation authorities. This for example, precluded the inclusion of sulphuric acid as a stopper in the kit.

(c) The box containing the kit should be relatively small but contain sufficient reagents for testing the number of sera that are likely to be collected in one year (an initial conservative estimate was 20,000). This precluded the dispatch of antigen-coated plates.

(d) The actual ELISA system adopted should be as simple and robust as possible. In this context the assay used in Tanzania [11] was indirect ELISA and used well-established reagents. However it was necessary to conduct trials on the stability of these reagents, and on their ability to withstand high temperatures and freeze-drying.

(e) The kit should contain all the necessary reagents. Thus all the buffers required must be included along with the more obvious conjugate and substrate.

(f) The kit should be supplied with a detailed manual. This should cover all aspects of the use of the kit as well as some practical information regarding buffer composition, interpretation of results, trouble-shooting, sera collection and references.

(h) The kit and the manual should be flexible enough to allow for the incorporation of changes as problems are encountered and solutions found. This was particularly relevant to reagent packaging (eg the later use of tablets instead of powders) and updating of the manual (ie a loose-leaf approach was essential).

(i) Components of the kit, including the plates should be available in bulk to ensure standardization. For example, the plates are obtained from NUNC (Nunc Ltd. Netherlands) as a single batch run of 10,000. Sixty plates from the run are initially sent to the FAO/IAEA Laboratory at Seibersdorf, for checking for defects prior to acceptance of the whole batch. This large batch run then provides a one-year supply of uniform plates to the rinderpest network.

Having taken into account these various factors and on completion of the reagent stability trials, the FAO/IAEA rinderpest indirect ELISA kit was ready for use in mid-1987. During the subsequent 4 years a great deal of experience was gained in the use of this kit, in problems relating to its dispatch to individual laboratories and in interpreting the results.

When examining problems relating to the use of the kit, it was found that in nearly all cases these related to the quality of the water used for reconstitution of the various reagents supplied. In particular, in reconstituting those components supplied freeze-dried (antigen, reference sera and conjugate) it was found essential that properly de-ionized water was used. Although in many cases the pH of the water is checked and found to be correct, other extraneous ions or pyrogens can interfere with the functioning of the reconstituted reagents. In 1990 sufficient water and glass vials for the reconstitution of all freeze-dried reagents were included in the kit.

The only other significant change to the kit was the supply of most reagents in tablet rather than powder form. Although this is more expensive, the reagents remain in better condition in tablet form and the use of tablets enables the reagent solutions to be prepared in smaller and more convenient volumes.

The kit is supplied as two distinct components. One component containing the antigen and positive and negative reference sera is dispatched from the Pirbright Laboratory, Institute for Animal Health, UK. The other component containing the remainder of the reagents is dispatched from the FAO/IAEA Laboratories, Austria.

It is pertinent to note that the rinderpest ELISA kit was designed to measure the level of rinderpest vaccination achieved in participating countries. The indirect ELISA which was developed was, and still is, ideal for this purpose. Nevertheless, as PARC moves towards a phase of serosurveillance to ensure the absence of circulating virus - and this will only be carried out after vaccination has ceased in a country - an assay is required with higher levels of sensitivity and specificity. To meet these needs an ELISA based around the use of a monoclonal antibody in a competitive assay was developed [3]. This new ELISA kit is already complete and participants in the programme have been trained in its use and have sufficient reagents to test the number of sera likely to be collected in the next twelve months. The network has thus now switched over to the routine use of this new assay.

Sera Sampling

A crucial factor influencing the validity of the results obtained, is the way in which the samples are collected. It is essential that the animals sampled are representative of the population as a whole and that sufficient data are collected with each sample to enable meaningful conclusions to be drawn.

In many countries, contract holders are not only responsible for the actual testing of the sera, but also for the collection procedure and it is essential to also provide support for this activity. In 1987 an FAO/IAEA consultants group was convened in Vienna to develop guidelines on the sampling protocol to be adopted. These guidelines took into account both the objectives of seromonitoring and the constraints that operate in Africa to restrict the use of ideal sampling approaches. In 1988, FAO/IAEA/SIDA published a booklet entitled "Guidelines for Seromonitoring of Cattle Conducted by PARC" giving epidemiological guidelines for the seromonitoring of cattle as envisaged under PARC. During subsequent research co-ordination meetings and training courses this acted as the basis for developing sampling strategies in each of the countries in the network. However, in all cases account has to be taken of local constraints and in no two countries is the sampling approach identical.

Support to national staff responsible for survey design and field work in the monitoring of the success of the mass-vaccination campaign has consisted of discussion at workshops, the preparation of training materials and consultancy visits. Assistance has also been given with analysis and presentation of results.

To some extent the survey design and implementation is a learning process for all concerned and is thus still evolving and indeed a new edition of the seromonitoring guidelines is under preparation.

Ancillary Support

Computerization

The PARC seromonitoring campaigns create a great deal of data concerning herd structures, their history of rinderpest vaccination and outbreaks, and details of ELISA test results from individual animals. A typical annual national survey which includes 100 herds, with an average of 40 animals sampled per herd, produces 100 herd records and 4000 test records every year. In a larger country with more than one ecological zone or system of animal management twice or three times this amount of data may be generated.

The records need to be analyzed in a variety of ways, to estimate the distribution of herd prevalences, to show the spatial distribution of herd prevalences, and to estimate prevalences in different age groups etc. To date, analysis has generally been fairly rudimentary but this area of work is expected to develop in the future as more countries produce data of high quality. The results must be presented clearly in tables and histograms and for between-country and between-year comparisons, some sort of standardized presentation is needed. Where very variable distributions are found there may be a need to investigate the effect of location, management system, vaccination history or herd structure on antibody prevalence.

To manage the volume of data and to allow flexibility in analysis, a computer is essential. Given the capabilities of modern microcomputers, one microcomputer with a hard disk in each participating country is sufficient to hold the national seromonitoring data, provided that the computer is not used for other tasks. It is not feasible for all the PARC data to be held centrally, since there is not sufficient manpower to deal with the data entry. In any case this would not be desirable since it would be almost impossible to verify the data and maintain a high level of data quality. Further, detailed data on ELISA tests can most conveniently be captured through a direct link between a computer and an ELISA reader. In the long term a centralized data processing system would lack flexibility and have limited use for the individual countries in PARC. The policy adopted has therefore been to supply each participating country with its own microcomputer, and to provide on-site training for the operators.

ELISA Data Information (EDI) Programme

Two types of software are used to capture the PARC seromonitoring data. To record details of ELISA tests and results, the computer and ELISA reader are directly linked by serial cable and the EDI programme is then used to control all the ELISA reader functions through an easy to use menu. Data generated from the testing of sera with the FAO/IAEA ELISA kit is automatically processed and transferred to the computer for storage and further manipulation if required.

Calculation of the results based on the negative and positive controls on each plate are automatically carried out and the programme calculates individual plate binding ratios and variation between duplicate samples. All this data can be immediately printed out using either the internal printer of the ELISA reader or an external printer connected to the computer. Finally, the results are stored in such a manner in the computer that they can be automatically transferred to the Serum Information Data (SID) programme containing all the details on each serum tested.

Serum Information Data (SID) Programme

For epidemiological analysis a combination of database and statistical functions is required. The Panacea programme which was chosen for this work combines the necessary functions and is not difficult to use. But for operators who use a computer only infrequently a database can be expected to present more problems than, for example, a word processor, or a spreadsheet used for financial calculations, because it is less "user friendly" and requires a greater understanding of the organization of data. For these reasons the decision was made to customize Panacea so that data entry and routine epidemiological analysis could be done easily and the programme could detect and draw attention to obvious errors during data entry. Participants in the seromonitoring are therefore now supplied with SID, which is a customized programme based on Panacea, and also with a full copy of Panacea, so that if they become sufficiently expert they can carry out a much wider range of analyses than is available through SID. Because the seromonitoring data are held at two levels (the herd and the individual animal), this requires a two-level database structure, but the partitioning of data is handled automatically by SID and is transparent to the user.

A data entry programme is of limited use without guidance in recording the data in the field. It is important that field forms match the contents of the computer database, and that the layout of field forms and data entry screens are as far as possible identical so that data entry can be fast and accurate. Two field forms are provided with SID and the manual which accompanies the programme contains some guidance on their use. To a great extent compatibility has been achieved between forms and screens. Some modifications are planned and any mismatches between paper and screen should then be removed.

Quality Assurance Programme

In utilizing a standardized protocol and set of reagents for conducting rinderpest seromonitoring in the many laboratories involved in PARC, it is hoped that a uniformity will be achieved in the ability of each laboratory to test cattle sera for antibodies to rinderpest virus. However, mere use of these reagents and adherence to the protocol does not ensure this and thus it is necessary to operate a quality assurance programme. Involvement in the programme will not only enable individual laboratories to ascertain if they are using the kit correctly, but also demonstrate to all interested parties that the results being obtained are reliable and comparative from one laboratory to another.

Although this assurance of the reliability of the seromonitoring data is important in the vaccination phase of the eradication campaign, it becomes essential in the various stages that a country must go through in declaring the disease eradicated. It is vital that outside regulatory bodies and indeed funding organizations are convinced of the reliability of such results from each laboratory.

The aim of the first quality assurance exercise in 1990 was to compare the reproducibility and sensitivity of the FAO/IAEA rinderpest ELISA system between laboratories. There was no element of criticism in this exercise and it was purely a means of quality control for the rinderpest seromonitoring network. It was agreed that the results would be treated in strict confidence and laboratories involved were asked to send a copy of the results including the actual optical density (OD) values, graphs and frequency distribution plots to FAO/IAEA, Vienna.

Of the 15 laboratories actively using the kit at that time, 9 submitted results. These revealed that the kit was working well although the overall binding ratio (an indication of the ability of the assay to separate positive from negative sera) was sub-optimal. The results also revealed that in every laboratory the local negative population gave a lower value than the kit reference negative sera. This was not unexpected, as the kit reference negative serum was never intended to be used for the calculation of negative/positive cut-off values and was included only as a reference. The examination of local negative sera and the establishment of the mean local population negative value is essential to the establishment of the test in any laboratory. An examination of individual laboratory results indicated that where problems were encountered it was invariably due to the use of poor water for reconstitution of reagents. This has confirmed the need to supply sterile de-ionized water for re-constitution of all kit reagents. The results from this quality assurance exercise proved vital in identifying problems with the kit itself and with the use of the kit in individual laboratories. In the most part these problems have now been resolved. However, in retrospect it is considered that the approach adopted was over-complicated and in future quality assurance will involve the testing of a panel of 44 sera distributed to all participating laboratories once a year.

Examples of Results Obtained

The rinderpest seromonitoring network is now generating a great deal of information on national vaccination campaigns and this is being used to monitor progress both on an annual basis and during the actual vaccination period. In this latter case information is being fed back to national co-ordinators continually enabling them to identify poorly vaccinated areas and even vaccination teams that are having difficulties.

This data is also being used on a regional basis to ascertain areas where levels of immunity are low and represent risks for the regional spread of the disease. For example, cases of rinderpest are still occurring in northern Uganda and southern Sudan. If the spread of disease westwards through Chad and the Central African Republic is to be prevented high levels of immunity must be achieved in these areas. Results from Chad would indicate that this is not at present the case and thus revaccination must be carried out along borders with infected countries [12].

In initially establishing the indirect ELISA it was necessary for each country to determine a local negative value (Fig 2) prior to testing sera from vaccinated animals. Once this has been carried out, then large numbers of sera can be rapidly tested and the results passed on to the national co-ordinator.

In analyzing the data it is imperative that details of the sampling frame are available. For example, if at the sera collection site it is not possible to randomly sample animals then this will produce a bias in the results and although these results may still be valid, care must be taken in their interpretation.

Examples of the types of the results that can be obtained using the recommended sampling frame are shown in Tables III and IV and Fig 2. It is possible to generate immunity levels on populations from region to region (Table III), from within different age groups (Table IV) or from year to year (Fig 3). Indeed, using the computer software programme SID it is possible to compare information from any combinations of the data fields being used.

In reality those supervising the vaccination teams wish to know which cattle populations from within a country are poorly vaccinated so that remedial action can be taken immediately. If seromonitoring is conducted as stipulated in the guidelines, then sera are collected approximately one month after a vaccination team has covered an area. Thus sera should be arriving at the laboratory on a continual basis, can be tested immediately and the results fed back to the national co-ordinator. Hence the national co-ordinator should be receiving seromonitoring data in an on-going fashion throughout his vaccination campaign and hence can continually monitor progress and take action where appropriate.

The more complex type of analysis with the full range of comparative statistics can then be produced annually to give information on immunity levels on a national basis.

Conclusions

Seromonitoring is an essential component of any vaccination campaign. It provides the final evidence that all elements of a programme are functioning correctly and can pinpoint problems as the programme is being carried out allowing corrective measures to be taken immediately.

Fig. 2. Optical density values for the local negative population

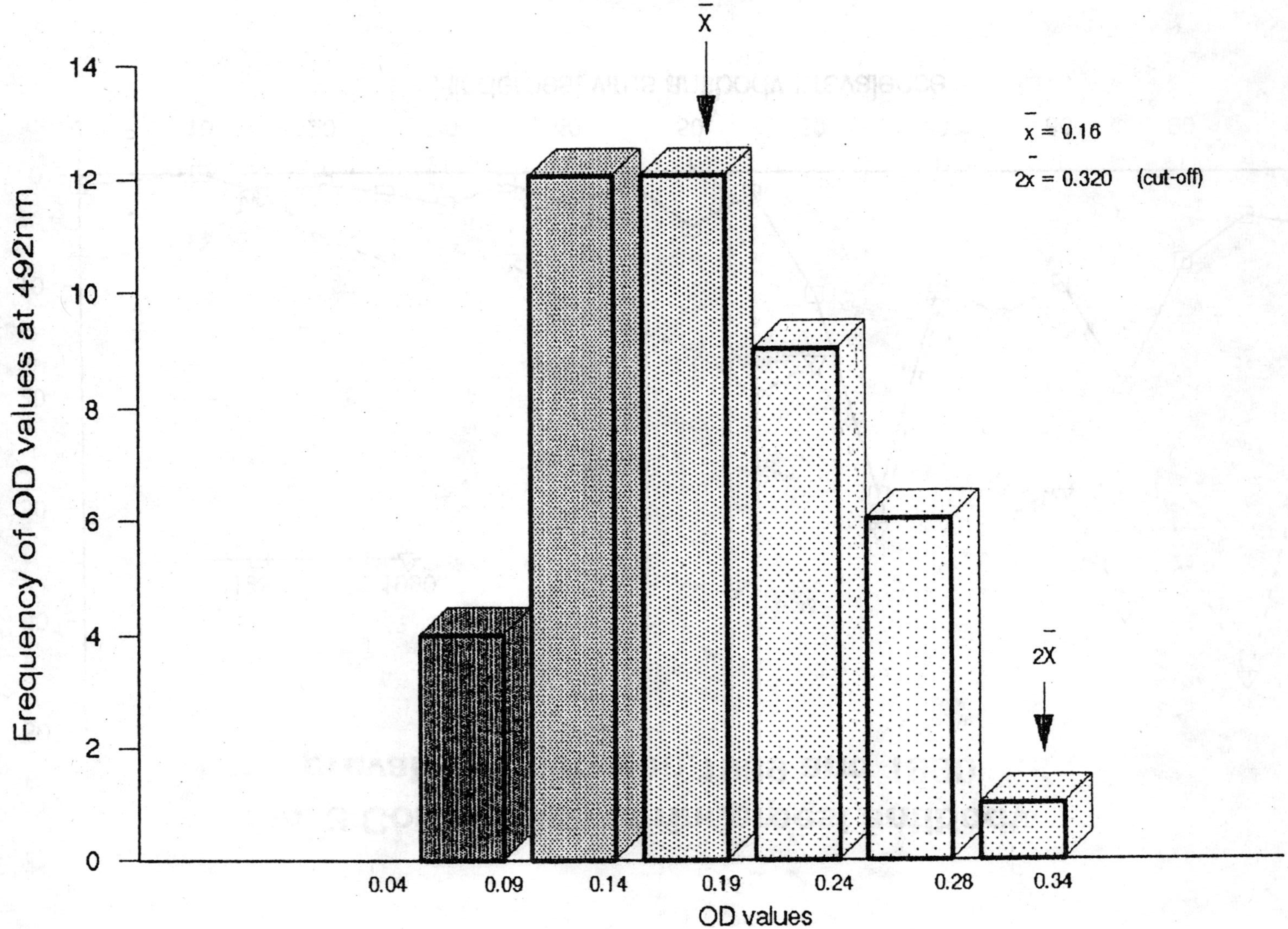

Fig. 3 Comparison of rinderpest antibody prevalence between 1989 and 1990

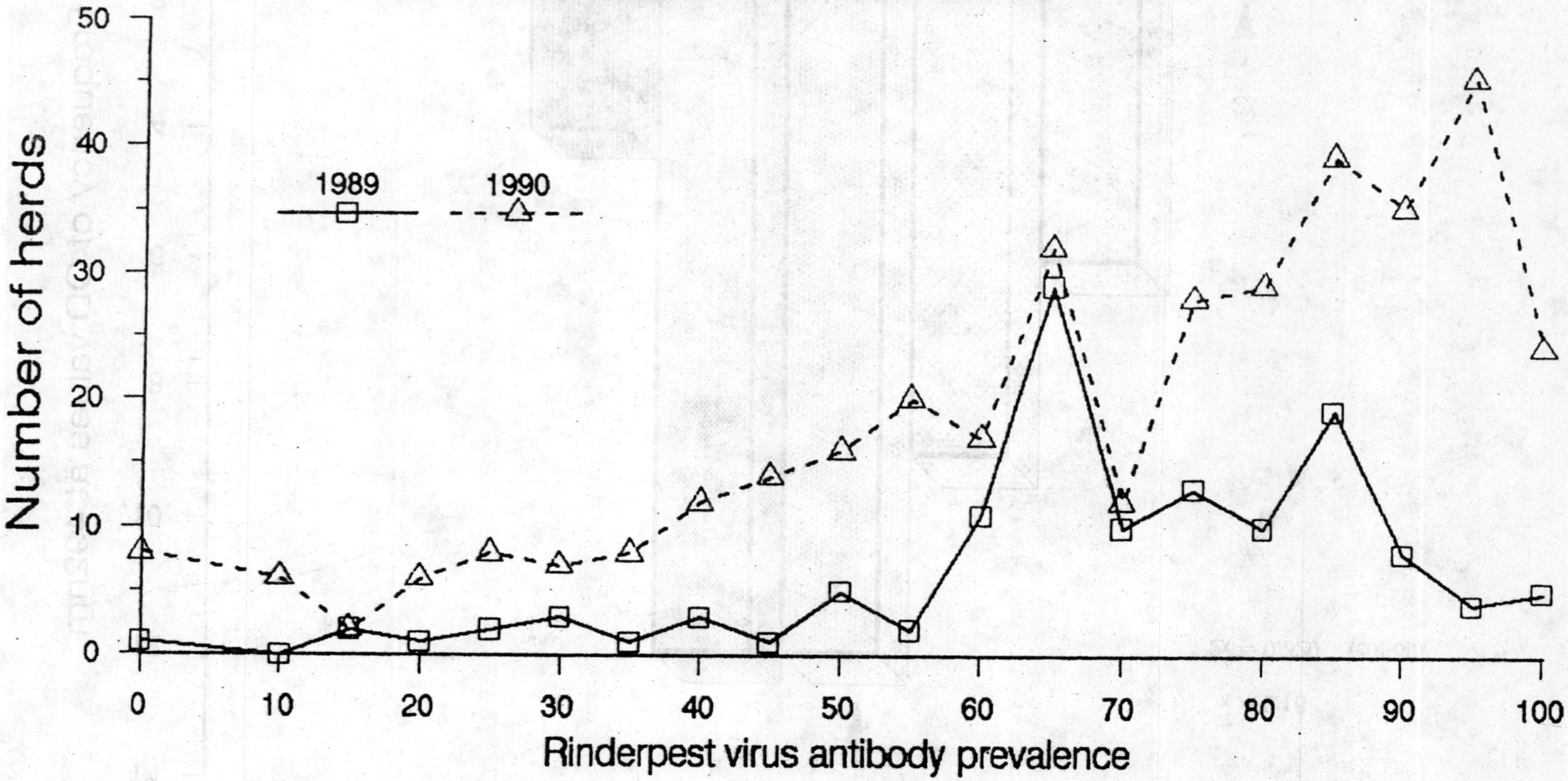

The seromonitoring component of the Pan African Rinderpest Campaign is an on-going example of how this activity can be integrated into a large multinational animal disease control programme. It serves to illustrate the advantages of seromonitoring as a means of determining the effectiveness of the vaccination programme and assuring that control and eventual eradication will be achieved.

This example also shows though, that at both the national and international levels, seromonitoring is a complex of many activities and to be successful the component parts must all be functioning. It is clear that a standardized approach with a fully validated assay is essential but that this alone will be unsuccessful without adequate training and technical backstopping. One further lesson from this programme is that establishing the capability at the laboratory for seromonitoring is meaningless without the inputs required to collect the sera. Even then, sera collection itself must be carried out in an epidemiologically acceptable manner for the final results to be valid.

Perhaps though, the most striking aspect of the PARC seromonitoring network has been its ability to retain in the majority of instances, the same counterpart in each testing laboratory. The continuity this has brought has ensured a progressive increase in the quality of the results coming out of the programme and should in the long run produce a real sustainability in the African region to conduct seromonitoring of this and other animal disease control programmes.

ACKNOWLEDGEMENTS

In the preparation of this manuscript considerable reference was made to information contained in the IAEA TECDOC-623 entitled "The Seromonitoring of rinderpest throughout Africa, Phase one" and in particular the author would like to acknowledge the contributions made by Dr J Anderson, Dr L Tyler and Miss A Macleod.

REFERENCES

1. CORBEL, M.J. (1985) Vet. Bull **55**:927.

2. KIT, S., AWAYA, Y., OTSUKA, H., KIT, M.J. (1990) Vet. Diagn. Invest. **2**:14.

3. The Sero-monitoring of Rinderpest throughout Africa Phase one, IAEA Publication (1991).

4. PLOWRIGHT, W. (1962) Bull. Off. Int. Epizoot. **57**:1.

5. ROSSITER, P.B., JESSETT, D.M. (1982) Res. Vet. Sci. **32**:253.

6. TAYLOR, W.P., ROWE, L.W. (1984) Res. Vet. Sci. **37**:155.

7. PLOWRIGHT, W., TAYLOR, W.P. (1967) Res. Vet Sci. **8**:118.

8. Recommended Diagnostic Techniques and Requirements for Biological Products, OIE publication, **II** Paris (1990) 10/10.

9. ANDERSON, J., ROWE, L.W., TAYLOR, W.P., CROWTHER, J.R. (1982) Res. Vet. Sci. **32**:242.

10. ANDERSON, J., ROWE, L.W. (1983) Res. Vet. Sci. **34**:77.

11. ANDERSON, J., ANDERSON, E.C., CHIDUO, F., JOSHUA, G.E., LORETU, K., MPELUMBE, I.E., KAVISHE, T.E. (1991) IAEA-TECDOC-623, Vienna 87.

12. DIGUIMBAYE, C. (1991) IAEA-TECDOC-623, Vienna 111.

Table I: FAO/IAEA/SIDA/PARC NETWORK FOR THE SERO-MONITORING OF RINDERPEST IN AFRICA

Name	Country	Related IAEA TC Project
Elamin A	Sudan	SUD/5/016
Wamwayi H	Kenya	KEN/5/010
Opoku-Pare G	Ghana	GHA/5/013
Ezeokoli D	Nigeria	NIG/5/014
Obi T	Nigeria	NIG/5/019
Majiyagbe K	Nigeria	NIG/5/019
Sidibie M	Burkina-Faso	n/a
Dialla I	Niger	NER/5/007
Sarr J	Senegal	SEN/5/019
Loretu K	Tanzania	URT/5/009
Tounkara K	Mali	MLI/5/011
Couacy-Hymann E	Cote DIvoire	IVC/5/016
Ngangnou A	Cameroon	RAF/5/006
Twinamasko E	Uganda	UGA/5/013
Mebratu Y	Ethiopia	ETH/5/009
Bedoura-Marboua E	Central African Republic	n/a
Dini A	Somalia	n/a
Nsabiyuma L	Burundi	n/a
Meberuka J	Rwanda	n/a
Touray E	Gambia	n/a
Karim I	Egypt	EGY/5/018

n/a - not applicable since not an IAEA member state

Table II: FAO/IAEA/SIDA/PARC NETWORK FOR THE SERO-MONITORING OF RINDERPEST; PHASE II.

Name	Country	Res. Con. No.	Related IAEA TCP
Elamin A	Sudan	6563/SD	SUD/5/016
Nduga E	Kenya	6578/SD	RAF/5/006
Opoku-Pare G	Ghana	6555/SD	GHA/5/018
Ezeokoli D	Nigeria	6560/SD	NIG/5/019
Obi T	Nigeria	6561/SD	RAF/5/006
Majiyagbe K	Nigeria	6559/SD	NIR/5/019
Sidibie M	Burkina Faso	6550/SD	n/a
Dialla I	Niger	6558/SD	NER/5/007
Sarr J	Senegal	6562/SD	RAF/5/006
Loretu K	Tanzania	6564/SD	URT/5/009
Couacy-Hymann E	Cote DIvoire	6556/SD	IVC/5/016
Ngangnou A	Cameroon	6551/SD	CMR/5/006
Twinamasko E	Uganda	6565/SD	UGA/5/013
Mebratu Y	Ethiopia	6552/SD	ETH/5/009
Guillaume K G	CAR	6751/SD	n/a
Touray E	Gambia	6554/SD	n/a
Tounkara K	Mali	6557/SD	MLI/5/011
Diguimbaye C	Tchad	6676/SD	n/a
Boubaccu Diallo	Mauritania	6579/SD	n/a
Karim I	Egypt	applied for	EGY/5/018

n/a not applicable since not an IAEA member state

Table III: RESULTS BY REGION FOR 1990

Region	No. of Sera	No. Positive	% Positive
Kayes	1240	878	70.8
Kuliboro	1182	790	66.8
Sikasso	2455	2143	87.2
Segou	1197	1070	89.3
Mopti	2510	1834	73.0
Timbouctou	1040	840	80.7
Gao	533	293	54.9
District	240	168	70.0
Overall	10,397	8016	77.0

Table IV: DISTRIBUTION OF SERO-POSITIVE ANIMALS TO RINDERPEST IN THE VARIOUS AGE CATEGORIES (1990)

Regions	No. of Sera	< 1 yr	1-2 yrs	2-3 yrs	> 3 yrs
Kayes	1240	64%*	65%	78%	73%
Koulikoro	1182	42%	60%	70%	77%
Sikasso	2455	57%	77%	92%	92%
Segou	1197	67%	83%	94%	94%
Mopti	2410	55%	69%	81%	82%
Timbouctou	1160	53%	76%	87%	89%
Gao	523	28%	48%	72%	76%
District	240	34%	56%	77%	93%
Overall	10,391	53%	68%	83%	86%

* % sera with antibodies to rinderpest virus

Vaccine Banks and Emergency Stocks of Vaccines Against Exotic Diseases

THE PLUM ISLAND (USA) MODEL

by

C A Mebus

History

After the devastating outbreak of foot-and-mouth disease (FMD) in Great Britain in 1967-1968, the British Government established a high-level commission chaired by the Duke of Northumberland (subsequently referred to as the Northumberland Commission) to examine the reasons for the outbreak and make recommendations for the future. One of the Commission's recommendations was to keep available a stock of FMD vaccine for use should similar outbreaks of FMD occur again. The Government purchased several hundred thousand doses of completely formulated FMD vaccine types A, O and C. Because of being completely formulated, most of the vaccine had to be discarded and replaced after 1 year.

During the mid-1970's, the technology was developed to concentrate and store FMD antigen. Concentrated antigen stored at ultra-low temperature remains stable for a long period and can subsequently be made into an effective vaccine. In early 1979, the United States Department of Agriculture (USDA) Secretary's Advisory Committee on Foreign Animal and Poultry Diseases recommended that a stockpile of FMD vaccine be established as an alternate source of protection for the livestock industry. The establishment of an FMD vaccine bank does not mean that the United States has changed its intention to eradicate the disease if it entered the United States. However, the size of the outbreak, and/or potential problems with environmental and animal welfare concerns may require the use of vaccination as part of the eradication procedures.

In September 1979, staff from the Biologics' Licensing and Standards, Veterinary Services, Animal and Plant Health Inspection Service, USDA, established a contract for the purchase of concentrated antigen for one million doses of serotype A5, O and C. This first contract also included additional storage costs of the antigen for 4 years and if needed, formulation, filling and packaging of the vaccine. Current contracts are for sufficient antigen to produce 2.5 million doses of vaccine.

In March 1981, a U.S.-Mexico meeting was held and a joint FMD vaccine bank was discussed. In January 1982, representatives of Canada, Mexico and the United States discussed establishment of a joint FMD vaccine bank. In August 1983, the text of the agreement for the establishment of the North American Foot-and-Mouth Disease Vaccine Bank was finalized.

Administration of the North American FMD Vaccine Bank

The Bank is administered by a two-level governing body. The top level is a commission comprised of the Chief Veterinary Officer or his representative from each country. The commissioners have full authority over establishing managements of the bank, cost-sharing and use of the bank.

The second level of the governing body is the technical committee which consists of one scientific and one regulatory representative from each country. This committee is responsible for advising the commissioners on all aspects of the vaccine bank, including cost-sharing, types and subtypes of antigen to be stored, methods of production and storage, changes in technology, appearance of new subtypes or explosive outbreaks which would increase the threat to the countries, utilization of the vaccine bank by each member country, and utilization by a non-member country.

The commission operates on a consensus basis.

The commission and technical committee meet annually or more often if needed.

The antigen is stored at the Foreign Animal Disease Laboratory, Plum Island. The USDA serves as administrator of the Bank and charges a 5 per cent overhead for its activities. These include handling contracts for purchase of antigen, testing of antigen, storage of antigen and maintenance of records on stored antigens.

Financing of the bank is based on the participating countries' percentage of the total cattle population, with Canada contributing 8 per cent, Mexico 20 per cent, and United States 72 per cent of the costs.

<u>Operation of the Bank</u>

The addition of a FMD serotype to the vaccine bank is based on the risk of its introduction to one of the member countries. Facts to be considered are (1) the country(ies) in which the serotype exists; (2) the serotype currently exits in a country(ies) where it was not known to exist in the recent past; and (3) whether a member country has significant trade with the country(ies) in which the serotype exists. If any of the above considerations exist, the serotype is tested for cross-reactivity with the antigens in the Bank and if insufficient protection is found, a commission meeting is held to consider purchase of the appropriate antigen.

If a new serotype is to be added to the Bank, a solicitation/contract is developed by the USDA. The solicitation is for production of the antigen and formulation of the vaccine from the antigen. Bidders are required to submit proposed methods of production of antigen and of vaccine and agree to inspection of production facilities by a team composed of representatives from the Ministry of Agriculture Canada, the Mexican Veterinary Service and the USDA. Outlines for antigen production, vaccine formulation and facilities must conform with Title 9, Code of Federal Regulations (CFR), Parts 101-123. If needed, the antigen will be formulated into a vaccine in a U.S. Biologics licensed facility.

In addition to the testing by the contractor during production of the antigen, the following samples must be submitted to the USDA:

Five 2 ml vials of the master seed strain.

Five 1 ml vials of both the master cell stock and the highest passage used in the production.

Ten ml of high titered reference antiserum produced from a virus seed of a different origin than the virus seed used to produce the master seed.

Five 1 or 2 ml vials of challenge virus with a known passage history.

Ten 2 ml samples of each lot or serial of concentrate with sufficient adjuvant for 200 cattle doses. (The antigen in these samples will be used by the U.S. vaccine-formulating firm to prepare at FADDL a pilot batch of vaccine, a portion of which will be used for the cattle potency test.)

Forty 2 ml samples for each lot or serial of concentrate for stability testing during storage.

Ten to 15 mg of sucrose or cesium chloride gradient purified vaccine virus stored in 1 ml amounts with 5 to 6 mg/ml.

The following additional tests may be conducted by the USDA before accepting the antigen concentrate:

(a) Potency test in cattle.

(b) Foot-and-mouth disease virus infection associated (VIA) antigen test on cattle used in the safety and potency tests.

(c) Antigen content by the complement-fixation test.

(d) Guinea pig potency test measuring serological response.

(e) Test for 140S particle content.

(f) Safety test by injection of 0.1 ml of virus concentrate into each of 20 sites in the tongue of each of 6 susceptible cattle.

(g) To assure stability, the USDA will conduct the complement fixation test or 140S particle determinations at 3 months, 6 months and yearly thereafter. If significant loss of stability is seen, a guinea pig potency test will be conducted. If reduction in serological response occurs, a vaccination-challenge test will be conducted in cattle. Failure in this test will require replacement of the serial. If failure occurs within the expiration period of 5 years, replacement will be at the manufacturer's expense.

The commission recognizes that 2.5 million doses of vaccine may not be sufficient in an outbreak of FMD. However, the cost of purchasing and storing large numbers of doses of vaccine antigen concentrates for a wide variety of FMD sub-types is prohibitive. In the face of an outbreak, the requesting of bids, and the negotiating and awarding of contracts would require a substantial period of time which could not be afforded. Vaccine producers estimate the time from obtaining an FMD isolate to production and availability of the final vaccine to be approximately 4 to 6 weeks. This time frame would include comparison of the isolate with currently available vaccine strains. Tests which could be used include complement fixation, virus neutralization, isoelectric focusing, monoclonal antibody studies and cattle inoculation. Because of the above factors, the technical committee felt that it was prudent to develop means of obtaining large numbers of doses of FMD vaccine in a timely manner and recommended that the Bank establish agreements with vaccine producers who could begin production upon request. Some requirements which would have to be met for such emergency vaccine production include:

1. USDA licensing requirements.

2. Mutually acceptable procedures for randomly inspection production facilities.

3. USDA acceptable, randomized quality control tests for currently produced FMD vaccines to maintain a constant level of confidence in the producer, and

4. Acceptable procedures for inactivation, biosecurity and recording of production since Bank member countries would have to agree to import such vaccine without safety testing.

The technical committee also recommended that Bank or member countries consider using the above policy to obtain other foreign animal disease vaccines such as African horse sickness and Rift Valley fever.

INTERNATIONAL VACCINE BANKS

by

T R Doel

INTRODUCTION

The concept of an emergency supply of vaccine to help in the control of an outbreak of foot-and-mouth disease has existed for many years. Following the 1967/68 epidemic in the United Kingdom, the Ministry of Agriculture purchased bulk vaccine at regular intervals for strategic control purposes. This type of reserve proved very expensive to maintain because of the need to purchase fresh vaccine when the previous batch had time-expired. A natural development of this approach is one in which highly concentrated, inactivated virus preparations are stored at very low temperatures until required. FMD antigen concentrates held at liquid nitrogen temperatures probably have shelf lives in excess of a decade. The operation of thawing and formulating a virus concentrate is not complex or problematical provided the principles of Good Manufacturing Practice are followed scrupulously.

The Pirbright Vaccine Bank

There are two international banks based on the storage of virus concentrates. The first of these was set up by Canada, Mexico and the United States. The second bank is run by the Pirbright Laboratory of the Institute for Animal Health, UK and represents Australia, Finland, Ireland, New Zealand, Norway, Sweden and the United Kingdom. The Pirbright facility comprises a dedicated building which contains liquid nitrogen vessels for the storage of virus concentrates, fermentation type vessels and equipment to allow the formulation of vaccine and packaging/storage facilities for finished vaccine. Six virus strains, each representing 500,000 cattle doses, are held in the Pirbright bank and may be drawn by a member country in the event of an emergency in their country. Each country has a maximum agreed drawing right and the contribution it makes to the purchase of an antigen batch and annual maintenance of the bank is adjusted to reflect this. For example, the UK is able to call on all of the 500,000 doses of a given strain of FMD and, correspondingly, makes one of the largest contributions. In the event that vaccine is required, up to 200,000 doses of $Al(OH)_3$/saponin vaccine can be provided within approximately 48 hours of the first notification to the bank and the remaining 300,000 doses produced over the next 48 hours. Although not possible at present, it is hoped that the Pirbright bank will be modified soon to allow the production of oil adjuvanted vaccines for cattle and pigs.

The E.C. Vaccine Bank

Following the cessation of vaccination against FMD within Western Europe, the E.C. intends setting up a vaccine bank similar to that at Pirbright. A major difference will be that five million cattle doses of each of nine virus strains will be purchased initially. This very much larger strategic reserve will be used to control any outbreaks of FMD within the 12 member states.

Advantages of a Vaccine Bank

The advantages of a bank of this type compared to the storage of bulk commercial vaccine are many and may be summarised as follows. Most importantly, there is complete flexibility of formulation at the time that the vaccine is required. Thus small quantities of very high potency vaccine can be made rather than the number of doses of standard vaccine specified originally by the bank. Such a vaccine could be used if the requirement was to suppress a relatively isolated outbreak in a small number of animals. On the other hand, it may be possible to dilute the vaccine further than the standard level to make more doses available for a large outbreak. In this respect it is worth noting that most of the vaccines made from the Pirbright virus concentrates are extremely potent and would tolerate a significant level of dilution beyond 500,000 doses without falling below the minimum PD_{50} stipulated by the bank.

Another reason for producing an extremely potent vaccine would be that the vaccine strain was not closely related to the outbreak strain. Whereas 'average' commercial vaccines may not give sufficiently high cross-protective antibody levels, vaccines made from virus concentrates may be adjusted accordingly. An example of this is to be found with the O_1 Manisa virus held in the Pirbright bank. While an 'average' O_1 Manisa vaccine might not be expected to protect against O_1 isolates from Western Europe, the potency of the Pirbright vaccine is such that significant levels of cross-protection should be possible.

Adjuvants may also be selected at the time the vaccine is required. For example, $Al(OH)_3$/saponin would still be the adjuvants of choice where a rapid development of immunity was required in cattle. If, however, it was necessary to immunise pigs or produce a longer lasting immunity in pigs and/or cattle the adjuvant of choice would be mineral oil. Should other adjuvants become available then these could be used with the concentrates.

There are also a number of operational advantages with virus concentrate storage. Unlike fully formulated vaccines, it is a simple matter to monitor the integrity of the virus at intervals following storage whereas whole vaccine can only be assessed effectively by potency testing in animals. Finally, virus concentrates require considerably less storage room and are relatively inexpensive to keep. For example, it is possible to store approximately 3 million doses or more in a single 330 litre liquid nitrogen vessel. The bank at Pirbright has the capacity to store at least 50 million cattle doses equivalent in a room with dimensions approximately 5 x 5 metres and with little more than a few minor modifications to the facility.

Conditions under which a Vaccine Bank might be used

Finally, there are a number of key questions regarding the conditions under which a vaccine would be used to control an outbreak and the qualifications required for membership of a bank.

Clearly, the veterinary authorities of a normally disease-free country would most probably consider first the quick, effective control of an outbreak by movement restrictions, zoosanitary measures and slaughter and destruction of diseased and contact animals. There are some circumstances, however, where vaccine use would be contemplated. In the first place, it might be deemed necessary to vaccinate valuable breeding animals. In the second place, vaccination would be a more likely option if there was a significant risk of the disease running out of control. Coupled to this last point is the ever increasing problem of the logistics of destroying large numbers of animals particularly in densely populated areas such as Belgium where West and East Flanders contain approximately five million pigs, Holland, Brittany and the Po Valley to mention only a few within Europe. To incinerate or render thousands of carcasses every day would probably be beyond the resources of many Western European countries. The alternatives of burial or burning on site may very well clash with environmental legislation and be unacceptable on animal welfare grounds. Vaccination would at least allow a breathing space during which circulating virus levels would be suppressed and vaccinated animals gradually removed from the population when the outbreak had been contained and time permitted.

Conditions for Vaccine Bank membership

It is important to stress the emergency nature of a vaccine bank and the reasons why it should be used accordingly. One strength of the Pirbright bank is the very high quality of the virus concentrates held and the unparalleled testing which occurs over the initial three or four year period. Many of the virus strains have been tested as vaccines in over 40 cattle since each was purchased. These features combine to create a high level of confidence that a bank vaccine will do the job required provided it is given every reasonable opportunity. This level of certainty also allows the manipulation of a vaccine to suit a particular field situation. It would be inappropriate, therefore, to waste such valuable, potent materials in situations where outbreaks were rife and would be best controlled by more extensive and repeated application of commercial bulk vaccine. This leads naturally to the question of membership of a bank.

In the first place, the quantities of virus concentrate purchased should reflect a reasonably worst case scenario. For example, sufficient virus/vaccine should be available in case of an outbreak in the border region between two members of the bank. Clearly, it would be politically and epidemiologically unfortunate if the first outbreak in country 'A' used all of the vaccine and was followed by a second outbreak just across the border in country 'B'. More importantly, a potential member country would need to have been free of FMD for a period of at least two years (possibly longer) during which time it would have allowed its disease-free status to be monitored by an independent authority. Anything less than these conditions could result in a bank which operated continuously for the benefit of one or several members and was never in the situation to recover sufficiently to respond to emergencies in the countries of the other members.

Clearly, such issues will provoke considerable discussion in the inevitable extension of FMD vaccine banks to countries not protected by the Pirbright bank, the U.S. bank and the proposed E.C. bank.

Discussion

During the discussions which took place after the two papers on vaccines banks, the following points were made:

Dr Lombard emphasised the differences between a vaccine bank and an antigen bank. In the case of the former, vaccine was immediately available for despatch, whereas antigen would have to be formulated into vaccine which would take valuable time. Also, the manufacturers responsibility ends at the hand over of the concentrated antigen, and subsequent contamination of it etc would be the responsibility of the bank managers.

Dr Doel countered these criticisms by pointing out that with a disease of the importance of FMD, there would be indications of the need to use the contents of the bank well in advance of the call for vaccine. This would give adequate time for the preparation of equipment and the subsequent formulation and bottling of the vaccine. Delay in getting vaccine to the field would therefore not be a problem. He also said that in his opinion the relatively limited shelf-life of fully formulated vaccines was something of a disadvantage - if, starting with a vaccine which was just over the minimum pass level for potency, what confidence could there be that the same vaccine towards the end of its storage period would still have an acceptable potency level? In contrast, the useful life of stored concentrated antigen was more or less unlimited!

Dr Lombard stated that in the EEC countries, the shelf-life of these products varied according to the manufacturer and was usually between 12 and 24 months. Manufacturers will normally guarantee the potency of the product at the end of the stated shelf-life.

In response to a question from the Vice-Chairman, Dr Doel said that there were no alternatives to assessing a stored vaccine other than by animal testing (cattle) - which would be expensive. With stored antigen it was a comparatively simple procedure to check the integrity of the material by bio-physical methods.

Dr Sizaret made the point that WHO does not use the term "shelf-life"but would prefer the "validity period" for indicating storage time. That would apply at the time of commencing cold storage, and not the time of manufacture, thus the validity period could be reduced by the interval between production and storage. He also enquired about the formulation and filling - making the comment that if not done by the producer, the vaccine bank must have equipment which stands idle for much of the time.

Dr Mebus thought that the 2 vaccine banks under discussion had taken opposite positions in that respect. The N American bank would prefer that the producer of the antigen should complete the work as and when necessary. The setting up of the equipment for the complete process would have required more financial investment and there were worries that when required in an emergency, the process might not work!

Dr Doel felt obliged to respond to that by stating the Pirbright bank had a permanent member of staff who was responsible for keeping the equipment in a state of permanent readiness. There was constant checking of the process and practise runs were made from time to time. The process in itself was not complicated, in that all that was needed, was the sterilisation of in situ stainless steel vessels and ancillary items, and formulation and bottling of the final product.

It was a simple process and there would be no difficulty in having ready 200,000 doses in 24 hours and continuing at the same rate of preparation.

Dr Mebus stated that another reason for not carrying out the full process at Plum Island was that a manufacturers licence would be required from the Federal Authorities and that would be difficult to obtain. The earliest material stored at Plum Island had been produced and concentrated there. When it was found to have deteriorated on storage, it was discarded and replaced by purchased material. The concentration process at Plum Island had been one of ultra-filtration, and it was assumed now that the protolytic enzymes normally present in such material had also been concentrated, resulting in digestion of the 146s antigen stored. The purchased antigen has been concentrated by precipitation with polyethylene glycol and has not suffered the same effect as before.

In response to questions concerning the time manufacturers will take to formulate the antigen and send off bottled vaccine, Dr Mebus said that these conditions had been defined

Special Presentations

ANTI-RABIES VACCINES - FEASIBILITY OF JOINT CONTROL OF MEDICAL AND VETERINARY VACCINES

by

O Thraenhart

INTRODUCTION

At present approximately 50,000 humans and millions of animals die from rabies every year. This is not necessary however, since the strategy exists to control rabies in man and animals. Rabies can best be prevented by vaccination, since vaccination against rabies is now highly efficient. Man and animal, vaccinated with potent and safe vaccines are usually protected against this otherwise fatal disease.

Almost 5 million Chinese, 1 million Indians and 1 million inhabitants of other Asian countries, as well as possibly another 5 to 8 million people in other continents are treated annually by vaccination against rabies.

Vaccines are only used in animals for prophylactic immunisation whereas humans receive vaccines both before exposure to rabies (pre-exposure vaccination) and after exposure.

Safety Aspects

Safety and potency of rabies vaccines implies protection against rabies infection and also against adverse reactions. Safe and potent vaccines are those which are produced from cell cultures. Brain tissue vaccines are not safe and not consistently potent. The use of brain tissue derived vaccines should therefore be stopped as soon as possible in all countries. This was one of the main recommendations of the Expert Committee on Rabies, which revised the seventh report from 1984 (Technical Report Series No. 709) in September 1991. The Committee reiterated:

> "the trend to limit or abandon completely - where economically and technically possible - the production of encephalitogenic brain-tissue vaccines, and strongly advocates the production and use of inactivated cell culture rabies vaccines in both developed and developing countries."

Brain tissue derived vaccines are dangerous for both man and animal, because the myelin which they contain may cause adverse complications. Repeated inoculations of homogenates of brain tissue evoke immune responses to some neural antigens in most recipients. In the case of Semple type vaccine, myelin basic protein and some of the gangliosides and phospholipids are responsible for these neurological complications. Though properly prepared suckling mouse brain vaccines contain virtually no myelin, neurological complications still occur, but at a much lower rate than with adult nerve tissue vaccines. The doctor who has only a brain tissue vaccine available and who has to decide, whether a post-exposure vaccination has to be given to an exposed person, has a most difficult decision to make since the vaccination may lead to a permanent neurological complication. Neurological reactions are observed not only in man but also in dogs. In general, complications in dogs and other animals may not be considered important. But many dogs are highly valued and such complications may have implications for the acceptance of mass vaccination campaigns. Moreover, the potency of these vaccines may be variable. If the vaccine for dogs is not potent, an uncertainty arises whether a vaccinated animal, to which a person has been exposed, is in fact immune. Therefore, all efforts should be made to eliminate the use of brain tissue vaccines and switch to the production of cell culture vaccines.

The Expert Committee on Rabies mentioned earlier recommended, that for countries, which initiate cell culture vaccine technology, substantial economies may be effected, if human and animal vaccines are produced jointly. There are only minor differences in the cell culture technology of vaccines produced for animals or man. It would be advantageous in the control of vaccines to have them made from the same substrate, namely cell culture derived antigen.

Vaccines

A. Vaccines for man now in use are always inactivated vaccines and intended for parenteral use.

Cell culture vaccines: These combine safety with high immunogenicity. Several types of cell cultures are used for rabies vaccine production: (i) primary cell cultures (hamster kidney, dog kidney or chick embryo fibroblasts); (ii) diploid cell lines (human or rhesus monkey origin); (iii) continuous cell lines (vero cells).

Advances in biotechnology, such as microcarriers in large scale bio-reactors have made possible the production of rabies vaccines at the industrial scale and reduced costs, although some problems of sterility may occur. Another procedure is the use of glass bottles, where smaller volumes may be easier controlled for sterility.

Continuous cell lines, such as BHK, give high yields of virus (thus not requiring concentration) and are presently used for the production of rabies vaccines for immunization of animals. These cell lines might be accepted for the production of low cost rabies vaccines for human use if they were to meet WHO requirements for human vaccines prepared in continuous cell lines. Investigations to solve the problem of eliminating cell DNA are currently being carried out.

Purified duck embryo vaccines: This is a preparation in which the fixed virus is grown on embryonated duck eggs and further purified. This vaccine offers the same immunogenicity and safety as modern cell culture vaccines.

New developments in brain tissue rabies vaccine production: The Fuenzalida-Palacios technique for the preparation of suckling mouse brain vaccine now uses mice not older than 1 day at the time of inoculation and centrifugation of the brain suspension at 17,000 g for 10 min., in order to reduce further the level of encephalitogenic substances in the final product.

B. Vaccines for animals now in use are those for parenteral or oral use. The parenterally used vaccines are mainly inactivated vaccines, although some modified vaccines are still produced. But increasing use of inactivated vaccines for animal immunization can be expected as a result of the improvements of vaccine production techniques.

Vaccines for parenteral use

Cell culture vaccines: The cell lines used are of canine, feline, porcine, hamster or monkey origin. Primary cell cultures such as chick embryo fibroblasts are used in addition. In fact the chick embryo fibroblast vaccines for man and animals use almost the same production technology.

Nerve tissue vaccines: Inactivated nerve tissue vaccine is prepared from fixed viruses in the brains of new-born sheep. The inactivated suckling mouse brain vaccines have shown their efficacy in mass immunization programmes in Latin America and the Caribbean.

Vaccines for oral use: There are several types of modified live viruses (ERA, SAD Bern, SAD B19, Vnukovo 32), all of which are derived from one rabid dog. These types of vaccines are produced on cell cultures only.

Recombinant vaccinia virus expressing the immunizing G glycoprotein of rabies virus has also been developed and is in use in limited areas.

Potency Requirements

Animal vaccines: Inactivated vaccines for parenteral use in animals with a potency value of not less that 1 IU per dose should not be approved unless an adequately designed challenge experiment has demonstrated a duration of immunity of at least one year in the species for which the vaccine is to be used.

Unlike vaccines for parenteral use, minimum potency requirements for vaccines intended for oral carnivore immunization have not been generally established. The minimum dosage required for immunization of a given species is now known. However the dosage for a fox cannot immunize dogs. No solution is currently available to solve the problem of dog vaccination with oral vaccine, since the amount of virus necessary to immunize dogs by the oral route with the presently available vaccine cannot be established.

Vaccines for man: Cell culture vaccines for human use should have a minimum potency of 2.5 IU/dose. For suckling mouse brain vaccine, a potency of 1.3 IU is required.

Necessity of Vaccine Control

The designation "rabies vaccine" - without proper control measures is not sufficient proof of safety and potency. This holds true for any type of vaccine. In the "Guidelines for Dog Rabies Control" (8) it is stated:

"Quality control of rabies vaccines is of utmost importance in any programme of rabies control: Vaccinations using uncontrolled vaccines should be avoided under all circumstances, because of the severe consequences of any false confidence in an animal's immunity.

No producer can assume that his produce is safe and potent: Every batch of rabies vaccine has to be controlled before release. This control comprises identification, safety, potency and stability of the vaccine."

Control Authorities

Quality control of rabies vaccines should be conducted at two levels: (a) by the manufacturer and (b) by a national control authority, e.g. the national rabies laboratory or national health service laboratory (Table 1).

Recommendations

The methods for quality control of rabies vaccines were revised by a WHO Expert Committee on Rabies in 1983 (7). They are summarized in the WHO Expert Committee on Rabies, 7th report, Technical Report Series 709, 1984 and in the Guidelines for Dog Rabies Control of WHO, 1987. Details of the methods are described by KAPLAN and KOPROWSKI (6). The revision of the Technical Report Series 709, 1984, was prepared in September 1991 and will be published most probably in 1992.

The Office International des Epizooties (OIE), WHO and FAO recommended in 1985, that in countries with a low incidence of rabies as in Europe only inactivated rabies vaccines should be used, MELENDEZ and BLAJAN (5). In 1985, 8 out of 16 European countries replied to a questionnaire of J. BARRAT (2) that they used live attenuated vaccines for parenteral use in animals. However, in 1991 live attenuated vaccines are only given for oral use in wildlife.

Priority will therefore be given to the evaluation of safety and potency of inactivated vaccines for inoculation of man and animals.

Modified Life vaccines

Modified live vaccines are tested for identification, safety and potency. Identification is carried out by protection of guinea pigs against a subsequent inoculation of rabies street virus or fixed virus. Safety is tested by injection of guinea pigs or target animals by the i.m. route; no local or systemic reaction should develop. The potency is tested by inoculation of the vaccine into guinea pigs. A sufficient potency is achieved, if 70% of vaccinated animals survive a challenge, which kills 80% of the unvaccinated controls.

Vaccines for oral immunization

Safety assessment has to be carried out for target and non target species before licensing of any oral vaccine by the administration of a 10 fold concentration of the dosage recommended for field use.

Inactivated Rabies Vaccines

Evaluation of Safety

Safety of Rabies vaccines is indicated by the absence of adverse reactions in the vaccinee.

The amount of non-specific protein per dose is one parameter which indicates the quality of a vaccine as shown in Table 2.

Purified inactivated tissue culture vaccines have the lowest content of non-specific protein. They consist almost entirely of rabies virus particles. This cannot be achieved with a rabies brain vaccine.

In addition, vaccines prepared from adult central nervous tissue contain neuroparalytic factors such as myelin. This hazard is reduced if vaccines are prepared from the brains of suckling mice and some additional steps such as ultracentrifugation are included in the production process. The amount of neuroparalytic factors in vaccines of avian tissue origin is lower, but they may still be allergenic.

Control of innocuity is carried out by injection of vaccine into mice or target species. Only vaccine batches can be considered for licensing, if they fulfil the criteria of microbiological sterility, rabies virus inactivation and absence of abnormal toxicity.

Evaluation of Potency

The potency of inactivated vaccines should be assessed by the measurement of protection after vaccination of the target species being exposed (man) or being challenged in nature with infectious virus (animal). Such protection tests are necessary for the development of new vaccines and vaccination schemes. However, it is impractical for the control of potency of serial batches. Alternatives therefore are necessary, which simulate the direct protection test in batch to batch control.

Potency may be evaluated in the target species, in laboratory animals or by in vitro methods.

In addition to protection tests either in the target species or in laboratory animals antibody induction tests are recommended especially for vaccines to be used in man, since the presence of antibodies, which neutralize the infectivity of the rabies virus (neutralizing antibodies), are strong indicators of immunity. Antibody kinetics, i.e. first appearance of antibodies after onset of vaccination, rate of increase, height of antibody titres and antibody persistence, correlate well with the potency of a vaccine.

Furthermore in vitro tests have been developed such as the antibody binding test (ABT), single radial diffusion test (SRD), radioimmune test (RIA) and enzyme immuno assay (ELISA). These are based on the determination of viral antigen, specifically the viral glycoprotein, by its binding to antibodies. The correlation of antigen content and potency can be established for inactivated tissue culture vaccines by this approach.

However, assessment of potency is essentially a biological problem. Therefore, in vivo tests cannot be totally done away with. So far, the NIH test is most important for the evaluation of potency. But depending on the purpose of the potency test (new vaccines, final product, production steps) and also factors such as level of animal protection, time needed and economics of testing and legal requirements, the appropriate tests are selected.

The control of the final product is carried out either by the NIH test, EP test or the simplified test.

In principal, these tests are similar to pharmacological ED50 tests: Animals are vaccinated with different doses of the vaccine. A challenge of a constant amount of infectious virus (50 LD50) is applied to all mice to assess the level of protection. In comparison to unvaccinated controls the mortality is reduced, due to immunity which depends on the dose of vaccine given. Its reduction to 50% (ED50) is a most useful parameter of protection, since the ED50 is the point of minimal variation.

If the mortality rates, which are observed with different vaccine doses, are plotted in a co-ordinate system of x = logarithm of dose and y = mortality rate, a sigmoid response curve can be drawn.

Due to the high degree of variation in the ED50 value from test to test and from laboratory to laboratory, a reference vaccine with known potency is tested in parallel to make the potency values comparable. By calculation of the ratio of the ED50 values or calculation of the distance between the dose response curves of the vaccines under test and the reference vaccine, the potency in IU values can be measured.

Effort for Joint Quality Control

The control testing of rabies vaccines is onerous and expensive. Firstly it is necessary to have well equipped laboratories and animal facilities. Also there is the necessity to establish safety protocols for work with highly infectious agents.

These initial steps require considerable investment and in addition, provision must be made for future running of the laboratories.

Joint control of vaccines for animal and human use at one location is now well established with some manufacturers.

Due to the division of the Ministries of Health and Agriculture in most countries, the control of vaccines is carried out according to their individual requirements and regulations.

However, national authorities should be encouraged to find a solution for the joint control of rabies vaccines for use either in man or animals. One should keep in mind that any rabies vaccine has to be controlled by the same procedures. It is therefore most cost effective to combine both veterinary and human rabies vaccine control.

In Germany, a joint control at the national level has been established within the Paul Ehrlich Institute - a Ministry of Health laboratory.

It is suggested that FAO and WHO should co-ordinate such joint vaccine control. Joint control may also enable the introduction of vaccine testing to those countries which do not have any control of rabies vaccines at present.

REFERENCES

1. BAHMANYARA, M., FAYAS, A., NOUR-SALEHI, S., MOHAMMADI, M. and KOPROWSKI, H. (1976) Successful protection of humans exposed to rabies infection. Post-exposure treatment with the new human diploid cell rabies vaccine and antirabies serum. J. Amer. Med. Ass. **13**: 2751-2754.

2. BARRAT, J. (1985) Report on replies to a questionnaire on rabies control in Europe. Rev. Sci. Tech. Off. Int. Epiz. **4**: 613-649.

3. KUWERT, E.K., MARCUS, I., WERNER, J., SCHEIERMANN, N., HÖHER, P.G., THRAENHART, O., HIERHOLZER, E., WIKTOR, T.J. and KOPROWSKI, H. (1977) Post-exposure use of human diploid cell culture rabies vaccine. Develop. Biol. Standard **37**: 273-286.

4. KUWERT, E., TRIAU, R. and THRAENHART, O. (1984) Innocuite et effets secondaires du vaccine rage obtenu en cellules diploides humaines. Les idees et les faits apres vaccination de plus de 500.00 personnes. Rec. Med. Vet. **160**: 1175-1177.

5. MELENDEZ, L.V. and BLAJAN, L. (1985) The role of the International Office of Epizootics (O.I.E.) in the adoption of new developments to control rabies at national and international levels.
   In: Kuwert, E., Merieux, C., Koprowski H., Bögel, K. (Eds): Rabies in the Tropics, Springer-Verlag Berlin-Heidelberg-New York-Tokyo, pp. 758-769.

6. WORLD HEALTH ORGANIZATION: Laboratory Techniques in Rabies, 3rd ed., editors Kaplan, M.M. and Koprowski, H. Wld. Helth. Org., Geneva (1973).

7. WORLD HEALTH ORGANIZATION: WHO Expert Committee on Rabies, 7th Report. Wld. Hlth. Org. Techn. Rep. Ser. **709** (1984).

8. WORLD HEALTH ORGANIZATION: Guidelines for Dog Rabies Control. Wld. Helth. Org. VPH/83.43 Rev. 1, Geneva, June 1987.

9. THRAENHART, O., KOPROWSKI, H., BÖGEL, K. and SUREAU, P. (Eds): "Progress in Rabies Control". Wells Medical, Royal Tunbridge Wells, Kent, England, 1989.

Table 1: FUNCTIONS OF VACCINE CONTROL AUTHORITIES

Manufacturer:	- Master seed virus
	- Serial lots of vaccines
	- Ingredients for vaccine production
	  - cells
	  - nutrient serum
	  - trypsin etc.

NationalAuthority:	- Master seed virus - Selected batches of vaccines (dependant on the reliability of the manufacturers controls) - Supply of reference vaccine

Table 2: REDUCTION OF NON-SPECIFIC PROTEIN IN RABIES VACCINES

Safety	Vaccine Type	Estimated Protein (mg) per Dose
Safe	tissue culture	0.05 - 0.50
	Duck embryo	5.0
	Suckling mouse brain	2.0 - 4.0
Unsafe	adult brain	20.0 - 70.0

THE ROLE OF MOLECULAR BIOLOGY IN QUALITY CONTROL OF VETERINARY VACCINES AND BIOLOGICALS

by

C A Mebus

Molecular biological techniques provide sophisticated ways to monitor the quality of conventional and recombinant DNA (r-DNA) biological products. Contrary to the beliefs of some of the general public, r-DNA derived biological products are not significantly different from similar products produced by conventional methods and thus are subject to the same regulations for development and licensing. The USDA places the emphasis on the product and its intended use, not the way the product was developed or is produced. In the USA in order to be licensed, a biological product must be pure, safe, sterile, potent and efficacious and not be worthless, contaminated, dangerous or harmful. In the Virus-Serum-Toxin Act of 1913, the term biological product includes viruses, sera, toxins and analogous products of natural or synthetic origin such as diagnostic reagents, antitoxins, vaccines, live micro-organisms, killed micro-organisms and the antigenic or immunizing components of micro-organisms intended for use in the diagnosis, treatment or prevention of disease of animals.

Production of biological products for veterinary use in the United States must be produced in accordance with the Master seed principle and where applicable Master cell principle as published in Title 9, Code of Federal Regulations. Molecular biological techniques can be used to confirm the uniformity and consistency of the products.

A master seed, constructed plasmids or transfected cells, deletions, or inserted genes can be characterized by nucleotide sequence, nucleic acid probes, base pair analysis, polyacrylamide gel analysis, restriction enzyme mapping, Western blotting, dot blots, drug resistance, and/or monoclonal antibodies. The same techniques can be used to determine if a nucleic acid change occurred in reverse-passage experiments.

Proteins and peptides in a product can be characterized by sodium dodecyl sulfate-polyacrylamide gel electrophoresis (SDS-PAGE), SDS-PAGE and immunoblotting using polyvalent or monoclonal antibody, radio-immunoassay using a panel of monoclonal antibodies, radio-immunoprecipitation and polyacrylamide gel electrophoresis, partial amino and carboxyl-terminal sequence analysis, isoelectric focusing, and/or High Performance Liquid Chromatography. The amino acid composition of a product can be determined and compared to the initiating gene sequence and/or the native compound. In a gene deletion vaccine, these techniques can be used to demonstrate the absence of gene product e.g. viral glycoprotein and thus identify a strain.

Normally immunogenicity testing in the host animal is correlated with the immune response in a laboratory animal which then can be used to test batches before release. The use of a characterized immunogen in a host animal immunogenicity test would permit immunogenicity to be correlated with in vitro qualitative and quantitative tests which then could be used to test the potency of batches before release. If the method of immunogen production were changed, complete characterization of the immunogens produced by the old and new procedures could be used to obtain approval of the new procedure without additional host animal immunogenicity testing.

Tests such as the BLUOGAL for detection of lactase can be used to detect insertion of a lactase gene as a marker into a genome.

If a gene that normally produces a specific product that induces an antibody response has been deleted from an agent in a modified live vaccine, the gene can be cloned and expressed to produce the product. This can then be used as an antigen in a serological test to determine if an animal's antibody response is to a wild or to a vaccine virus. The same determination can be done when vectored vaccines are used; an animal's serum can be tested for antibodies to a cloned viral protein other than those vectored in the vaccine. Some inactivated vaccines do not induce the same spectrum of antibodies as is produced when an agent replicates in the animal. In these cases, again a specific protein could be used to distinguish vaccinated from infected animals.

In situ hybridization, immuno-labelling and detection of nuclei acid by the polymerase chain reaction can be used to study the replication and persistence of a vaccine in an animal or cell culture.

Safety testing can be more extensive when in addition to the targeted host, drugs e.g. dexamethasone, and a variety of laboratory animals including immuno-deficient ones such as the athymic (nu/nu) nude mouse and severe combined immuno-deficient (SCID) mouse can be used. The rationale for using immuno-deficient mice is that they can be considered as a "worst case" scenario for the relative safety of a recombinant vaccine. Today, the extent of AIDS infection lends creditability to extremes in testing.

The immune response to an immunogen can be compared with another immunogen by a neutralization, ELISA, lymphocyte blastogenesis, cytotoxic T-cell and/or macrophage migration inhibition tests.

Molecular biological techniques not only enable us to do a better job of quality control of biological products, but more significantly, allow us to understand the mechanism behind earlier procedures, used simply because they worked. For example, conventional attenuated vaccines were developed by multiple serial passages in cell culture until by chance they naturally mutated to an attenuated state. A possible reason for the attenuation may have been a point mutation or single base change. Today, attenuation can be accomplished by deleting a whole gene whose structure, location and function in the ability of the agent to replicate and cause disease is known. The chance of reversion can be predicted by knowing what would have to be recreated and the availability of a similar piece of genome from another agent or host cell.

REFERENCES

BACHRACH, H.L. (1982) Recombinant DNA technology for the preparation of subunit vaccines. JAVMA. Vol 181 pp 992-999.

CALLIS, J.J. (1986) Vectors of animal Vaccines. Proc. 90th Annual Meeting of the United States Animal Health Association pp 127-133.

ESPESETH, D.A., JOSEPH, P.L., SHIBLEY, G.P., GAY, C.G. (1987) Current USDA licensing requirements for R-DNA derived animal biological products. Proc. 91st Annual Meeting of the United States Animal Health Association pp 182-195.

ESPESETH, D.A., SHIBLEY, G.P., JOSEPH, P.L., VAN DEUSEN, R.A. WHETSTONE, C.A. (1985) USDA licensing policy for biologicals produced by R-DNA. Develop. Biol. Standard. Vol 59 pp 167-173.

JOSEPH, P.I., ESPESETH, D.A., SHIBLEY, G.P., GAY, C.G. (1988) Environmental considerations for field testing and licensing of live genetically-engineered veterinary biologics, Rev. Sci. Tech. Off. Int. Epiz. **7** (2), pp 282-291.

DEVELOPMENT AND TRANSFER OF VACCINE TECHNOLOGY TO THE THIRD WORLD: LONG-TERM CHALLENGES AND STRATEGIES - BIOFORCE 95

by

A Atger

Since 1984, the United Nations Industrial Development Organisation's (UNIDO) work to promote industrial production of vaccines in developing countries has been guided by its Advisory Panel on Preventive Medicine. Its members - no more than 16 - are specialists in various aspects of preventive medicine and can call on other additional experts if necessary. Representatives of UN sister organizations (particularly WHO and FAO) can serve as members and technical advisers.

With the advice of the Panel the UNIDO Secretariat prepared a background paper for the Third Consultation on the Pharmaceutical Industry held in Madrid, 1987 entitled: "The challenge of biological technology transfer to developing countries" (ID/WG.466/20 (Spec). This document gives a good reflection on the challenging supply situation in developing countries.

The strategy of the UNIDO programme on industrial production of biologicals (IPB) is based on an industrial approach characterised by the concept of unit processing and a homogenous culture system. This approach also secures consistency in consecutive production lots by means of built-in quality assurance. It advocates the necessary transfer of technology through a long-term support programme, enabling the recipient to adopt and assimilate the technology, as well as assisting in the promotion of new products.

To make production more efficient even at the small scale, UNIDO promotes the production of human and veterinary vaccines and other biologicals, in an existing facility with sufficient capacity either sharing only the same services and infrastructure or even using the same production equipment on a time sharing basis. The introduction of human vaccines in an existing production unit for veterinary vaccines, or vice versa, should be carried out by the application of good manufacturing practices and quality assurance, in line with the requirements of WHO.

This innovative idea has been realized in the establishment of a pilot plant for the Production of Vaccines for Africa which is under implementation in Garoua/Cameroon.

In the months before its formal inauguration, the plant produced over one million doses of tetanus vaccine. Annual production is expected to be 7.2 million doses. The ambition of Dr Charles Merieux (Chairman of UNIDO's advisory panel and president of the Fondation Marcel Merieux) for the pilot unit is that, its vaccines having reached WHO's demanding standard of excellence, it will play a significant part in a drive to eradicate neo-natal tetanus by 1995, the centenary of Louis Pasteur's death.

The facility can be expanded to produce other biologicals and UNIDO sees it not only as the nucleus of Central Africa's human vaccine production but as a training centre in modern biological science and technology.

BIOFORCE 95

The concept of Bioforce (bio=biologicals) is based on the principle that when different energies are pooled the effect is greater than the sum of the separate parts.

UNIDO's biologicals programme coined the word to describe its own motivation. Bioforce is the driving power of UNIDO's industrial production of biologicals programme, which it regards as its specific input to a global effort energized by the UN family against all disease controllable by immunization.

In January 1991, when the pilot plant to produce tetanus vaccine was formally inaugurated in Garoua, Cameroon, BIOFORCE 95 was born - specifically to eradicate tetanus in Africa by 1995, but with other diseases also targeted.

Bioforce measures aimed at eliminating cholera and measles were launched soon after.

Against cholera, UNIDO is working in close co-operation with UNICEF and WHO, and with FAO and UNDP, sent out a task force to central Africa in late 1991, to investigate the possibilities of attacking this dreadful disease.

Similarly against measles, a joint UNDP.UNICEF.UNIDO/WHO team began assessing worldwide vaccine production potential and global needs, as a preliminary to developing a bioforce that would reduce deaths by 95 per cent from this disease by 1995.

Constraints to Vaccine Production

CONSTRAINTS IN VACCINE PRODUCTION AND QUALITY CONTROL IN DEVELOPING COUNTRIES

by

F G Davies

INTRODUCTION

The constraints to production in developing countries relate principally to the intermittent failure of the basic services, such as water and electricity. They are also the cause of many indirect costs as damage to equipment is regularly a consequence of their failure. Buildings are not generally inadequate for much of the vaccine production work, but new investment is required to effect the changeover to the use of specific pathogen free poultry flocks for vaccine production and quality control testing purposes.

The dependence upon imported media and biologicals is unavoidable at present and a drain on foreign exchange. Political and economic factors are highly significant for a variety of reasons, but the availability of competent trained local staff is not generally a problem.

TECHNICAL CONSTRAINTS

Services

Basic services such as water, electricity and steam supplies for autoclaves etc are liable to be taken for granted in the developed world. This is by no means the case in many developing countries.

Electricity

Electricity supplies are frequently interrupted by failures induced by a wide variety of problems. The breakdown of main supply systems, silting of turbines in hydroelectric schemes, fuel shortages etc, are all liable to be the cause of problems at different times. Storm damage and faults following the overloading of transformer systems as laboratories grow larger, without stepping up the supplies are additional common faults.

They are particularly unwanted at critical times during egg incubation, harvesting and during freeze drying, when batches may be readily lost. Stand by generators are essential, and should be programmed to cut in only after attaining the required voltage. Further problems may follow the return of the mains supply which often cuts in with a lower voltage and greater current, and wavers up and down below and above the required levels. This is accompanied by the smell of burning insulation, as incubator motors, refrigerator systems, solenoid switches etc suffer damage. The safety cut outs do not always save equipment in these circumstances.

Water Supplies

Variable and failing water supplies are a further common cause of time out from production in many developing countries. These are subject to failures due to a variety of causes, the principle one being the inadequacy of supplies to a rapidly expanding urban and industrial city complex. These greatly interfere with production. Steam boilers essential for most washing, cleaning and autoclaving functions come to a standstill. Steam distillation becomes impossible, water cooled freeze drier compressors cut out unless cooling circuits are available, and batches of vaccine can be lost.

Much time out is due to steam boiler problems in addition to the water failures, as fuel pumps, burners and control systems fail. Spare parts may be difficult to obtain or may take a long time when ordered through the Government Supply systems. Regular servicing contracts are often cancelled by cash deprived departments. Steam piping and boilers may become heavily scaled as a result and become dangerous and inefficient.

Water supplies may contain quantities of particulate matter which causes a variety of problems. Distillation apparatus, and automatic washing machines all fail to function properly. Efforts to cope with the main supply problems by using private bore hole water can be a mixed blessing. These may be high in sediment or salts. The valuable switchgear which is necessary to control the borehole pump has been known to attract undue attention and in one instance was stolen time after time by thieves.

Buildings

The buildings and facilities for production are not normally a major constraint to vaccine production in developing countries. While those available may not be perfect, and may have been built many years ago, they have often been altered and adapted by resourceful people to provide adequate conditions. Many developing countries have custom built facilities.

Good basic hygiene, discipline and technique can achieve a great deal. The advent of laminar flow technology has been of considerable help in raising standards and reducing contamination during production processes. A great deal has been achieved however in the field of vaccine production in developing countries without the benefit of the advanced technology available in production laboratories in the developed world.

The greatest current building requirement for vaccine production in the developing countries is to provide the facilities for Specific Pathogen Free egg supplies. These are necessary for vaccine production and quality control and safety testing. Such a complex requires a considerable investment, which may not be possible with the budgets available for animal health and disease control today.

Equipment

Much equipment which was purchased 20-30 years ago is still the mainstay of production laboratories in many parts of the world. It is possible to see rows of freeze drying machines which are more than 30 years old still virtually in daily use. Centrifuges, microscopes, waterbaths, refrigerators, incubators, freeze driers and the like are found to be in good working order. Many additions, replacements and new equipment are also to be found - for the Supplies Officers appear to give a reasonably high priority to the purchase of equipment.

The vagaries of the electrical supplies in many developing countries is a strong argument against the current trend to fit electrical switchgear and solenoid type valves to much laboratory equipment where manual operation was previously used. This results in much time out for centrifuges and freeze driers as these burn out following electrical problems. It is not uncommon to find the new generation of freeze driers idle for such reasons when the old ones with manual valves are perfectly satisfactory.

An increased demand for and the increase in the range of vaccines produces, is the reason why many laboratories in the developing countries now require new equipment plant and buildings.

The storage facilities for biologicals, media and vaccine both in preparation and bottled ready for use, are a continuing source of problems. Cold room breakdowns in climates with high ambient temperatures are the rule, and in the absence of revolving operational funds, not permitted by Treasuries in most countries. Rapid repairs are difficult to carry out through the Government servicing systems. There are delays while tenders are offered and examined. There is often no facility to cope with such emergencies. Surplus capacity cold storage should be available if possible.

Supplies of dry nitrogen, oxygen and acetylene cylinders for use in vaccine production may be influenced by local supply problems and reserve cylinders should be held in the department. Vaccine vials are usually obtained from abroad, and as the ordering and supply interval can be prolonged and there are many steps in the procedure, hold ups in such orders may not be detected for very long periods of time. Shortages of vaccine vials has occurred at most laboratories and it is not difficult to understand how this has happened.

<u>Media and Biologicals</u>

Nearly all developing countries will largely rely on international suppliers for these. They make a persistent demand for foreign exchange. Media, chemicals and specific reagents are expensive and laboratory consumables are also liable to be costly. An FAO project in Turkey many years ago set up a spray drying system for the preparation of bacteriological media components from readily available cheap local components. This allowed very considerable savings of between 60-80% of the costs of purchase in the international market. Similar plant could be established in many countries with the prospect of considerable savings.

Tissue culture media formulations and other tissue culture reagents are a special problem. The technology demands that high quality freshly prepared media be used. In house preparation from components demands regular replenishment of stocks, and many laboratories have now come to rely upon the commercially prepared media which are highly satisfactory but expensive. No practical alternative is available at present.

The relatively low cost and availability of labour on an intensive scale in developing countries should support systems which employ glassware and washable equipment rather than disposable items. The use of disposable pipettes, petri dishes and bottles is difficult to justify in such situations. Plastic laboratory ware is expensive although it can be reused many times by cleaning and sterilising in microwave ovens. The failure of services often creates situations when the use of plastic ware is a necessary alternative.

However, problems often arise when the material support provided by FAO or other donor project is withdrawn and the comparable help is not maintained by the Institute. This is a regrettable but regular fact of life in developing countries.

The dependence of laboratories in poorer countries upon the importation of so much of their requirements, makes them vulnerable to foreign exchange and political problems. This is an undesirable situation but it is difficult to see how it can be avoided at the moment.

SOCIO-ECONOMIC CONSTRAINTS

Political Stability

Political instability has been a recurring disruptive factor for laboratories in recent decades. One has only to look at the situation in Uganda or Mozambique to appreciate this. The destruction of laboratory facilities, the loss of equipment, loss of services, loss of staff and their technical ability can completely destroy an effective and successful laboratory establishment. These consequences are usually followed by periods of economic disaster when resources to rebuild are not available.

Staffing

The quality of staff available in production laboratories is the result of the operation of many factors. The status and local reputation of the laboratory, its general standards or morale and the quality of its products are surprisingly important. Professional staff and their levels of competence are not usually a weakness in most developing countries, and are not a constraint to production, in comparison with the service and supply problems already mentioned. Professional staff have generally been well trained at home and abroad, and constitute a valuable resource.

A satisfactory but unfortunate consequence of this is that such competent staff with a track record of production and competence in vaccine production, are highly marketable. They are liable to be snapped up exceedingly quickly by commercial concerns operating in fields such as vaccine production, poultry management or animal production related business. This is not a loss of resource to the country but is an unfortunate loss of trained staff to the government service. Government is traditionally a bad employer and the attraction of big salary increases with perquisites is sufficient to make such moves all too common.

A consistently weak area in many Institutes is the absence of a fully trained refrigeration engineer, with his tools of trade to maintain freeze driers, cold rooms and the like. Huge savings would be achieved in servicing alone, if he could be maintained with supplies of spares and gas. The ability to cope with emergency situations would be invaluable.

The core strength of many Production Laboratories is to be found amongst the relatively underpaid and undervalued ranks of the technological and technician grades. Frequently these people represent a huge reservoir of valuable experience in all aspects of vaccine production, freeze drying, dispensing and equipment maintenance. They are invaluable but often have poor conditions of employment.

Conditions of service and remuneration in Government Laboratories are usually less satisfactory than those in commercial employment. These must be brought up to those offered elsewhere if the staff are to be retained.

Political Influences

In some countries, the career structure is liable to be influenced by factors other than competence in a particular area of work. Nepotism and the godfather principle may act to the general detriment of the service. As a result, opportunities for training and promotion may be determined by less than honourable motives. Such realities are the source of some disaffection and dissatisfaction with the system. Work and morale suffers.

The reality of the administrative inefficiency which is an indirect consequence of this, causes great disruption in continuous on-going laboratory production schedules. The interminable journeying which may be required to obtain long overdue allowances of various sorts, greatly interferes with the worktime of staff at all levels. Much time is spent on servicing and supply work which should not be the province of the laboratory staff. Effective supply officers should be carrying out such tasks. Regrettably this is rarely the case.

Technical Training

This has not always been readily available in the field of production, quality control and safety testing of vaccines. A basic training in laboratory technology has largely sufficed, together with the hands-on training of the routine production laboratory staff. FAO has made considerable efforts over recent years to remedy this by running numerous training courses.

Some have been held at Regional Quality Control Laboratories - for which they are well suited.

Individual vaccine production laboratories in both developing and developed countries have been enormously helpful over a period of many years by having people attached to their laboratories for training purposes. This has been a great help to many people and due acknowledgement must be made for this courtesy. Commercial concerns are clearly reluctant to extend this service.

The ability acquired by years of service at the technical level is a valuable training resource, and is applied at the non professional level with hands-on training for all newly recruited staff. This is generally extremely valuable, and the main method for the training of staff newly recruited to a vaccine production laboratory. It is probably the most valuable and appropriate.

There is a need to provide further training in the latest safety and quality control methods applicable to SPF produced poultry vaccines. This new advancement is now becoming more relevant to developing countries, many of whom see the need to apply this to their own poultry industry. Much of the SPF production in the developed world is in the hands of the commercial producers and unavailable for training purposes. A variety of serological reagents are also required for this purpose and may not be readily available.

Economic Factors

These express themselves through some of the means discussed in earlier paragraphs. The general status of the animal production industry in a country has an important influence. If there is a good market for livestock with rewarding prices and possibly an export market, this is usually reflected in a more aggressive approach to animal health and disease control. Vaccine campaigns are actively pursued, disease surveillance is improved and in general all areas associated with the industry are supported. Vaccine production laboratories receive good support and service.

The converse is true when there is a depression in the industry, when persistent failures in plant and equipment are associated with poor servicing and maintenance. Field services may fail as vehicles break down and are not repaired, cold chains are not maintained and funds are not available to mobilise vaccination teams in the field.

These facts have been well recognised by the PARC/EEC rinderpest project, which, while focusing upon the eradication of rinderpest, is also designed to restore the field veterinary services. This will furnish vehicles, refrigerators, and establish mobile refrigerated facilities for vaccine transport. Hopefully this will go some way to restore the veterinary services in many developing countries, which have suffered considerably in the economic climate of the last decade. This is a totally realistic approach, much to be applauded.

TECHNICAL, FINANCIAL AND SOCIO-ECONOMIC CONSTRAINTS ON VACCINE PRODUCTION IN AFRICA

by

L E Carmichael and D Sylla

1. FINANCIAL

(a) Shortage of foreign/local currency for construction, equipment, supplies for vaccine production, transportation and maintenance of facilities.

- *This requires long-term planning to anticipate needs and problems in order to avoid lengthy breakdowns in production and distribution of products.*

(b) Dependence on supplementary donors upon termination of funded projects.

- *Sustainability has been a sanguine goal, but it has been rarely achieved - especially with livestock or animal health projects.*

(c) Production/distribution is too frequently on a national rather than regional basis.

- *A 'non-competitive' environment is commonly subject to influences that do not favour the maintenance of sustained quality or best use of limited resources. Can lead to variable quality of products.*

(d) Delays in process of bidding, ordering and receipt of essential materials.

(e) Lack of financial incentives to attract people in country/region.

- *Qualified personnel often disenfranchised in favour of foreign technicians - sometimes less qualified than available nationals.*

- *Low salaries of government employees.*

(f) Ponderous bureaucracies.

- *Often poor mechanism for payment of laboratories for vaccines or other services. Payments should be made promptly to provide funds for continued production and facilities maintenance.*

- *<u>Autonomy</u>: Laboratory Directors should be able to have direct access to bank accounts in order to obviate delays (government bureaucracies) and to quickly replenish critical supplies and meet short term obligations.*

2. TECHNICAL

(a) Need for assistance in management support

- *Management Development and Support Team (MSDT) was a successful model established by USAID in Mali. Project implementation and effectiveness benefited immensely from the accounting, financial analysis, logistics and work planning/control systems installed by the MSDT. Joint management committees (JMC) established between donors/recipients (at the Ministerial level) also were positive innovations, resulting in reduction in management costs and sources of professional advice, improved communications between projects and ministries involved on policy issues. The MSDT also reduced the preoccupation of JMC with project details.*

- *Assist in planning, procurement, logistics support of production and distribution.*

- *Remedy ineffective mechanisms for cash recovery by producers.*

  - Producers not always 'paid' by governments.

  - A 'privatized' or 'quasi-privatized' basis for conducting business might offer some relief.

(b) Managements problems: Lack of infrastructure for maintenance of facilities; separation of production from research and diagnostic facilities and from quality control laboratories to comply with GMP rules.

- *Total separation of quality control from other services is critical.*

(c) Critical lack of engineers (especially national) with equipment maintenance training.

- *Absence of 'technological environment'.*

(d) Communications: ordering, receiving, maintenance of inventories, distribution to areas of greatest need; maintenance of proper inventories.

- *Lack of basic communications on regional basis affects some areas. It is common for a period of 3 to 6 months to elapse for engineers to respond to breakdowns in essential equipment such as freeze-dryers. In such instances, the visit, DFA and fees must be paid.*

(e) Transportation: vehicles, maintenance, unavailability of spare parts and fuel.

(f) Lack of essential equipment: water purification; air filtration systems; low temperature freezers; freeze-drying equipment; egg incubators, etc.

(g) Lack of documentation - protocols, technical libraries, manuals for equipment maintenance and repair, textbooks and scientific journals to keep up to date with contemporary developments.

(h) Unavailability of reagents: Sera for vaccine production, SPF eggs for seed; eggs for production; small animals (mice, guinea pigs, etc) for safety tests; media components; glassware; washing facilities etc.

(i) Absence of 'raw materials' available locally (to save money) viz, protein hydrolysates or sources of sera from within country/region.

(j) Inadequate production and quality control staff and facilities to test and monitor vaccines.

(k) Integrity of the "cold chain" could be improved - research on better methods of stabilization and lyophilization.

(l) Shortage of personnel with expertise in vaccine production and quality control and training programmes.

(m) Availability of vaccines - sometimes unobtainable when need is greatest - especially in times of unexpected outbreaks. Lack of proper inventory records also may lead to overstocking and maintenance of out-dated vaccine.

3. SOCIO-ECONOMIC

(a) Lack of commitment of governments to animal health needs of country/region, especially in time periods where priority diseases seem 'under control'.

- *It is essential that governments, or their representatives (eg OAU/IBAR in Africa) take on a more formal directorial role, commencing with joint representation of both governments and donors.*

(b) Lack of permanent regional organizations with a high degree of commitment and managements skills to oversee management, production, quality control and distribution of vaccines.

- *Governments should promote regional approach; only those laboratories with the demonstrated ability or potential to compete (produce good vaccines) should be supported.*

(c) Loss of trained staff to private sector as a consequence of low salaries and frustration (2 b,c,d).

- *Lack of incentives for laboratory workers has resulted in highly qualified technical staff leaving a service in favour of higher paying jobs.*

(d) Networking of labs has improved, but should be enhanced. Meetings of biologics producers: A "PanAfrican Biological Producers Association" meeting should be held annually to share problems, views and explore ways to improve vaccine quality, quantity, modes of distribution and integration of efforts.

- *Support could come from national governments or regional institutions, if established.*

(e) Diffusion of information on animal health activities and requirements, are needed to better inform the beneficiaries of the value of animal health programmes.

- *Such publications as the "Panvac Bulletin", Progress Reports of PARC (OAU/IBAR/PARC), the excellent brochure by LANAVET (Cameroun), and dissemination of information to the popular media.*

(f) Integration of vaccine production with satisfactory mechanisms of national or regional distribution is needed eg the "PARC" model.

(g) Lack of regional determination of vaccine costs and <u>ability to pay in local currencies</u>.

- *There is lack of acceptance of local currencies by several regional countries.*

(h) Lack of confidence in some "locally-produced" products.

(i) Import-export laws/restrictions/requirements (customs problems).

(k) 'National pride'.

- *Some laboratories are not economically justified, yet sustained by governments.*

Licensing and Quality Control

LICENSING AND QUALITY CONTROL OF DNA TECHNOLOGY PRODUCTS

by

C A Mebus

The objective of a licensing procedure for a biological product is to establish that the product is pure, safe, potent and efficacious, and not to be worthless, contaminated, dangerous, or harmful. Some of the general public are concerned that new recombinant DNA (rDNA) derived micro-organisms or products could have adverse effects on the environment and therefore should be rigidly controlled or prohibited from release. The majority of the scientific community, on the other hand, takes the position that properly characterized and evaluated products developed through biotechnology pose no risk to public health or the environment. The USDA has taken the stance that r-DNA derived products are not significantly different from similar products produced by conventional methods and thus are subject to the same regulations for development and licensing. The USDA places the emphasis on the product and its intended use, not the way the product was developed or produced.

Products derived through biotechnology, as those developed by conventional means, are classified into three broad categories based upon the biological characteristics and safety concerns for the new product.

<u>Category I</u> consists of inactivated recombinant DNA-derived vaccines, bacterins, bacterin-toxoids, and viral subunits, and bacterial subunit products to be used as immunogens; and monoclonal antibodies to be used prophylactically, therapeutically or as components of diagnostic kits. These products are non-viable and thus pose no risk to the environment and require no new or unusual safety concerns.

<u>Category II</u> contains live organisms modified by deletion or addition of one or more genes. The deletion may remove a gene coding for virulence, oncogenicity, enzyme activity, or some biochemical function required for virulence. An added gene may cause attenuation by interference with the function of a resident gene or mark an organism by the addition of a gene that produces a unique marker antigen or enzyme.

In this category, it must be shown that the deletion or the addition of one or more genes does not increase the virulence, pathogenicity, or survivability of the new organism over the parent or wild-type organism. Field testing and/or licensing may also require presentation of sequence information, base pair analysis, restriction endonuclease sites for the insertion, a comparison of the phenotypic characterization and biochemical pathways of the parent and new organism, and an Environmental Assessment or decision document.

Two diseases for which vaccines in this category have been developed are pseudorabies and Rift Valley fever.

<u>Category III</u> consists of products using live organisms (vectors) genetically-engineered to carry genes coding for immunizing antigens and/or immune stimulants from different organisms or different strains of the same organism. Examples of vectors currently being

used include (but are not limited to) polyoma and SV-40 viruses (lytic viruses), retroviruses (shuttle viruses), vaccinia virus, other pox viruses, adenoviruses, herpesviruses, papilloma virus, salmonella, and E. coli.

For field testing and/or licensing, organisms in this category must be fully characterized and compared to the parent organism. Characterization includes but is not limited to presentation of sequence information, base pair analysis and restriction endonuclease sites for the insertion, comparison of the phenotypic characterization and biochemical pathways of the parent and new organism, comparison of the virulence, pathogenicity, and survivability of the new organism over the parent or wild-type organism, and an Environmental Assessment or Environmental Impact Statement.

Two products which have been developed in this category are the vaccinia-vector recombinant rabies vaccine and the vaccinia-vector recombinant rinderpest vaccine.

In the United States, development, testing and licensing of genetically-engineered live biological products (Categories II and III) intended for use in animals is done in four closely controlled stages. The following is an example of the procedures which have to be followed.

The initial <u>in-vitro</u> and <u>in-vivo</u> development and experiments not involving release into the environment can be done with the approval from the appropriate Institutional Biosafety Committee. This initial work should be done in Veterinary Services (VS) level 4 and level 3 containment facilities (equivalent to biosafety levels 4 and 3 as described in Appendix G-III of the National Institutes of Health Guidelines). Veterinary Services (VS) containment level 4 requires air exhaust to be filtered or treated so as to prevent release of the agent into the environment; effluents and sewage decontaminated; and bedding, manure, and solid wastes incinerated or effectively disinfected; and all test animals destroyed and incinerated or effectively disinfected. After satisfactory completion of the initial developmental work, studies can then proceed at VS containment level 3. At this level the Master Seed is characterized, studies on shedding, spread and fate of the organism, and reverse-passage/reversion to virulence are done in the host animal. If needed, nontarget hosts are studied at level 3. The difference between levels 4 and 3 is that after approval by the VS/State authorities, the experimental animals can be removed for slaughter or rendering.

In the United States, Title 9 Code of Federal Regulation part 103.3 requires authorization from the Deputy Administrator, APHIS, prior to any intrastate, interstate, or export shipment of any experimental veterinary biological product. The movement of an experimental veterinary biological from strict containment (VS containment level 4 and 3) to field use is usually done in stages. Before the agent can be moved from containment level 3 to VS quarantined field testing (level 2), information generated at level 3 plus the proposed field experiment must be submitted to VS for evaluation. From this information, VS prepares an abbreviated Environmental Assessment, which includes information on the biological properties and potential environmental effects of the parent and modified organisms, for the authorised shipment of the product and initiation of quarantined field testing. The submission to VS must include the following:

1. A description of the product and its intended use;

2. Characteristics of the modified agent which include but are not limited to: description of the vector, source and function of the DNA insert, expression of the insert, and genetic stability of the modified organism;

3. A comparison of the phenotypic characterization and biochemical pathways of the parent;

4. Construction of the modified agent which includes but is not limited to: synthesis of the insert, sequence information, comparison of the native gene and the insert, construction of the plasmid, construction of the recombinant, restriction endonuclease sites for the insertion, selection of the recombinant, restriction enzyme analysis of the recombinant, and analysis of the expressed antigen;

5. Results of studies on shedding, spread and fate of the organism, reverse-passage/reversion to virulence, and if needed, the effect on nontarget hosts;

6. Description of the master cell stock, master seed stock, production of the vaccine, and testing of the vaccine for purity, safety, sterility, potency and efficacy;

7. Proposed procedures and methods to be used in the field evaluation of the product, to include but not limited tc maintenance of records on the quantity of the product prepared, shipped and used, and methods for biological or physical control and retrieval in the event of an adverse effect of the product;

8. The names and locations of the proposed test sites and the quantity of material to be shipped to each site; and,

9. A letter of permission to conduct the test from the regulatory authority in each state involved.

The requirements for a quarantine facility (VS containment level 2) for a restricted field test are:

1. The facility should be so located and constructed so as to prevent the test animals from having contact with any other animals - domestic or wild;

2. The facility should be constructed of materials that will permit washing and decontamination;

3. Doors, windows and other openings should be screened to prevent the entrance or exit of insects;

4. A program for the control of insects, ectoparasites, and mammalian pests;

5. Be of sufficient size to prevent overcrowding;

6. Meet Federal, State and local regulations relating to pollution control and protection of the environment;

7. Have an adequate water supply;

8. Have a procedure acceptable to the Deputy Administrator of VS for the disposal of any test animal that dies or is killed;

9. Have facilities to incinerate or effectively disinfect bedding and soil waste at the termination of the experiment.

At the termination of the restricted field trial, experimental animals can be slaughtered if there is no evidence of survival of the recombinant agent and that the agent poses no environmental risk.

The next step in development of a genetically-engineered live biological product is a request to APHIS for authorization to conduct a limited field trial outside of quarantine (VS containment level 1). Before such a trial is authorized, APHIS reviews all of the sponsor's safety data (including human safety), the field testing protocol, alternatives to the genetically engineered product, affected environment, environmental consequences, and consults with other agencies to assess the impact of the field trial on the environment and prepares the Environmental Assessment document. The purpose of the Environmental Assessment is to provide the public with documentation of APHIS's assessment of the environmental effect of the product. If the conclusion from this assessment is that there is no significant impact, a notice of the availability of the Environmental Assessment and the intention of initiating the field trial within 30 days is published in the Federal Register.

Upon completion of a successful field trial, the license applicant submits all required additional data to show that the product is pure, safe, potent, and efficacious. Using this information, an amended or supplemental Environmental Assessment is prepared and its availability and the intention to issue a license is published in the Federal Register. Licensing of the product removes any geographical restraints on the product.

REFERENCES

BACHRACH, H.L. (1982) Recombinant DNA technology for the preparation of subunit vaccines. JAVMA. Vol **181**. pp 992-999.

CALLIS, J.J. (1986) Vectors of animal vaccines. Proc. 90th Annual Meeting of the United States Animal Health Association. pp 127-133.

ESPESETH, D.A., JOSEPH, P.L., SHIBLEY, G.P., GAY, C.G. (1987) Current USDA licensing requirements for R-DNA derived animal biological products. Proc. 91st Annual Meeting of the United States Animal Health Association. pp 182-195.

ESPESETH, D.A., SHIBLEY, G.P., JOSEPH, P.L., VAN DEUSEN, R.A., WHETSTONE, C.A. (1985) USDA licensing policy for biologicals produced by R-DNA. Develop, Biol. Standard. Vol **59**. pp 167-173.

JOSEPH, P.I., ESPESETH, D.A., SHIBLEY, G.P., GAY, C.G. (1988) Environmental considerations for field testing and licensing of live genetically-engineered veterinary biologics. Rev. Sci. Tech. Off. Int. Epiz. **7** (2), pp 285-291.

LICENSING OF VETERINARY VACCINES AND BIOLOGICALS

by

J M Rutter

INTRODUCTION

The main purpose of veterinary medicines is to treat or prevent diseases of food producing or companion animals. In this respect medicines make a major contribution to improvements in animal health and welfare as well as increasing the availability of protein for the world's human population. Extensive research is carried out during the development of veterinary medicines and extensive testing is now required prior to licensing to ensure their safety and efficacy. During the last two decades consumers in many countries have become particularly conscious of the quality and safety of food, and the need for food to be free of potentially harmful chemical additives and residues. At the same time, the regulatory requirements for veterinary medicines have become increasingly stringent in the light of new scientific knowledge and this is reflected in the developments highlighted in this paper.

Legislation

A legislative framework is required as the basis for the regulation of veterinary medicines and such frameworks are in place in many countries. In the United Kingdom, all medicines, whether human or veterinary, are controlled by the same primary legislation set out in the Medicines Act of 1968. Associated legislation is directed at the specific requirements for veterinary medicines. European Community (EC) Directives covering veterinary medicines, residues of veterinary medicines, feed additives and products derived by biotechnology are implemented by legislation in each Member State of the Community. These laws are designed to ensure that all medicines can be used safely, are of good quality and are effective through a system of licences and controls placed on their manufacture and distribution. The legislation makes it an offence to import, sell or supply a veterinary medicine without an appropriate licence or certificate.

The Licensing Authority for veterinary medicines in the UK is the Agriculture and Health Ministers, who are advised by two independent statutory committees of independent scientific experts, the Veterinary Products Committee and the Medicines Commission. These Committees act as sources of advice and as apellate bodies. The Veterinary Medicines Directorate (VMD) is the executive arm of the Licensing Authority for veterinary medicines and is responsible for all aspects of the administration of animals medicines legislation, including assessment of applications, the issue of licences and post-licensing surveillance, and policy advice.

The Licensing Criteria and Procedures

The key feature of the UK Medicines Act is the product licence. No veterinary medicinal product may be marketed without a licence which is granted only after the product has undergone rigorous assessment on the criteria of safety, quality and efficacy. Safety is interpreted widely to include the animal being treated and in-contact animals; the user, including the veterinarian, farmer or pet owner administering the medicine; the consumer of livestock products from treated animals; and the environment. Quality means that medicines must be manufactured with appropriate quality control procedures in premises that are inspected and licensed; the ingredients must be of appropriate purity, in the correct proportions and correctly processed; the containers must be robust with secure closures, and the labelling must be accurate and informative. Efficacy means that the medicines must be effective against the diseases, in the species of animals, at the dose rate, frequency and duration of treatment, and by the route of administration claimed by the manufacturer.

Data supporting all aspects of safety, quality and efficacy must be provided by the applicant. Only after these requirements have been rigorously examined and met will a product licence be issued. The approval process for a simple application which satisfies current standards can be dealt with quickly. For new medicines and more complex applications assessment takes longer. Appeals procedures are built into the UK licensing system whereby the applicant has the right to request oral or written hearings before the expert Committees assessing the applications if the licensing criteria have not been met. An important part of the approval process is the agreement of a published data sheet, which summarises the details of the product and its conditions of use.

Licensing Safeguards

The rigorous and independent assessment of applications, and conditions attached to the product licence provide the major safeguard for the public and for users of veterinary medicines. Additional safeguards are provided by the licensing of manufacturing premises and regulation of distribution systems for veterinary medicines, by post licence surveillance for residues of veterinary medicines and by notification to the Licensing Authority of suspected adverse reactions, including lack of efficacy. For vaccines and biologicals, additional safeguards may include pre-licence testing during assessment of the application to ensure that safety criteria can be met, batch control testing to ensure that successive batches of the licensed product meet the required standards, and inspections of quality control procedures to provide quality assurance of the production procedure and the finished product.

Consumer safety is addressed during the assessment of licence applications and by post licence surveillance for residues. All applications for product licences must contain data to satisfy the Licensing Authority that use of the product will not leave potentially harmful residues in food. Companies must provide residue data from animal products from which withdrawal periods can be calculated. This is the period following cessation of treatment during which an animal or its products should not be used for food. Legislation in the UK provides for the taking of almost 50,000 samples each year to allow testing for the presence of potentially harmful residues of veterinary medicines and the results of the surveillance are published.

Post-licensing surveillance covers not only testing for residues of veterinary medicines, but also surveillance of suspected adverse reactions to licensed veterinary medicines. This includes adverse reactions in animals receiving veterinary medicines and in humans administering or handling the products. If the reactions are serious and are confirmed, amendments may need to be made to the product literature or batches of product may need to be withdrawn from the market. Suspension of the licence would be the final step.

Product licences are valid in the UK for five years and after this period licences may be reviewed before they are reissued to ensure that they continue to meet current standards. However, the Licensing Authority has the power in legislation to remove products from the market at any time should the need arise.

Support for The Licensing Functions

In order to operate effectively the Licensing Authority needs to be supported by an efficient executive and enforcement body. In the UK this is provided by the VMD, which is a multidisciplinary group of some 90 veterinarians, biologists, pharmacists, administrators and support staff, in co-operation with other Government Departments and bodies. The aims of the VMD are to ensure the safety, quality and efficacy of veterinary medicines in the UK and its staff are divided into three multidisciplinary teams covering the main areas of its work - Feed Additives, Pharmaceutical Products and Recombinant and Biological Products.

The VMD is responsible for the licensing of veterinary medicines, the establishment, monitoring and enforcement of controls in co-operation with bodies such as the Royal Pharmaceutical Society of Great Britain, and the provision of policy advice on UK and EC animal medicines matters to Ministers. It also provides UK delegates to the EC Committee for Veterinary Medicinal Products, the Committee of Experts on Feed Additives, and to numerous national and international working groups.

Under UK requirements the VMD must recover the full costs of its licensing work from fees charged to companies for licence applications, inspections of manufacturing premises and for inspection of procedures for quality assurance. The VMD must also process licence applications as efficiently as possible to meet targets set by Ministers. An important requirement is to increase public knowledge and understanding of the rigorous licensing procedure for veterinary medicines and the consequent safeguards for consumers of food from treated animals. In order to do this the VMD publishes an Annual Report, brochures and bulletins that contain full details of its activities.

Current Requirements and Future Developments

The continuing increase in scientific knowledge and technological advances means that the licensing process is evolving to meet ever higher standards for veterinary medicines. The main areas of information required to be covered in current applications for veterinary medicines are summarised in Table 1. A summary of the proposed standards and protocols required for dossiers supporting licence applications for veterinary immunological products within the European Community are summarised in Table 2, and specific information required in the UK for vaccines in Tables 3 - 5. All applications need to satisfy the Licensing Authority that a pharmaceutical product, medicated feedstuff or vaccine - whether it be a live virus vaccine, an inactivated virus vaccine, a bacterial vaccine, a toxoid vaccine or a subunit vaccine derived by biotechnology, meets the stringent requirements of safety, quality and efficacy. The developments in biotechnology have meant that new criteria have had to be developed for the assessment of such products. In particular, the introduction of live vaccines consisting of genetically-manipulated organisms have to be assessed with great care to ensure that there are no harmful effects arising from their release.

Codes of practice setting out Good Laboratory Practice, Standard Operating Procedures and Good Manufacturing Practice are being implemented to ensure that there is a continuing commitment by manufacturers to quality during the whole of the research, development and manufacturing process for veterinary medicines. Training programmes to ensure that staff in research, manufacturing and licensing activities keep up to date with modern technological advances are also essential. Furthermore, the design of new manufacturing facilities that meet modern safety standards need to be discussed with licensing authorities at an early stage.

With the introduction of the single European market in 1993 proposals are being implemented to increase mutual recognition of licensing requirements in Member States. A procedure is also proposed for the issue of Community licences that will permit companies to market products in all 12 of the Member States. Increasing agreement on common standards is being sought internationally within the Community as well as between Europe, USA and Japan so that companies do not have to meet different requirements in different countries. However, all such agreements need to ensure that there is no weakening of the protection and safeguards afforded by the licensing system to animals and to the public.

Table 1: INFORMATION REQUIRED FOR LICENSING VETERINARY MEDICINES

Name	Form	Composition
Manufacturer	Importer	Preparation
Indications	Side-effects	Contra-indications
Safety precautions	Dose	Dosage schedule
Administration	Shelf life	Withholding period
Quality Control	Experimental studies	Clinical trials
Data sheet	Package insert	Label

Table 2: PROPOSED STANDARDS AND PROTOCOLS REQUIRED FOR THE TESTING OF VETERINARY IMMUNOLOGICAL PRODUCTS IN DOSSIERS SUPPORTING LICENCE APPLICATIONS

Summary of data

Summary of product characteristics

Expert Reports on documentation for safety, quality and efficacy

Analytical tests (all to be validated and state of the art)
- Qualitative and Quantitative Particulars
- Development Pharmaceutics
- Method of Preparation of Finished Product
- Production and Control of Starting Materials
  - biological
  - non-biological

Control tests during Production

Control tests on Finished Product
- General Characteristics
- Identification and assay of active ingredients
- Identification and assay of adjuvants
- Identification and assay of excipients
- Safety Tests
- Sterility and Purity
- Inactivation
- Residual humidity
- Batch Consistency

Stability Tests

Safety Tests
- Laboratory requirements
- Special requirements for live vaccines
  - spread
  - reversion to virulence
  - recombination
  - residues
  - interactions

Field Studies

Ecotoxicity

Efficacy

Table 3: INFORMATION REQUIRED FOR LICENSING VACCINES

Starting materials/manufacturing process	
Seed material	Antibiotics
Attenuation	Preservatives
Cell substrates	Inactivation
Substances of animal origin	Methods of manufacture
Other substances	Consistency of manufacture
Eggs	Plant/Site location and inspection
Harvesting	

Table 4: INFORMATION REQUIRED FOR LICENSING VACCINES

Final Vaccine
Safety
Reversion to virulence
Virus spread
Efficacy
Duration of immunity
Stability
Compatibility

Table 5: INFORMATION REQUIRED FOR LICENSING VACCINES

Final Lot/Batch Testing
Safety
Sterility
Extraneous agents
Potency
Titre
Diluent
Inactivation
Freedom from abnormal toxicity or pyrogenic substances

Discussion

This commenced with the Chairman asking for information about the availability of seed stocks for the preparation of the attenuated Rift Valley Fever vaccine mentioned by Dr Mebus in his talk.

Dr Mebus responded by stating that the vaccine had been developed by the medical services of the US army for the protection of its troops, and the vaccine was now in the final stages of testing and certification, and should be available soon.

Dr Lombard told the meeting that Rhone Poulenc had signed an agreement with the US authorities for use of the vaccine both in humans and animals, but at present the master seeds were still in the US.

Dr Rweyemamu asked for Dr Sizaret to comment on the possibility, if not desirability, of joint production of rabies vaccine for human and animal use in the developing countries.

Dr Sizaret replied by saying that while he could not give the official view of WHO, his own attitude to this was that he was in favour of schemes which would prove cost-effective in the developing countries. He knew of situations where Institutes were producing the 6 vaccines for the Extended Immunisation Programmes along side the production of veterinary vaccines, and this arrangement had proved successful and cost-effective.

Dr Bhat pointed out that in the developing countries the budget for rabies control was usually in the keeping of the health authorities for whom rabies was a human problem and little provision was made for paying for control of rabies in animals. Who should pay for the latter? - veterinary budgets were more concerned with diseases such as rinderpest.

Dr Mannathoko thought that it was wrong to generalise about policies in the developing countries, and suggested that each country had its own approach to such problems. Dr Mannathoko asked about WHO's stipulation that producers supplying vaccines for the EPI's should provide 10% - what did that mean?

Dr Sizaret explained that such a producer was concerned with manufacture at a significant scale of operation, ie 10% of the global requirement for a particular vaccine. He also stated that the recipient countries of these vaccines did not receive a manufacturers protocol unless it was specifically requested. Guidelines are mostly intended for countries where there are virtually no control structures, and the WHO guidelines are to ensure minimum safety and efficacy. If there are problems with specific vaccines WHO will react very quickly to investigate and take action. Also if there are indications of low efficacy, WHO will again take rapid action to correct the situation, but mainly its policy is to promote high standards for these products so that such problems will not arise. There is no specific policy of WHO on joint production of human and veterinary vaccines by the same producer. It is for individual countries to make their own policies.

Dr Atgar returned to the subject of rabies raised by Dr Bhat. He made the point that rabies is a topic of great importance for both the human and animal disease control authorities in most countries. The most significant point was that rabies vaccines are comparatively expensive and very large amounts of it are needed for effective control. The question is therefore an economic one. WHO stresses the need for close collaboration between those involved in the human and animal aspects of controlling the disease. In his opinion there is need for the setting up of a special fund directed to supporting joint action by human and veterinary services to control the disease.

Dr Rutter returned to the subject of post-licensing surveillance which he had described in his paper. He said that investigation of suspected adverse reactions following the use of a biological product was a crucial part of post-licensing surveillance in the UK and the EEC. In the UK there is a mandatory requirement for manufacturers to report to the licensing authority any suspected adverse reaction after the use of its products. The definition of adverse reactions includes not only the lack of safety but also the lack of efficacy. The licensing authority also relies to some extent on voluntary reporting of adverse reactions by vets in practice, farmers and pet owners, in addition to the statutory requirements of the legislation. A short pro-forma has been distributed to every veterinary practitioner in the UK. It is also available to farmers, pet owners and the public at large as a means of notifying the Veterinary Medicines Directorate of suspected adverse reactions, which the Directorate subsequently follows up.

Reports are sent to the Veterinary Products Committee for assessment and appropriate action. The findings are published annually in the Veterinary Record giving details of the type of product, the adverse reactions observed and the species involved. This aspect of licensing is developing, particularly in relation to reports of lack of efficacy and will be of increasing importance in the future.